Mechanisms in Respiratory Toxicology

Volume II

Editors

Hanspeter Witschi, M.D.

Senior Research Staff Member
Biology Division
Oak Ridge National Laboratory
Oak Ridge, Tennessee

Paul Nettesheim, M.D.

Chief
Laboratory of Pulmonary Function and Toxicology
National Institute of Environmental Health Sciences
Research Triangle Park, North Carolina

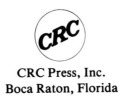

CRC Press, Inc.
Boca Raton, Florida

Library of Congress Cataloging in Publication Data

Main entry under title:

Mechanisms in respiratory toxicology.

   Includes bibliographies and indexes.
   1. Lungs--Diseases. 2. Respiratory organs--Diseases.
3. Toxicology. I. Witschi, Hanspeter.
II. Nettesheim, P. [DNLM: 1. Lung--Pathology. 2. Lung
diseases--Chemically induced. WF 600 M486]
RC732.M43   616.2'4   81-2135
                                  AACR2

Direct all inquiries to CRC Press, Inc., 2000 N.W. 24th Street, Boca Raton, Florida 33431.

© 1982 by CRC Press, Inc.

International Standard Book Number 0-8493-5690-3

Library of Congress Card Number 81-2135
Printed in the United States

PREFACE

This second volume of *Mechanisms in Respiratory Toxicology* is not meant to stand by itself. Rather much of the material discussed can only be fully appreciated in the context of the subjects treated in Volume I. Volume I deals with the structural elements of the lung, the ways toxic agents gain access to the lung, and the way the lung reacts to chemical injury.

This volume discusses endogenous modulating factors, pulmonary defense mechanisms, bioactivation of toxic agents as well as the many long-term consequences of pulmonary injury, namely emphysema and fibrosis. Again emphasis is placed on the general principles underlying injury and disease development rather than on discussion of individual toxic chemicals.

Hopefully, the two volumes will provide useful information as well as an incentive to the experimental toxicologist to study further the many fascinating aspects of lung damage produced by chemicals.

THE EDITORS

Hanspeter Witschi, M.D., is a Senior Research Staff Member at the Biology Division, Oak Ridge National Laboratory. Dr. Witschi received his M.D. degree from the University of Bern, Switzerland, in 1960. He worked as a research fellow in the MRC Toxicology Research Unit in Carshalton/England, the Kettering Laboratory at the University of Cincinnati, and in the Department of Pathology, University of Pittsburgh. From 1969 to 1977 he was at the Department of Pharmacology, Faculty of Medicine, University of Montreal before moving to Oak Ridge National Laboratory. His present research concerns mechanisms of acute and chronic lung damage.

Paul Nettesheim, M.D., is Chief of the Laboratory of Pulmonary Function and Toxicology at the National Institute of Environmental Health Sciences, National Institutes of Health, Department of Health and Human Services. Dr. Nettesheim received his M.D. degree from the University of Boun Medical School in 1959. His professional experience includes training in Pathology at the University of Freiburg i Br. and the University of Pennsylvania between the years 1960 to 1963. He was a member of the research staff at the Biology Division of Oak Ridge National Laboratory from 1963 to 1978. In 1978 he became a member of the National Institute of Environmental Health Sciences. His present research concerns pulmonary cell biology and respiratory tract carcinogenesis.

CONTRIBUTORS

Michael R. Boyd, M.D., Ph.D.
Chief, Molecular Toxicology Section
Clinical Pharmacology Branch
National Cancer Institute
Bethesda, Maryland

Kathryn H. Bradley
Chemist
Pulmonary Branch
National Heart, Lung, and Blood
  Institute
National Institutes of Health
Bethesda, Maryland

Arnold R. Brody, Ph.D.
Head, Pulmonary Pathology Group
Laboratory of Pulmonary Function and
  Toxicology
National Institute of Environmental
  Health Sciences
Research Triangle Park, North
  Carolina

Carroll E. Cross, M.D.
Professor
School of Medicine
Departments of Physiology and
  Medicine
University of California
Davis, California

Ronald G. Crystal, Ph.D.
Chief, Pulmonary Branch
National Heart, Lung, and Blood
  Institute
National Institutes of Health
Bethesda, Maryland

Gerald S. Davis, M.D.
Chief
Division of Pulmonary Medicine
University of Vermont
Burlington, Vermont

Michael J. Evans, Ph.D.
Associate Director
Medical Sciences Department
SRI International
Menlo Park, California

Victor J. Ferrans, M.D.
Chief, Ultrastructure Section
Pathology Branch
National Heart, Lung, and Blood
  Institute
National Institutes of Health
Bethesda, Maryland

Joan Gil, M.D.
Associate Professor of Medicine and
  Anatomy
Cardiovascular-Pulmonary Division
Department of Medicine
University of Pennsylvania
Philadelphia, Pennsylvania

Arnold B. Gorin
Assistant Professor in Medicine
School of Medicine
University of California
Davis, California

Kaye H. Kilburn, M.D.
Ralph Edgington Professor of Medicine
Director
Environmental Sciences Laboratory
University of Southern California
  School of Medicine
Los Angeles, California

Charles Kuhn, M.D.
Professor of Pathology
Washington University School of
  Medicine
Associate Pathologist
Barnes Hospital
St. Louis, Missouri

Jerold A. Last, Ph.D.
Associate Professor of Internal
  Medicine and Biological Chemistry
University of California
Davis, California

Lee V. Leak, Ph.D.
Professor of Anatomy
Director
Ernest E. Just Laboratory of Cellular
  Biology
College of Medicine
Howard University
Washington, D.C.

Marvin Lesser, M.D.
Chief of Pulmonary Medicine
Bronx Veterans Administration Medical
  Center
Assistant Professor of Medicine
Mount Sinai Hospital
Bronx, New York

Gibbe H. Parsons, M.D.
Director
Medical and Respiratory Intensive Care
  Unit
University of California Davis Medical
  Center
Sacramento, California

John A. Pierce, M.D.
Director, Pulmonary Disease Division
Professor of Medicine
Washington University
St. Louis, Missouri

Otto G. Raabe, Ph.D.
Associate Adjunct Professor
Department of Radiological Sciences
School of Veterinary Medicine
University of California
Davis, California

Stephen I. Rennard, M.D.
Senior Staff Fellow
Pulmonary Branch
National Heart, Lung, and Blood
  Institute
National Institutes of Health
Bethesda, Maryland

Sami I. Said, M.D.
Chief, Pulmonary Disease Section
Veterans Administration Medical
  Center
Professor of Internal Medicine and
  Pharmacology
University of Texas Health Science
  Center
Dallas, Texas

Robert M. Senior, M.D.
Associate Professor of Medicine
Washington University School of
  Medicine
Co-Director, Pulmonary Disease and
  Respiratory Division
The Jewish Hospital
St. Louis, Missouri

Alan G. E. Wilson, Ph.D.
Senior Research Toxicologist
Metabolism Section
Environmental Health Laboratory
Monsanto Company
St. Louis, Missouri

TABLE OF CONTENTS

Volume I

Volume II

Modifying Factors and Events

Chapter 1

ALVEOLAR MACROPHAGE TOXICOLOGY

Arnold R. Brody and Gerald S. Davis

TABLE OF CONTENTS

I. INTRODUCTION

The pulmonary alveolar macrophage (AM) utilizes its phagocytic and lytic properties to provide effective defense of the respiratory membrane against inhaled particles and microorganisms.[1] The AM participates in lung defense, inflammation, and immune responses by

1. Isolating ingested particles by means of phagocytosis
2. Acting as a vehicle for physical transport of substances out of the lung
3. Detoxifying inhaled and phagocytized material
4. Presenting antigens to lymphocytes
5. Releasing factors which attract other inflammatory cells
6. Responding to immunologic signals from sensitized lymphocytes

There is a growing body of evidence suggesting that abnormal macrophage function or macrophage death can mediate certain pulmonary diseases.[1-3] In this chapter, we will consider the toxic responses of macrophages to a variety of inhaled particles and gases and discuss the known mechanisms of macrophage toxicology as they relate to pulmonary disease.

II. ORIGIN, FATE, AND VARIABLE MORPHOLOGY OF THE PULMONARY MACROPHAGE

It is now well understood that pulmonary macrophages originate from bone marrow-derived, blood-borne monocytes which differentiate into large aerobic cells upon arrival in the lung. Recent reviews by Brain et al.,[3] Sorokin,[4] and Green et al.[1] describe in detail the origin and fate of lung macrophages and their role in pulmonary host defenses. Briefly, it has been shown that dividing promonocytes of the bone marrow give rise to circulating monocytes which leave the bloodstream at a rapid rate (8.4 hr half-time in man[5]) and enter perivascular connective tissues. The macrophages of the alveolar airspace may originate directly from blood monocytes[3,6-8] or from a local proliferating cell population within the lung.[9] It appears that these interstitial macrophages may or may not divide, depending on a variety of stimuli such as increased load of phagocytized particles, with some of the progeny migrating to the air spaces and others remaining in the interstitium.[3,10] This hypothesis requires further confirmation.

Morphologic studies of normal and pathologic tissues have shown that interstitial macrophages and monocytes move through alveolar basement membranes and between alveolar lining cells during migration to the air spaces,[11,12] as shown in Figure 1. It is not clear whether the different morphologic and functional types of AMs which comprise this heterogenous population all arise from a single type of monocyte precursor and whether the different cell types represent intermediate sequences or final stages of differentiation. The factors governing macrophage proliferation and differentiation also are unknown.

Once a macrophage has entered the alveolar space, the choices for its pathway out of the lung are limited. The particles, gases, and other substances which the AM confronts in the alveolus may, in part, determine its lifespan and fate. Most AMs exit from the lung by way of the mucociliary escalator to be ultimately swallowed or expectorated. It remains unknown whether particle-laden macrophages can reenter the interstitial space from the alveolus in reverse of the interepithelial migration route. The question then arises as to how particle-laden macrophages collect in the pulmonary interstitium and lymph nodes if they did not carry the dust there. Animal and in vitro

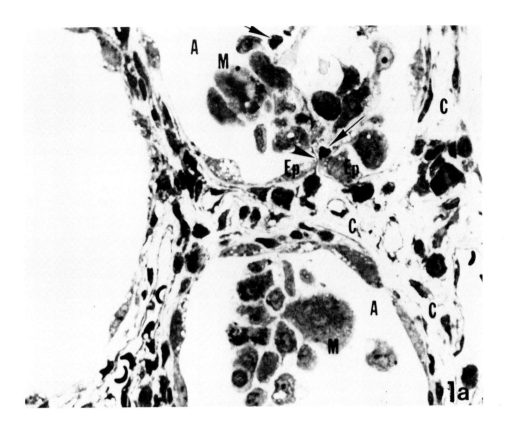

FIGURE 1A.   Light micrograph of plastic-embedded lung tissue from an individual with interstitial fibrotic lung disease. Macrophages (M) and lymphocytes (arrows) are in the small airspaces (A) lined by epithelial cells (Ep). Increased connective tissue (C) is seen in the interstitium. An interstitial macrophage has a cytoplasmic process (arrowhead) extending between two epithelial cells and into the airspace. Perhaps this cell is migrating into the alveolar space. (Original magnification × 320.)

models of particle exposure have shown that particulates can cross the alveolar and bronchial epithelium directly, thus entering the interstitium without transport by macrophages.[13,14] Thus, particle-laden interstitial macrophages which accumulate following exposure could have phagocytized the dust in the interstitium. They may have carried the dust with them from the air spaces, although morphologic evidence has not yet been presented to confirm this hypothesis. Furthermore, Lauweryns and Baert[15] demonstrated that particles may move from the pulmonary interstitium to small lymphatics without the aid of macrophages. Adamson and Bowden[16] found no evidence of carbon-laden macrophages moving from the air spaces to interstitium. Our work has shown consistently that migrating macrophages have a configuration suggestive of movement toward the air spaces (see Figure 1). Thin pseudopods appear to lead the larger mass of the cell which contains the nucleus and most of the organelles.

There seems to be little doubt that the majority of AMs are cleared by means of the mucociliary escalator. The mechanism by which the macrophages move onto the escalator is poorly understood, and it is not known if different subpopulations of cells (e.g., necrotic or particle-laden) are cleared at different rates.

There is no evidence that pulmonary macrophages migrate back into the vasculature. Again, the presence of particle-laden macrophages in the blood and lymphatic vessels as well as in lymph nodes and subpleural connective tissue could reflect the phagocytosis of extracellular particles by resident or circulating phagocytes. It is likely that many such particles were ingested by macrophages which subsequently died, thus re-

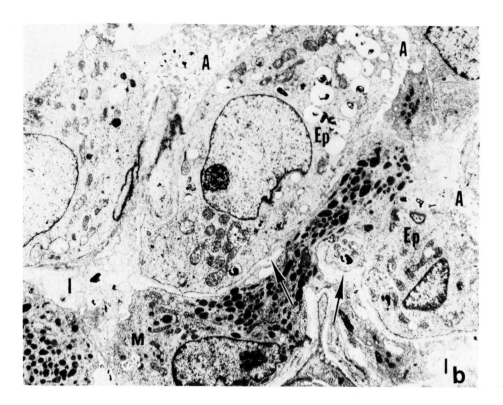

FIGURE 1B.   Transmission electron micrograph from lung tissue similar to that described above. A macrophage (M) with numerous electron-dense lysosomes is in the process of migrating from the interstitium (I). It has passed through the basement membrane (arrows) and between cuboidal epithelial lining cells (Ep) on the way to a small airspace (A). (Original magnification × 7000.)

leasing the particles for phagocytosis by new cells at different sites. This is a common event caused by toxic particulates and will be discussed in more detail below.

Some populations of macrophages may remain in the lung for long periods of time. It is known that exposure to a diffuse-dust aerosol results in focal accumulations of the particulates,[17] and certain tissue macrophages appear to sequester particulates in various anatomic compartments in the lung (see Figure 2). The ultimate fate of these cells and intracellular particles and how long they remain in the lung are not known. It is likely that the pathogenic nature of some particles is altered by increased residence time in the lung. Some particles could be rendered inert, while others might exhibit enhanced cytoxic properties.

AMs are cells of varying morphology and states of activation. Light and electron microscopic techniques have shown that they generally are large cells (15 to 30 μm) with a single kidney-shaped nucleus, numerous lysosomes, and a well-developed rough endoplasmic reticulum (see Figure 1). These internal features are quite variable, depending upon the phagocytic activity and environment of the cell. There seem to be several subpopulations of macrophages, although we know very little about this phenomenon.[3] It is difficult to study AMs *in situ*, as most fixation techniques displace the cells from their normal position on the alveolar walls. Within these limitations, it is possible to recognize macrophages *in situ* as being flat or round, ruffled or smooth, and in varying combinations of these conditions (see Figure 3). Interestingly enough, AMs collected from human and animal lungs by bronchoalveolar lavage show similar surface variability in vitro (see Figure 4). We do not know the significance of this morphologic variance, but studies are in progress to address the basic question of how

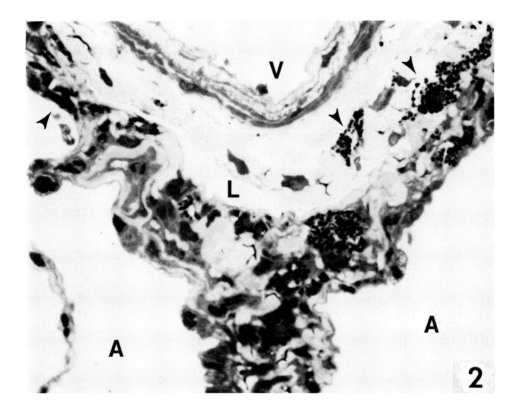

FIGURE 2. Light micrograph of plastic-embedded lung tissue from a cigarette smoker. It is not unusual to find accumulations of anthracotic pigment (arrowheads) in macrophages and connective tissue of perivascular and perilymphatic regions. The lumens of a small arterial vessel (V), a lymphatic channel (L), and air spaces (A) are seen. (Original magnification × 320.)

macrophage form relates to function. For example, human AMs which are flat in vitro phagocytize more iron particles than do round cells[18] (see Figure 4).

The AM resides in a unique microenvironment. It functions in the humidified gas phase of the alveolar space, adherent to the surface and bathed in the lipoproteins and serum constituents of the alveolar lining material. It is a highly aerobic cell, dependent on oxidative phosphorylation and relatively high oxygen tensions.[19] It cannot metabolize or phagocytize effectively in an hypoxic liquid environment[20] in which polymorphonuclear (PMN) leukocytes perform normally. It is distinctly different from the PMN or the peritoneal macrophage, and studies using these latter cell types may not accurately predict AM behavior.

In summary, available data indicate that most AMs originate from the bone marrow and are borne by the blood to the lung where they migrate to the interstitium. Here the cells may or may not divide, depending upon various stimuli, and those phagocytes destined to be AMs migrate through basement membranes and between epithelial cells to the small airspaces. A variety of morphologic and functional types of AMs may be recovered from the airspaces. An apparently distinct population of phagocytes remains in the pulmonary interstitium where they undergo mitotic division. Macrophages generally are cleared from the lung by the mucociliary escalator of the airways. Other clearance pathways may be operative, but are poorly understood.

III. ALVEOLAR MACROPHAGES AND PARTICLES

The AM confronts and ingests a variety of particles in its role as the primary phagocyte of the lung (see Figure 5). The events which accompany phagocytosis and the

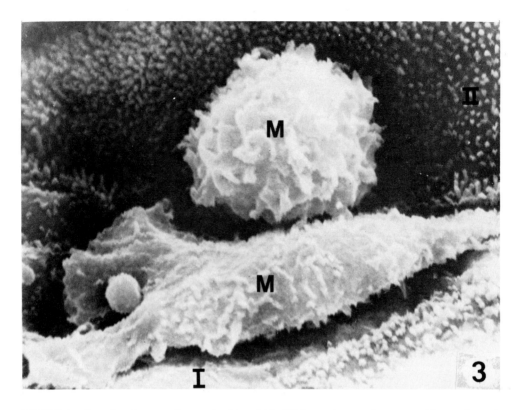

FIGURE 3.   Scanning electron micrograph of two AMs (M) in an air space from normal human lung. A cuboidal Type II epithelial cell (II) with numerous microvilli is seen in the background. The migrating macrophage in the foreground is on an attenuated Type I (I) cell. These macrophages appear healthy with numerous surface ruffles and intact membranes. (Original magnification × 8600.)

effects of ingested particles on the macrophages may be indirect determinants of respiratory disease. The AM contains a rich store of lysosomal enzymes with proteolytic, elastolytic, and inflammatory properties.[21,22] Digestive enzymes and other factors derived from macrophages produce emphysema,[23,24] pulmonary fibrosis,[25-27] and inflammation.[25,28] It is well known that the AM is responsible for initial defense of the lung against inhaled microorganisms.[29]

Both organic and inorganic particles which reach the respiratory surface are ingested rapidly by AMs. Many toxic particles can express their effects through macrophages inasmuch as phagocytosis results in the release of lysosomal enzymes and other substances. Such active substances may be released from macrophages consequent to cell disintegration, as is seen following silica ingestion (see discussion below), or may be selectively released without cell injury, as occurs during phagocytosis of starch granules.[30] We have studied the release of cell contents from AMs during phagocytosis of a variety of particles. The appearance of certain marker enzymes was measured in the medium surrounding cells in monolayer tissue culture. Beta-glucuronidase (β-G) and other enzymes were used as markers of lysosomal enzyme release, while lactic dehydrogenase (LDH) activity was used as an index of leakage of cytoplasmic contents, resulting from loss of cell membrane integrity. Appearance of β-G in the supernatant medium without increase LDH activity was interpreted as selective lysosomal enzyme release without cell injury. Parallel increases of both these enzymes in the medium was interpreted as indicating cytotoxicity. Table 1 summarizes the effects of phagocytosis of several crystalline, organic, and mineral particles on guinea pig AMs.

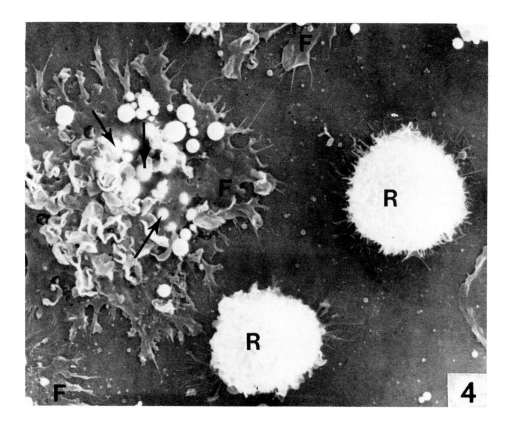

FIGURE 4. Scanning electron micrograph of normal human AMs in vitro. Two shapes are recognized, flat cells (F) and round cells (R). The flat cells have phagocytized numerous iron oxide particles (arrows). It has been shown that the flat cells are more avid phagocytes in vitro. (Original magnification × 2000.)

Three distinct patterns of response were seen with different types of particles. Calcium pyrophosphate crystals and carbon dust had no significant effect on enzyme release. The organic particles zymosan and *Staphylococcus albus* caused selective release of lysosomal enzymes without cell injury. Kaolinite, silica, asbestos, and urate caused cell injury and release of both marker enzymes.

The release of lysosomal enzymes during phagocytosis is not an obligatory response to all particulates. Calcium pyrophosphate salt crystals caused no cell injury and no selective release of lysosomal enzymes, although monosodium urate crystals were highly cytotoxic. Carbon dust was phagocytized without cytoxicity or enzyme release, but silica was injurious to the macrophage. This demonstrates that certain particulates are inert and may be phagocytized without significant pathological consequences. Within the spectrum of cell effects caused by various particles under uniform conditions, the asbestos fibers demonstrated less cytotoxicity than the highly injurious silica or urate particles, but more activity than kaolinite.

Henson[31] and Weissmann et al.[32,33] have summarized current theories of enzyme release from PMN leukocytes and have postulated that lysosomal enzymes may be selectively released either by leakage from open phagolysosomes or by direct exocytosis of lysosomal contents. Both "regurgitation during feeding" and "reversed endocytosis" have been captured in a single electron micrograph of an AM.[30] Lysosomal enzymes may leak from an open phagolysosome if lysosome fusion occurs prior to phagosome closure or if a closed particle-containing phagolysosome reopens to admit a second particle.[31] This regurgitation could occur either during invagination or pseu-

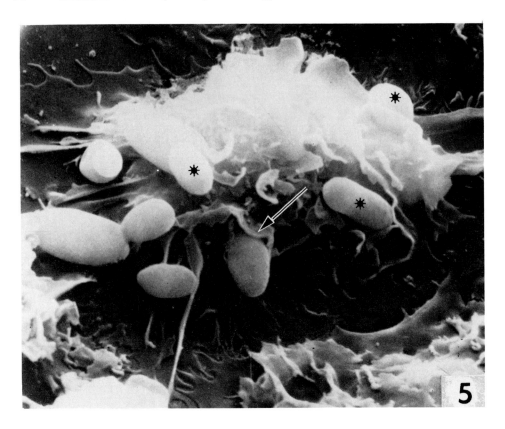

FIGURE 5.   Scanning electron micrograph of a human AM in vitro. This cell is in the process of in-gesting a number of yeast particles (*). One particle is being taken into a phagocytic cup (arrow) formed by the macrophage. (Original magnification × 4000.)

dopodial extension of the cell membrane to form phagocytic cups.[32] Lysosomal con-tents may also be directly emptied into the external milieu of the macrophage by fusion of the lysosomal membrane with the plasma membrane and exterior opening of the lysosome. The "reversed endocytosis"[32] may be seen during ingestion of particles at membrane locations near phagocytic cups or during "frustrated phagocytosis"[31] of immune complexes adhered to an uningestable surface.

Ingested particles need not injure the phagocyte for liberation of lysosomal enzymes to occur. This selective release of lysosomal contents into the surrounding tissues takes place during the phagocytic event. Selective release has not been reported to cause any recognized cell or tissue defects.

On a day-to-day basis, easily digested and/or inert particles are the most common type inhaled into the lungs. Thus, we are unaware of ongoing particle-cell interactions under normal circumstances. On the other hand, certain particulates are toxic to AMs and cause irreparable harm and irreversible lung injury. It has been shown that inhaled particles smaller than 20 μm are deposited in alveolar spaces.[34] There are many circum-stances in which individuals are exposed to toxic particles in this size range, e.g., min-ing, industry, ambient environment. The interactions of macrophages with toxic par-ticles, such as crystalline silica (SiO_2) and asbestos, are partially understood and will be considered here.

A. Silica

Marks[35] initially reported that silica dust is toxic to AMs in vitro. Allison and co-workers[36] extended these observations by demonstrating cytotoxicity and release of

Table 1
RELEASE OF MARKER ENZYMES FROM AMs
DURING PHAGOCYTOSIS

Particle added[a]	Percent total cell enzyme released	
	β-G (lysosomal)	Lactic dehydrogenase (cytoplasmic)
Resting cells	6	4
Calcium pyrophosphate crystals	6	5
Carbon dust	8	5
Staphylococcus albus	10	4
Zymosan starch granules	17	4
Kaolinite dust	21	17
Amosite asbestos	25	22
Silica dust	37	44
Urate crystals	28	89

[a] Particles were added to monolayers of guinea pig AMs (particle: cell = 10:1), and the supernatant medium was harvested after 2 hr of incubation.

lysosomal enzymes during phagocytosis of silica. They suggested that macrophage injury might be the mediator of fibrosis in silicosis and postulated that the silica particles injure macrophages from within. The authors hypothesized that silica particles are ingested and sequestered normally in phagolysosomes. Subsequently, silicic acid or other residues within the crystal matrix bond with lipid and protein constituents of the phagolysosomal membrane, deforming it and allowing escape of lytic enzymes into the cytoplasm with consequent autolysis and ultimate leakage of cell contents into the surrounding tissues. This process has been observed with the electron microscope through release of electron-dense lysosomal markers into the cytoplasm of macrophages following silica ingestion.[37]

The biochemical mechanism of lysosomal membrane injury in AMs which have phagocytosed silica is not fully understood. It has been proposed, although not proven, that highly reactive hydroxyl groups (OH^-) of silicic acid residues on the surfaces of crystalline silica act as hydrogen donors and combine with as yet undefined components of the phagolysosome membrane.[2,38] The cytotoxicity of silica is largely blocked by the addition of poly-2-vinyl-pyridine-N-oxide (PVPNO) to either the particles or the culture medium.[38] Apparently, the hydrogen binding properties of the PVPNO compete for reactive sites on the crystalline silica, thus sparing the phagolysosomal membranes. Coating silica with serum will delay the cytotoxic reaction while lysosomal enzymes digest the serum proteins, but toxicity soon ensues.

As well as injuring the macrophage, silica must qualitatively or quantitatively change it in other ways since extracts of silica-treated macrophages promote fibrosis and collagen synthesis in animal models[25,39] and fibroblast cultures.[26,27,40,41] Silica-damaged AMs also stimulate in vitro fibroblast proliferation.[42] It is assumed that macrophage particle interactions described above occur upon inhalation of crystalline silica into alveolar ducts and air spaces. There is no question that humans and animals exposed to inhaled silica develop significant pulmonary disease which can follow one of several pathogenetic patterns:

1. Diffuse fibrosis and chronic inflammation
2. Nodular fibrosis and chronic inflammation
3. Acute alveolar edema and diffuse fibrosis

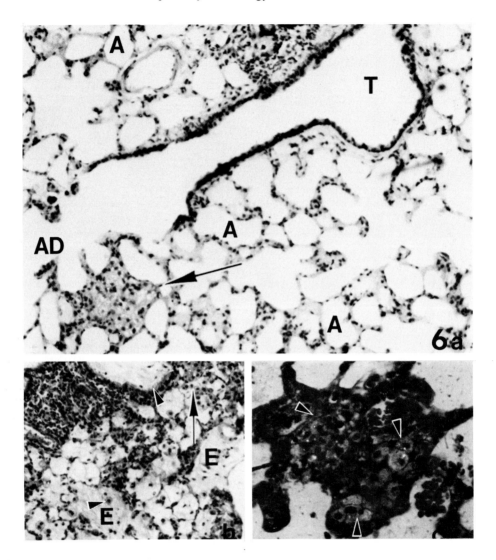

FIGURE 6.   Lung tissue from a rat dusted with crystalline silica for 4 days and then sacrificed 60 days after the exposure period. A terminal bronchiole (T) and alveolar spaces (A) are seen. The predominant lesion in these animals is a nodular accumulation of dust-containing macrophages (arrow) adjacent to alveolar ducts (AD). (Original magnification × 80.) A less common form of lesion in these animals is a diffuse alveolar exudate (E) containing necrotic macrophages (arrow heads). A nodular lesion (arrow) is seen. (Original magnification × 80.) The lesions from the silica-dusted rats contain large numbers of necrotic macrophages (arrowheads) containing birefringent silica particles. (Original magnification × 320.)

Perhaps all of these lesions are associated with macrophage toxicity and the release of lysosomal enzymes and other substances. This hypothesis needs much additional study.

A rat model of silica dust inhalation in our laboratory has shown that small (2 to 10 μm) particles of crystalline quartz are deposited along the small airways and alveolar ducts 9 days after the initial exposure. Ninety days after a 1 week exposure to 100 mg/ m^3 of dust, small nodular lesions develop in the pulmonary parenchyma adjacent to alveolar ducts (see Figure 6A). The most prominent feature of the lesions is large numbers of necrotic macrophages containing silica particles (see Figures 6B and C). These studies provide supporting evidence for the role of macrophage toxicity in the pathogenesis of dust-related pulmonary disease and raise a number of important questions to be pursued.

B. Asbestos

Another, perhaps even more important, class of particles which exhibits clear toxicity for AMs is the fibrous silicate, asbestos.[38] The two classes of asbestos, serpentine and amphibole, possess different degrees of cytoxicity and cause varying forms of pulmonary disease, e.g., diffuse fibrosis, bronchogenic carcinoma, and mesothelioma. Asbestos apparently is phagocytized more slowly than silica,[42] but clearly causes increased permeability of cell membranes.[43] Even though such cytotoxic events occur, there is some question as to whether or not this plays any role in the formation of asbestosis inasmuch as the fibrogenic effects of asbestos are reduced to practically nothing in the presence of serum proteins.[38] In addition, PVPNO fails to suppress the fibrogenic effects of asbestos in vivo, and there is no correlation between degree of macrophage cytotoxity seen in vitro and in vivo fibrogenicity to man and animals.[38] However, there is evidence that longer fibers (>20 μm) are more fibrogenic than shorter ones. As mentioned above, this has little to do with toxic potential of the fiber, but is more likely associated with selective enzyme release of macrophages attempting to phagocytize the long particles. They do so with a great deal of difficulty, often with several macrophages gathered around a single fiber for long periods of time, thus providing ample opportunity for enzyme leakage and consequent tissue damage.[44] It is known that serpentine asbestos, i.e., chrysotile or "white asbestos", is the most toxic form studied, although the mechanisms(s) of its cytotoxicity is not very clear. There are suggestions that the crystalline silica component of the fiber exerts a deleterious influence on phagolysosomal membranes, much like that which occurs after ingestion of silica (SiO_2). Interestingly enough, the elemental components of chrysotile are Mg, Si, and O_2, but the cytotoxic potential of the fiber has been shown to correlate with its magnesium content.[45]

Since the onset of clinical asbestosis is usually delayed for years following dust exposure, the initial cytotoxicity of asbestos for AMs may be of less importance than its ability to stimulate production of AM factors which promote fibroblast growth or collagen synthesis.[25-27] It is possible that long-term residence in the lung alters asbestos fibers to make them more fibrogenic, even if less acutely toxic. The ways in which asbestos and macrophages interact to produce fibrosis clearly deserves further investigation.

C. Other Toxic Dusts

There are other particulates which have been implicated in the pathogenesis of fibrotic pulmonary disease consequent to industrial or environmental exposures. Dusts, such as kaolinite (aluminum silicate), mica (potassium aluminum silicate), and talc (magnesium silicate), are among these. They are rapidly phagocytized by AMs and clearly are hemolytic in vitro.[46] The mechanism of macrophage toxicity is not known, although experimental evidence suggests that hydroxyl radicals on the surface of the crystalline complexes exert a strong binding potential with cell membranes.[46] The degree of particle hydration seems to be an important variable in the extent of cell injury created. Kaolinite which has been heated sufficiently to drive off most of the OH radicals bound in surface water causes little hemolytic activity.[47] Dissolution of silicic acid residues from kaolinite, mica, and talc mitigates the toxicity of these particles, suggesting again a role for hydrogen-donating complexes which may interact with lysosomal membranes. Data in Table 1 demonstrate that in vitro kaolinite is toxic to the alveolar macrophages of guinea pigs.

IV. ALVEOLAR MACROPHAGES AND TOXIC GASES

Environmental, occupational, or medical exposure to a variety of gases can produce increased susceptibility to respiratory infection which may, in part, be attributed to

AM dysfunction. Air pollution,[48] therapeutic oxygen, and cigarette smoke[49,50] commonly cause impaired pulmonary host defenses because of their toxic nature. Animal model and isolated lung cell studies suggest that macrophage toxicity may account for a major portion of these effects. The role of the macrophage in host defense against infection has received almost exclusive attention in such studies. Unfortunately, the effects of toxic gases on other macrophage functions has not been examined.

Exposure to toxic gases may be acute and intense, as with general anesthesia, or chronic at low concentrations, as with air pollution. Since gases do not persist in the lung as particles generally do, tissue exposure is limited largely to the time of actual ambient exposure. Studies related to macrophage toxicity have focused on relatively short-term exposure of hours or days. Local alveolar concentrations of gases are related in a complex fashion to ambient gas levels, aqueous gas solubility, and ventilatory patterns, as reviewed in detail by Morgan and Frank.[51] Thus, highly toxic gases such as sulfur dioxide may rarely reach the macrophage to cause injury because of dissolution in more proximal respiratory fluids. Several gases very likely of importance to phagocyte function are ozone, nitrogen oxides, oxygen, chlorine, metal fumes, anaesthetic gases, and the vapor phase of cigarette smoke.

Major problems remain in assessing the importance and clinical relevance of potentially toxic effects of gases. Animal studies show genuine effects which may not be due to reputed AM toxicity, while studies utilizing isolated AMs (in vitro) may omit critical components contributed by the interactions between multiple lung cell types and body fluids in vivo. Species and age variation in susceptibility to toxic gas effects are a major obstacle to extending laboratory observations to the human condition. Thus, studies on young rodents may not accurately predict effects on industrial workers. Toxic gases may actually produce injury to AMs, but these effects may be trivial and clinically inapparent in the face of overwhelming injury to more sensitive cell types such as the Type I alveolar epithelial cell. Toxic gases affect macrophages primarily by means of oxidant injury, as with oxygen, ozone, and the oxides of nitrogen, and by nonoxidant mechanisms, as with acids, metal fumes, or anesthetics.

A. Oxygen Toxicity

Oxygen toxicity serves as a model for macrophage oxidant injury and has been more extensively studied than the effects of other toxic gases. Oxygen toxicity is relevant to the many patients requiring supplemental oxygen in the treatment of cardiopulmonary diseases, with major effects on lung structure and function.[52]

A well-known model using aerosol exposure of mice to radiotracer-labeled bacteria demonstrates the bactericidal function of the resident AM.[29] This system has been used to test the effects of hyperoxia on pulmonary microbicidal function. Sturin et al.[53] showed no impairment of intrapulmonary bacterial killing following 24 hr of 100% oxygen exposure, while Huber and LaForce[54] demonstrated significant impairment of bacterial killing after 48 and 72 hr of similar oxygen exposure. Diminished phagocytosis of inhaled gold particles by hamsters after 4 days of oxygen exposure has also been described.[5] These studies indicate that prolonged hyperoxia impairs pulmonary defense mechanisms in vivo.

Studies evaluating the effects of hyperoxia on AM function directly have been more equivocal. Murphy et al.[56] found no impairment and slight enhancement of in vitro bacterial phagocytosis by AM obtained from rabbits exposed to hyperoxia for 3 days. Murine AM exposed to oxygen in vitro for 2 days, however, demonstrated impaired phagocytosis,[57] and guinea pig macrophages have demonstrated a similar functional impairment after 24 hr of in vitro oxygen exposure.[130]

An important mechanism of oxygen injury may involve stimulation of the endogenous production of superoxide anion (O_2^-,), but cellular superoxide dismutase (SOD) may protect against injury caused by this high-energy oxygen radical.[58] Oxygen exposure for 7 days produced a significant rise in the level of SOD in the lungs of adult rats.[59-61] Similar adaptive changes were not seen using guinea pigs, hamsters, or mice.[59] Autor and co-workers[62,63] observed increased whole lung SOD levels following only 24 hr of oxygen exposure using neonatal rats, with no change in adult rat lung over this short exposure. They postulated that the rapid inducibility of this enzyme in neonates might explain their relative resistance to oxygen toxicity. These studies did not identify the cell types responsible for the increased SOD activity, but ongoing research suggests that O_2 induces SOD in AMs. The variability of results caused by animal age and species differences are notable in this series of experiments. Similar variation has been found when examining the SOD response of isolated AMs after 4 days of in vivo oxygen exposure. Simon[64] found a similar response in mouse macrophages after 1 day of in vitro exposure. In contrast, Deneke[61] found no change in rat macrophage SOD levels after 7 days of in vivo exposure or 2 days of in vitro exposure to high oxygen tensions. Despite considerable disagreement among the results of various investigators, some general conclusions about the effects of hyperoxia on macrophage function may be drawn. Relatively brief (1 to 7 days) exposure to clinically relevant oxygen tensions appears to impair pulmonary host defense in general, and AM phagocytic function in particular. The resident or recruited AM may respond to hyperoxia by increased production of the antioxidant enxyme SOD, but this response is probably inadequate to completely prevent injury. Further investigation is required to determine whether lower levels of oxygen exposure (30 to 60%) which generally do not cause overt lung injury can impair AM function and pulmonary resistance to infection to a clinically significant degree. Studies are also required to determine the effects of hyperoxia on the macrophage as an immunoregulatory cell, a source of proteolytic enzymes, and a stimulus to fibrosis.

B. Toxicity of Other Gases

Other important oxidants which may be toxic for AMs include ozone, the oxides of nitrogen, and cigarette smoke. This last all-too-common pollutant will be discussed in more detail below, although some of its mechanisms of injury may be through oxidant pathways. Oxidants are thought to mediate pulmonary injury primarily through peroxidation of the lipids which form external and intracellular membranes.[65] In the lung, peroxidation of surfactant lipids also may be of major importance. Studies similar to those discussed above have been carried out using oxidant air pollutants to evaluate the effect of these substances on alveolar macrophages. For example, relatively brief exposure to ambient concentrations of ozone (O_3) or nitrogen dioxide (NO_2) achieved in urban environments produced dose-related depression of pulmonary bactericidal activity in mice.[54,66] Surprisingly, these two gases did not act additively, although a similar mechanism of injury might be postulated for them.[67] Coffin[68] observed that exposure of rabbits to ozone for up to 24 hr produced an infiltration of leukocytes into the lung and a decrease in the ability of AMs to phagocytize streptococci. Similar suppression of AM phagocytic activity and resistance to virus infection have been observed following NO_2 exposure.[69] Alterations in macrophage metabolism[70] and morphology[71] have also been described. It remains unclear whether the abundance of extracellular surfactant lipids which surround the macrophage in vivo might serve to absorb oxidants and protect it or conversely could enhance its injury. Most available reports concur that impairment of pulmonary microbicidal function occurs with levels of air pollutant exposure below those which can produce other detectable respiratory abnormalities. Thus, AM dysfunction might be a subtle, but clinically important consequence of chronic air pollution.

Nonoxidant mechanisms of macrophage injury have been less extensively studied.

Inhalation of large quantities of gases which dissolve to form acids (e.g., NO_2 and chlorine) might cause macrophage injury, but as discussed above these substances are also potent oxidants. Inhalation of gases to a degree sufficient to cause direct acid injury to the AM might be expected to cause severe generalized pulmonary parenchymal injury with little selective effect on the macrophage. Several commonly used general anesthetic agents have been observed to impair murine pulmonary bactericidal activity, an effect believed to be mediated through the AM.[72] Direct effects of general anesthetics on AMs have not been extensively studied, but might be of clinical importance. Metal fumes, particularly cadmium, can impair macrophage metabolism,[73] and the emphysema produced by chronic cadmium exposure might be partially mediated by effects on the Am. Preliminary studies have demonstrated alterations in the macrophage population,[74] decreased AM viability,[75] and impaired phagocytosis[76] following in vivo or in vitro exposure to a variety of trace metals.

The effects of toxic gases on the AM deserve more study. All the known literature relates to high-dose, short-term exposure of animals and the subsequent assessment of macrophage bactericidal function. The effects of long-term, lower-dose exposure of humans to potentially toxic gases may not be accurately predicted from these studies. Effects on the macrophage other than its microbicidal function may be of equal or greater importance to human disease.

V. CIGARETTE SMOKE — A MODEL OF MACROPHAGE TOXICITY

Cigarette smoke serves as a useful and clinically relevant model of AM toxicity, inasmuch as it represents one of the most common universal insults to lung defenses. Moreover, it's effects on human AMs have been extensively studied. In response to chronic smoke exposure, the macrophage population undergoes hyperplasia (increased cell numbers), hypertrophy (increased cell size), and multiple changes in microbicidal function, metabolism, and immunologic responsiveness, as reviewed by Martin.[77]

The previous sections of this chapter have considered the reactions of AMs to toxic gases and particulates. Cigarette smoke offers unique advantages in studying various combinations of these inasmuch as it has been shown by several groups of investigators that both toxic gases (e.g., acrolein)[78] and inorganic particles (e.g., kaolinite)[79] are components of main stream smoke. Very little is known about the physicochemical associations of inorganic dust and tobacco smoke. However, it is quite clear that the pathogenesis of neoplastic pulmonary disease is accentuated in individuals who smoke and simultaneously are exposed to asbestos dust[80] or uranium ore.[81] In addition, inorganic particles, such as talc and ferric oxide, prolong the clearance time of carcinogens from the lungs of experimental animals, thus causing increased incidence of respiratory tract tumors.[82]

A. Smokers' Macrophages

The role of the macrophage is obscure in this question of gas-particle synergism. However, it is interesting to speculate that phagocytes could play an important part in modifying the influence of toxic materials, For example, we know that inorganic particles found on the surface of cigarette tobacco travel in mainstream cigarette smoke and are phagocytized by AMs.[79] These smokers' macrophages (see Figure 7) have picked up cytotoxic aluminum silicates which very likely are covered by varying amounts of adsorbed gases and tars. When the particles are phagocytized, the adsorbed materials could be digested and rendered harmless or alternatively could exert strong influences on the behavior of the macrophages themselves. There is virtually no data on these important questions. To understand the role of the macrophage in many lung diseases consequent to cigarette use, we must pursue this question of particle-gas syn-

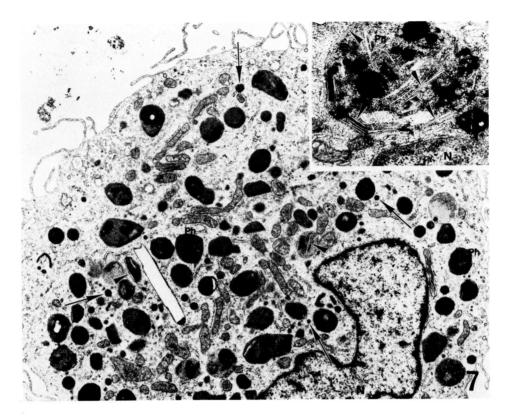

FIGURE 7. Transmission electron micrograph of an AM from a cigarette smoker. The cell contains numerous primary lysosomes (arrows) and phagolysosomes (Ph). Peculiar linear inclusions characteristic of smoker's macrophages are illustrated here (arrowheads). The higher magnification inset shows the fine structural nature of the smokers' inclusions in a phagolysosome. (Original magnification × 10,250; inset × 27,200.)

ergism as others have for particle-carcinogen combinations.[83] Since it has been shown that certain inorganic particulates and gases have profound influences on macrophage viability and consequent disease as discussed above, it is likely that such particles and gases combined in cigarette smoke will cause important reactions.

It is known that changes in the macrophage population are evident in lung tissue and isolated cells of cigarette smokers. Large numbers of pigmented macrophages are seen filling alveoli and small bronchioles in early respiratory bronchiolitis caused by tobacco smoking,[84] and increased numbers of macrophages can be enumerated in the airspaces of histologically normal lung tissue from cigarette smokers.[12] It is unclear to what extent this increase in the airspace macrophage population represents an influx of new cells from the blood stream, increased replication of a macrophage population within the lung, or a decrease in the rate at which cells exit and are cleared from the lungs. All three processes may be operating in concert.

Subsegmental saline pulmonary lavage using a flexible fiberoptic bronchoscope or balloon-tipped catheter allows rapid safe access to alveolar cells and secretions in normal human subjects and patients with lung diseases. This technique has allowed detailed study of the human macrophage, and typical results from healthy nonsmoking and smoking volunteers have been reported by a number of investigators.[77,85,87,88] Pulmonary lavage is performed by gentle wedging the tip of the bronchofiberscope in the lumen of a descendent or horizontal subsegmental bronchus of matching size, instilling 30 to 60 cc of isotonic saline solution, immediately withdrawing this solution, and repeating this "washing" procedure up to 5 or 6 times. Representative values for vol-

Table 2
PULMONARY LAVAGE OF NORMAL
HUMAN VOLUNTEERS[a]

Parameter	Nonsmokers	Smokers
Number of subjects	25	26
Instilled lavage fluid recovered[b] (%)	73	72
Total cells recovered[c] (in millions)	17	40
Macrophages[c] (%)	93.9	95.8
Lymphocytes (%)	4.3	3.4
PMN leukocytes[c] (%)	1.8	0.8

[a]   Average age 26 years.
[b]   Bronchofiberscopic subsegmental lavage was performed by the instillation and immediate withdrawal of four 60 cc boluses of 0.9% saline solution.
[c] p Value <0.02 by student's nonpaired t test.

ume recovery, cell numbers, and cell types are shown in Table 2. All investigators have reported a three- to fivefold increase in the number of cells recovered by lavage from smokers in contrast to nonsmokers, thus reflecting the increased numbers of cells seen in the airspaces of the lungs studied.

A variety of morphologic, metabolic, and functional comparisons have been made between macrophages derived from tobacco smokers and nonsmokers, as summarized in Table 3. These comparisons highlight the wide variety of effects which chronic cigarette smoke exposure has on human macrophages. As described above, smoker's macrophages are larger, and most of them contain distinctive brown pigment as well as numerous cytoplasmic inclusions which distinguish them from nonsmokers' cells.[79] The macrophages of mice and dogs smoking under experimental conditions have identical inclusions.[89,90] The quantity of total cell protein measured on an average per cell basis is also increased as might be expected with increased size. It should be noted that not all cells in the smokers' macrophage population are enlarged, but rather that there is a greater proportion of very large cells as well as many cells which are morphologically indistinguishable from those of nonsmokers.

Degradative lysosomal enzymes are also increased in smokers' macrophages. Both "internal" lysosomal enzymes which may participate in the digestion of phagocytized particles, such as β-glucuronidase, and "secreted" lysosomal enzymes which are released into the environment around the cell, such as elastase and lysozyme, are increased 2- to 25-fold in smokers' cells. The increased total burden of potentially tissue-damaging enzymes incurred by the increased number of macrophages and increased enzyme content per cell has been emphasized.[91]

Smokers' macrophages are metabolically more active than nonsmokers' cells. Oxygen consumption, as measured in our laboratory by electrode methods, is slightly higher at rest in smoker's cells, and the smokers' macrophages show a substantial increase during the phagocytosis. Glucose consumption is also increased.

Despite the increase in cell size, lysosomal enzyme armamentarium, and metabolic activity, the performance of smoker's AMs as phagocytes appears comparable or slightly worse than that of nonsmoker's cells. As can be seen in Table 3, rates of ingestion of yeast particles were similar regardless of smoking status, as measured in two laboratories. Martin and Warr[77] observed slightly depressed rates of ingestion of

Table 3
CHARACTERISTICS OF HUMAN AMs FROM SMOKERS AND NONSMOKERS

Parameter tested[a]	Nonsmokers' cells	Smokers' cells	Ref.
Brown pigmented cells (%)	14	83	114
Flat cells by SEM (%)	55	74	18
Large cells by SEM (%)	1.6	4.5	18
Cell protein ($\mu g/10^6$ cells)	185	278	114
β-G (μg phe/hr/10^6 cells)	35	150	91
Elastase ($\mu g/10^6$ cells)	7.8	16.9	92
Lysozyme ($\mu g/10^6$ cells)	1.2	2.7	92
Aryl hydrocarbon hydroxylase ($\mu m/10^6$ cells)	10	95	128
Peroxidase ($\mu m/10^6$ cells)	13.8	18.0	130
Oxygen consumption: rest	3.6	3.7	130
($\mu l/hr/10^6$ cells) phagocytosis	4.4	5.7	
Glucose consumption: rest ($\mu mol/hr/10^6$ cells)	0.5	1.4	86
Phagocytic cells (%)			
Staphylococcus aureus	95	70	77
Candida krusei	90	86	
Candida organisms/100 cells	320	315	20
Staphylococcus albus Phagocytosis:			
Uptake (%)	39	35	20
Killing (%)	54	43	

[a] Studies reported were performed on normal volunteer human PAMs.

Staphylococcus aureus, while we observed no difference in the rates of uptake of *Staphylococcus albus*. The rate of killing of ingested bacteria was, however, slightly decreased in smokers' cells.

B. Pulmonary Defense

The effects of tobacco smoking on pulmonary defense mechanisms have been extensively studied using animal models and isolated lung cells. Smoking increases both the frequency and severity of lower respiratory tract infections in otherwise healthy adults.[49,50,92] Clearance of bacteria from lungs following aerosol challenge is primarily a reflection of the effectiveness of AM macrophage function,[29] as described above. Mice exposed to acute doses of cigarette smoke and then challenged with aerosolized bacteria demonstrate impairment of pulmonary bacterial killing.[93-95] Dose-related impairment of bacterial ingestion and killing by animal AMs in vitro has been observed following exposure to cigarette smoke,[96] cigar smoke,[97] marijuana smoke,[98] and synthetic tobacco substitutes.[99] These effects may, in part, be attributed to acrolein and other oxidant gases,[100,101] and this effect may be partially mediated through inhibition of glycolysis.[100] Interestingly, the toxic effect of the filtered gas phase of cigarette smoke on AM bactericidal function can be blocked by the antioxidant sulfhydryl agents glutathione and cysteine.[102] Chronic exposure to cigarette smoke in vivo does not produce tolerance to this acute in vitro effect or to protection by cysteine. Human smokers' macrophages remain susceptible to in vitro toxicity with the gas phase of cigarette smoke as shown in Table 4.

An overview of the clinical significance of chronic cigarette smoke toxicity on the microbicidal function of the AM is somewhat difficult because of the conflicting hu-

Table 4
EFFECTS OF CIGARETTE SMOKE IN
VITRO ON HUMAN PULMONARY
AMs

Macrophage cell source	Number of subjects	Percent bacteria phagocytosed[a]	
		Control	Smoke[b]
Nonsmokers	8	39	29
Smokers	6	35	25

[a] ^{32}P- labeled *Staphylococcus albus* (10^5 bacteria) were added to macrophage monolayers (10^6 cells) in Hanks Balanced Salt Solution with 10% autologous serum and incubated for 45 min at 37°C.
[b] Filtered gas phase of cigarette smoke, 4 cc/20 cc tissue culture tube.[96]

man and animal, in vivo and in vitro, results summarized above. Smoking produces profound changes in the size and constituency of the macrophage population of the lung and in the physical and metabolic characteristic of individual AMs. However, the antibacterial function of these cells appears to be normal or only minimally impaired. Acute exposure of animals to large doses of tobacco smoke produces measureable impairment of overall lung bacterial clearance, but it remains unclear whether such an effect occurs with clinically relevant doses of smoke or whether tolerance to this effect develops with chronic smoking. Studies with isolated AMs in vitro provide further difficulties in interpretation because of

1.   High doses of smoke are required to produce effects
2.   The most toxic components are water soluble and may dissolve in respiratory secretions before reaching the alveolus
3.   Alveolar lipids and proteins may absorb the brunt of toxic gases and thus protect the macrophage
4.   Sulfhydryl compounds, similar to cysteine, may be available in vivo to protect against the observed effects

Further work in this area must await better definition of the alveolar microenvironment and its response to cigarette smoke exposure.

In addition to the functional effects observed on phagocytosis, acute in vitro cigarette smoke exposure has been reported to have a variety of other toxic effects on AMs.[103] For example, animal macrophages exposed to smoke demonstrate decreased oxygen consumption,[104] decreased viability,[105] and peroxidation of cell lipids.[65] Reduced amino acid transport[106] and diminished protein synthesis also have been recognized. It is not certain to what extent these effects occur in the lungs of human tobacco smokers, or the extent to which smokers' macrophages might adapt to the influences of tobacco smoke.

C. Altered Immunologic Responses

The AM participates actively in the multiple immunologic responses of the lung. The lung should be viewed as an independent immunologic organ which may have local responses without generalized systemic responses and in which local responses may be absent despite systemic sensitization. A full discussion of the immune responses of the lung is beyond the scope of this chapter, but has been reviewed by Kaltreider.[107]

The role of the AM in pulmonary immunologic responses has also been reviewed recently.[108,109] The evidence for involvement of macrophages in initial immune sensitization, humoral immune responses, and cell-mediated immune responses is summarized here so that the effects of cigarette smoke toxicity on these systems can be evaluated.

The macrophage participates in the processing of antigenic materials inhaled into the lung primarily by disposing of them and rendering them nonantigenic. Thus, toxic effects could alter the potential antigenic load to which immunocompetent cells become exposed. A small portion of the antigen processed by macrophages may be conveyed directly to uncommitted lymphocytes. It appears likely that the AM may at least participate in, if not be essential for, appropriate presentation of antigens to lymphocytes for immune sensitization.[110]

The function of the AM as a phagocyte is enhanced by humoral immunity against challenge particles. Coating of bacteria or yeast particles by specific antibody potentiates their phagocytosis by AMs. This enhancement occurs with immunoglobulin G (IgG) antibody, but not with IgM antibody.[111] Cell membrane surface receptors have been identified on human AMs for the Fc portion of IgG and the third component of complement, but not for IgM.[112-114] These surface binding receptors may increase attachment of target particles to phagocytic cells. In addition, it appears that the event of an IgG-coated particle binding to an appropriate membrane receptor stimulates internalization of that particle by the macrophage, although similar stimulation after binding does not occur at the complement receptor site.[115]

The macrophage is an important effector of cell-mediated immunity in the lung. Sensitized T lymphocytes secrete "lymphokines" following antigen stimulation, and AMs are responsive to these signals.[109,116] This responsiveness has been demonstrated most extensively in systems which demonstrate inhibition of random macrophage movement and test for "migration inhibition factor" (MIF). AMs also respond to substances from sensitized stimulated lymphocytes by undergoing "activation". The activated macrophage enlarges, becomes a more aggressive phagocyte, increases its consumption of oxygen and glucose, and increases its lysosomal enzyme content.[117] In response to signals from T lymphocytes, the AM becomes capable of killing intracellular infectious agents, such as Lysteria, Mycobacteria, or Toxoplasma, which it could not otherwise dispose of. This activation is not immunospecific, and the activated macrophage can kill in vivo or in vitro organisms of the same species used to sensitize the lymphocytes as well as different species of intracellular parasites. Thus, the immunologically activated cell is a far more potent defender of the lung against infectious diseases than the resident macrophage at rest.

The macrophage also functions as an orchestrator of the inflammatory response in the lung. As well as being receptive to signals from lymphocytes, AMs also elaborate "monokines" which signal other inflammatory cells to multiply and congregate in an area of macrophage activity. Human macrophages elaborate colony-stimulating factor which promotes bone marrow granulocyte and mononuclear cell proliferation.[118] AMs elaborate a small molecular weight chemotactic factor which attracts PMN leukocytes.[119,120] They also elaborate a leukocyte chemotactic factor in response to phagocytosis of latex bends or immune complexes. These studies indicate that the macrophage plays a pivotal role in immunospecific as well as nonspecific lung defense.

The macrophage functions as an antigen processor, an effector cell of humoral and cell-mediated immunity, and as an amplification and modulation system in pulmonary inflammation. The important point to be made here is that tobacco smoke has a variety of toxic effects on the pulmonary immune response and the immunologic role of the AM. It has been shown that smoking impairs antibody-forming cell production in laboratory animals,[121] and human smokers have a less intense and less prolonged immune response to influenza infection of immunization then do nonsmokers.[122] Antigen processing by smokers' macrophages probably is altered regarding phagocytic function (see above). A smaller proportion of the smokers' macrophage population has receptors for complement (C3b) than in nonsmokers, although the frequency of IgG receptors is unchanged.[114] Smokers' AMs demonstrate increased random movement and responsiveness to nonimmunologic chemoattractants or increased "chemokinesis".[116] However, true immunologic responsiveness of these same cells appears depressed since they do not respond to immunologically stimulated lymphocyte MIF as intensely as do cells from nonsmokers.[123]

D. Activated Macrophages

Smokers' macrophages are sometimes referred to as "activated macrophages", and share some characteristics with immunologically activated AMs such as those obtained from Bacille Calmette Guerin (BCG) immunized rabbits.[124] Table 3, which contrasts features from smokers' and nonsmokers' cells, may be used to address the issue whether smokers' macrophages are activated. Smokers show an increase in the number of macrophages in the lung and an increased proportion of cells which assume a flat shape in monolayer culture, as do activated macrophages.[18] In contrast, smokers' cells show decreased rather than increased cell membrane complexity and have many intracellular inclusions.[79] Both activated and smokers' AMs show increased oxygen consumption, glucose consumption, and lysosomal enzyme content. These morphologic and metabolic features of smoker's cells encompass most of the similarities, although important functional differences can be identified as well. Activated macrophages show increased rates of phagocytosis of a variety of particles, but smokers' macrophages generally show decreased rates or no change from nonsmokers' cells. Smokers' AMs appear to demonstrate decreased, rather than enhanced responsiveness to lymphocyte immunologic signals. The ability of smokers' and nonsmokers' macrophages to kill *Lysteria* or other intracellular pathogens, a hallmark of the activated macrophage, has not been tested. Although morphologic and metabolic similarities exist, the smokers AM is not functionally equivalent to an activated macrophage and probably should not be viewed as an equal.

In summarizing briefly, we can say that cigarette smoking provides a complex and relatively well-studied model of macrophage toxicology. The changes in cell population, morphology, metabolism, and function observed with smoking probably are representative of similar changes which occur with a wide variety of potentially toxic gases and particles. Continuing research efforts are required to characterize macrophage responses to a variety of toxic exposures. Efforts also should be directed towards a better understanding of how individual smoke components cause specific alterations in macrophage form and function. In this way, tobacco smoke serves as a probe for better understanding the basic cell biology of the AM.

E. Carcinogenesis

It is very likely that the AM bears a major responsibility for the disposal of inhaled cancer-causing substances. For example, carcinogenic particulates such as asbestos initially are ingested and transported by macrophages as discussed earlier. Nonparticulate carcinogens also may be ingested by macrophages from the fluids lining the alveolus. Condensation of carcinogens on particulates such as tars absorbed onto respirable kaolinite particles in cigarette smoke might be an important mechanism by which these substances reach the AM. Ideally, the disposal system should be enlarged to meet the challenge of an increased load of carcinogens. Perhaps the increased number and size of AMs which result from cigarette smoking might be viewed in this light. Conversely, impaired AM function might lead to impaired disposal and consequently to increased exposure to carcinogens. Although the number of AMs available for particle phagocytosis is increased in smokers, the ability of individual cells to phagocytize is not increased and actually may be impaired. The relative importance of these conflicting responses in carcinogenesis is unclear.

Macrophages might potentiate the effect of inhaled carcinogens, either by concentrating them in local areas of the lung or by converting them into compounds of higher carcinogenicity. It seems plausible that macrophages may collect potentially carcinogenic substances for storage in phagolysosomes, thus concentrating those materials within cells. When macrophages aggregate and then disintegrate in the respiratory bronchioles of smokers,[79,84] high concentrations of carcinogens might be applied to local areas within the lung. Processing of debris by macrophages might contribute to carcinogenesis by converting a relatively innocent substance into a carcinogenic one. Polycyclic hydrocarbons such as benzo[α]pyrene are present in high concentrations in cigarette smoke and are known to cause lung cancer in experimental animals.[125] The microsomal enzyme aryl hydrocarbon hydroxylase (AHH) is present in most mammalian cells to process polycyclic hydrocarbons.[126] This enzyme may convert benzo[α]pyrene and other similar substances to more carcinogenic epoxides during their degradation to hydroxides.[127] Thus, exposure to benzo[α]pyrene and high levels of AHH might lead to increased carcinogenic potential. A tenfold increase in AHH is found in smokers' macrophages and increased AHH can be induced in nonsmokers' AMs by smoking.[128] Interestingly though, lung cancer patients appear to have appropriate macrophage AHH levels for their smoking status. Variability between individuals at different times, and the rapid inducibility and decline of AHH make clinical interpretation of these findings difficult. The alveolar location of most macrophages and the predominance of proximal bronchial carcinomas[129] suggest that the AM may not be of major importance in the instigation of many lung cancers. On the other hand, metabolic conversion of environmental substances by AMs from acutely toxic to less toxic but carcinogenic forms and the ultimate delivery of these substances to targets such as the bronchial epithelium deserve further investigation. The smoker appears to be continuously subjected to

1. An increased load of carcinogenic substances in smoke
2. Altered processing mechanisms which may possibly enhance carcinogenic effects
3. Altered immunologic responsiveness which might impair tumor rejection once established

The role of the macrophage in the processing and disposal of carcinogens is an area of extreme importance where little data are available.

VI. SUMMARY

The AM is an important participant in many normal pulmonary functions and a significant mediator of a variety of lung diseases. Available evidence has shown that AMs originate as monocytes of the bone marrow and migrate from the pulmonary vasculature into the interstitium. To reach the small air spaces, the cells migrate through basement membranes and between alevolar lining cells. The air spaces contain a variety of morphologic and functional types of macrophages, most of which are cleared from the lung by the mucociliary escalator of the airways.

The AM provides the first line of defense against inhaled microorganisms and inorganic particles. In attempts to phagocytize, package, digest, and export these materials, the cell releases into its milieu a variety of enzymes with proteolytic, elastolytic and inflammatory properties. These enzymes are associated with the formation of pulmonary emphysema and fibrosis through mechanisms which are poorly understood. It seems that silica and asbestos in particular are potent promoters of fibrotic lung disease. The pathogenesis of disease may be mediated by toxic events which occur between the inhaled particles and lysosomal membranes of the macrophages.

Toxic gases are inhaled and can produce increased susceptibility to respiratory infection. This could be attributed to macrophage dysfunction inasmuch as death is caused by toxic events consequent to oxidant injury by commonly encountered gases, such as O_2, NO_2, and O_3. AMs exhibiting toxic injury from gas exposure are compromised of phagocytes in both animals and man.

Cigarette smoke is a common insult to the AM and is considered a combination of particles and gases which are known to cause cell toxicity. Indeed, the AM exposed to cigarette smoke is altered in a variety ways, including its morphology, microbicidal function, and immunologic responsiveness. Cigarette smoke contains inorganic particulates, oxidant gases, and carcinogens which may act synergistically to compromise normal macrophage function and consequently could mediate a variety of lung diseases associated with cigarette use.

The AM is an important, dynamic, and rather exciting resident of the lung. We have much to learn about its normal functions as well as the roles it may play in pulmonary disease.

REFERENCES

1. **Green, G. M., Jakab, G. J., Low, R. B., and Davis, G. S.,** Defense mechanisms of the respiratory membrane, *Am. Rev. Respir. Dis.,* 115, 479, 1977.
2. **Allison, A. C.,** Mechanisms of macrophage toxicity in relation to the pathogenesis of some lung diseases, in *Respiratory Defense Mechanisms,* Vol. 2, Brain, J. D., Proctor, D. F., and Reid, L. M., Eds., Marcel Dekker, New York, 1977, 1075.
3. **Brain, J. D., Godleski, J. J., and Sorokin, S. P.,** Quantification, origin, and fate of pulmonary macrophages, in *Respiratory Defense Mechanisms,* Brain, J. D., Proctor, D. F., and Reid, L. M., Eds., Marcel Dekker, New York, 1977, 849.
4. **Sorokin, S. P.,** Phagocytes in the lungs, in *Respiratory Defense Mechanisms,* Vol. 2, Brain, J. D., Proctor, D. F., and Reid, Eds., L. M., Marcel Dekker, New York, 1977, 711.
5. **Meuret, G. and Hoffman, G.,** Monocyte kinetic studies in normal and disease states, *Br. J. Haematol.,* 24, 275, 1973.
6. **Ungar, J. and Wilson, G. R.,** Monocytes as a source of alveolar phagocytes, *Am. J. Pathol.,* 11, 681, 1935.
7. **Van Furth, R. and Cohn, Z. A.,** The origin and kinetics of mononuclear phagocytes, *J. Exp. Med.,* 128, 415, 1968.
8. **Virolainen, M.,** Hematopoietic origin of macrophages as studied by chromosome markers in mice, *J. Exp. Med.,* 127, 943, 1968.
9. **Golde, D. W., Finley, T. N., and Cline, M. J.,** The pulmonary macrophage in acute leukemia, *N. Engl. J. Med.,* 290, 875, 1974.
10. **Bowden, D. H. and Adamson, I. Y. R.,** The pulmonary interstitial cell as immediate precursor of the alveolar macrophage, *Am. J. Pathol.,* 68, 521, 1972.
11. **Murphy, G. F., Brody, A. R., and Craighead, J. E.,** Monocyte migration across pulmonary membranes in mice infected with cytomegalovirus, *Exp. Mol. Pathol.,* 22, 35, 1975.
12. **Davis, G. S., Brody, A. R., and Craighead, J. E.,** Analysis of airspace and interstitial mononuclear cell populations in human diffuse interstitial lung disease, *Am. Rev. Respir. Dis.,* 118, 7, 1978.
13. **Mossman, B. T., Adler, K. B., and Craighead, J. E.,** Interaction of carbon particles with rodent tracheal epithelium in culture, *Environ. Res.,* 16, 110, 1978.
14. **Crapo, J. D., Brody, A. R., Barry, B. E., and O'Neil, J.,** *Morphologic, Morphometric and X-ray Microanalytical Studies on Lung Tissue of Rats Exposed to Chrysotile Asbestos in Inhalation Chambers,* Proc. IARC Symp. Biological Effects of Mineral Fibers, Lyon, France, 2, 273, 1980.

15. Lauweryns, J. M. and Baert, J. H., Alveolar clearance and the role of the pulmonary lymphatics, *Am. Rev. Respir. Dis.,* 115, 625, 1977.
16. Adamson, I. Y. R. and Bowden, D. H., Adaptive responses of the pulmonary macrophagic system to carbon. II. Morphologic studies, *Lab. Invest.,* 38, 430, 1978.
17. Brain, J. D., Kruidson, D. E., Sorokin, S. P., and Davis, Y. A., Pulmonary distribution of particles given by intratracheal instillation or by aerosol inhalation, *Environ. Res.,* 11, 13, 1976.
18. Davis, G. S., Brody, A. R., and Adler, K. B., Functional and physiologic correlates of human alveolar macrophage cell shape and surface morphology, *Chest,* 75, 280, 1979.
19. Bowden, D. H., The alveolar macrophage, *Curr. Top. Pathol.,* 36, 1971.
20. Cohen, A. B. and Cline, M. J., the human alveolar macrophage: isolation, cultivation *in vitro,* and studies of morphologic and functional characteristics, *J. Clin. Invest.,* 50, 1390, 1971.
21. Cohn, Z. A. and Wiener, E., The particulate hydrolases of macrophages. I. Comparative enzymology, isolation and properties, *J. Exp. Med.,* 118, 991, 1963.
22. Cohen, Z. A. and Wiener, E., The particulate hydrolases of macrophages, II. Biochemical and morphological response to particle ingestion, *J. Exp. Med.,* 118, 1009, 1963.
23. Mass, B., Ikeda, T., Meranze, D. R., Weinbaum, G., and Kimbel, P., Induction of experimental emphysema: cellular and species specificity, *Am. Rev. Respir. Dis.,* 106, 384, 1972.
24. Janoff, A., Anatomic emphysema produced in mice by lysosome-containing fractions from human alveolar macrophages, *Fed. Proc. Fed. Am. Soc. Exp. Biol.,* 31, 254, 1972.
25. Kilroe-Smith, T. A., Webster, I., Van Drimmelen, M., and Marasas, L., An insoluble fibrogenic factor in macrophages from guinea pigs exposed to silica, *Environ. Res.,* 6, 298, 1973.
26. Heppleston, A. G. and Styles, J. A., Activity of a macrophage factor in collagen formation by silica, *Nature (London),* 214, 521, 1967.
27. Nourse, L. D., Nourse, P. N., Botes, H., and Schwartz, H. M., The effects of macrophages isolated from the lungs of guinea pigs dusted with silica on collagen biosynthesis by guinea pig fibroblasts in cell culture, *Environ. Res.,* 9, 115, 1975.
28. Turino, G. M., Rodriguez, J. R., Greenbaum, L. M., and Mandl, I., Mechanisms of pulmonary injury, *Am. J. Med.,* 57, 493, 1974.
29. Green, G. M. and Kass, E. H., The role of the alveolar macrophage in the clearance of bacteria from the lung, *J. Exp. Med.,* 119, 167, 1964.
30. Ackerman, N. R. and and Beebe, J. R., Release of lysosomal enzymes by alveolar mononuclear cells, *Nature (London),* 247, 475, 1974.
31. Henson, P. M., The immunologic release of consituents from neutrophil leukocytes. II. Mechanisms of release during phagocytosis, and adherence to non-phagocytosable surfaces, *J. Immunol.,* 107, 1547, 1971.
32. Weissman, G., Zurier, R. B., Spieler, P. J., and Goldstein, I. M., Mechanisms of lysosomal enzyme release from leukocytes exposed to immune complexes and other particles, *J. Exp. Med.,* 134, 149, 1971.
33. Weissmann, G., Zurier, R. B., and Hoffstein, S., Leukocytic proteases and the immunologic release of lysosomal enzymes, *Am. J. Pathol.,* 68, 539, 1972.
34. Morrow, P. E., Alveolar clearance of aerosols, *Arch. Intern. Med.,* 131, 101, 1973.
35. Marks, J., The neutralization of silica toxicity *in vitro, Br. J. Ind. Med.,* 14, 81, 1957.
36. Allison, A. C., Role of lysosomes in oxygen toxicity, *Nature (London),* 205, 141, 1965.
37. Nadler, V. and Goldfischer, S., The intracellular release of lysosomal contents in macrophages that have ingested silica, *J. Histochem. Cytochem.,* 18, 368, 1970.
38. Harrington, J. S., Allison, A. C., and Badani, D. V., Mineral fibers: chemical, physiochemical and biological properties, *Adv. Pharmacol. Chemother.,* 12, 291, 1975.
39. Halme, J., Uitto, J., Kahanpaa, K., Karhunen, P., and Lindy, S., Protocollagen proline hydroxylase activity in experimental pulmonary fibrosis of rats, *J. Lab. Clin. Med.,* 75, 535, 1970.
40. Burrell, R. and Anderson, M., The introduction of fibrogenesis by silica-treated alveolar macrophages, *Environ. Res.,* 6, 389, 1973.
41. Leibovich, S. J. and Ross, R., A macrophage-dependent factor that stimulates the proliferation of fibroblasts *in vitro, Am. J. Pathol.,* 84, 501, 1976.
42. Miller, K., Handfield, R. F., and Kagan, E., The effects of different mineral dusts on the mechanism of phagocytosis: a scanning electron microscope study, *Environ. Res.,* 15, 139, 1978.
43. Chamberlain, M. and Brown, R. C., The cytotoxic effects of asbestos and other mineral dust in tissue culture cell lines, *Br. J. Exp. Pathol.,* 59, 183, 1978.
44. Davies, P., Allison, A. C., Ackerman, J., Butterfield, A., and Williams, S., Asbestos induces selective release of lysosomal enzymes from mononuclear phagocytes, *Nature (London),* 251, 423, 1974.
45. Morgan, A., Davies, P., Wagner, J. C., Berry, G., and Holmes, A., The biological effects of magnesium leached chrysotile asbestos, *Br. J. Exp. Pathol.,* 58, 465, 1977.

46. **Narang, S., Rahman, Q., Kaw, J. L.,and Zaidi, S. H.,** Dissolution of silicic acid from dusts of kaolin, mica and talc and its relation to their hemolytic activity — an *in vitro* study, *Exp. Pathol.,* 13, 346, 1977.

47. **Manyai, S., Kabai, J., Kis, J., Suveges, E., and Timar, M.,** The effect of heat treatment on the structure of kaolin and its *in vitro* hemolytic activity, *Environ. Res.,* 3, 187, 1970.

48. **Shy, C. M., Creason, J. P., Pearlman, M. E., McClain, K. E., Benson, F. B., and Young, M. M.,** The Chattanooga School children study: effects of community exposure to nitrogen dioxide. II. Incidence of acute respiratory illness, *J. Air Pollut. Control Assoc.,* 20, 582, 1970.

49. **Haynes, W. F., Jr., Krestulovic, V. J., and Loomis, A. L., Jr.,** Smoking habit and incidence of respiratory tract infections in a group of adolescent males, *Am. Rev. Respir. Dis.,* 93, 730, 1966.

50. **Parnell, J. L., Anderson, D. O., and Kinnis, C.,** Cigarette smoking and respiratory infections in a class of student nurses, *N. Engl. J. Med.,* 274, 979, 1966.

51. **Morgan, M. S. and Frank, R.,** Uptake of pollutant gases by the respiratory system, in *Respiratory Defense Mechanisms,* Vol. 1, Brain, J. D., Proctor, D. F., and Reid, L. M., Eds., Marcel Dekker, New York, 1977, 157.

52. **Clark, J. M. and Lambertsen, C. J.,** Pulmonary oxygen toxicity: a review, *Pharmacol. Rev.,* 23, 37, 1971.

53. **Sturin, P. A., Permutt, S., and Riley, R.,** Pulmonary antibacterial defenses with pure oxygen breathing, *Proc. Soc. Exp. Biol.,* 137, 1202, 1971.

54. **Huber, G. L. and LaForce, F. M.,** Comparative effects of ozone and oxygen on pulmonary antibacterial defense mechanisms, *Antimicrob. Agents Chemother.,* 10, 129, 1970.

55. **Brain J. D., and Feldman, H. A.,** Exposure to 100% oxygen affects pulmonary macrophage adhesion and endocytosis *in vivo, Am. Rev. Respir. Dis.,* 117, 315a, 1978.

56. **Murphy, S. A., Hyams, J. S., Fisher, A. B., and Root, R. K.,** Effects of oxygen exposure on *in vitro* function of pulmonary alveolar macrophages, *J. Clin. Invest.,* 56, 503, 1975.

57. **Raffin, T. A., Braun, D., Simon, L. M., Theodore, J., and Robin, E. D.,** Impairment of phagocytosis by relatively low level O_2 exposure (40% O_2) in alveolar macrophages, *Clin. Res.,* 25, 422a, 1977.

58. **McCord, J. M. and Fridovich, I.,** Superoxide dismutase, *J. Biol. Chem.,* 244, 6049, 1969.

59. **Crapo, J. D. and Tierney, D. F.,** Superoxide dismutase and pulmonary oxygen toxicity, *Am. J. Physiol.,* 226, 1401, 1974.

60. **Kimball, R. E., Reddy, K., Pierce, T. H., Schwartz, L. W., Mustafa, M. G., and Cross, C. E.,** Oxygen toxicity: augmentation of antioxidant defense mechanisms in rat lung, *Am. J. Physiol.,* 230, 1425, 1976.

61. **Deneke, S. M., Bernstein, S., and Fanburg, B. L.,** Absence of inductive effect of hyperoxia on superoxide dismutase activity in rat alveolar macrophages, *Am. Rev. Respir. Dis.,* 118, 105, 1978.

62. **Autor, A. P., Frank, L., and Roberts, R. J.,** Developmental characteristics of pulmonary superoxide dismutase: relationship to idiopathic respiratory distress syndrome, *Pediatr. Res.,* 10, 154, 1976.

63. **Stevens, J. B. and Autor, A. P.,** Induction of superoxide dismutase by oxygen in neonatal rat lung, *J. Biol. Chem.,* 252, 3509, 1977.

64. **Simon, L. M., Liu, J., Theodore, J., and Robin, E. D.,** Effect of hyperoxia, hypoxia, and maturation on superoxide dismutase activity in isolated alveolar macrophages, *Am. Rev. Respir. Dis.,* 115, 279, 1977.

65. **Lentz, P. E. and DiLuzio, N. R.,** Peroxidation of lipids in alveolar macrophages, *Arch. Environ. Health,* 28, 279, 1974.

66. **Goldstein, E., Eagle, M. C., and Hoeprich, P. D.,** Effect of nitrogen dioxide on pulmonary bacterial defense mechanisms, *Arch. Environ. Health,* 26, 202, 1973.

67. **Goldstein, E., Warshauer, M. A., Lippert, W., and Tarkington, B.,** Ozone and nitrogen dioxide exposure, *Arch. Environ. Health,* 28, 85, 1974.

68. **Coffin, D. L., Gardner, D. E., Holzman, R. S., and Wolock, F. J.,** Influence of ozone on pulmonary cells, *Arch. Environ. Health,* 16, 633, 1968.

69. **Acton, J. D., and Myrvik, Q. N.,** Nitrogen dioxide effects on alveolar macrophages, *Arch. Environ. Health,* 24, 48, 1972.

70. **Vassallo, C. L., Domm, B. M., Poe, R. H., Duncombe, M. C., and Gee, J. B. L.,** NO_2 gas and NO_2 effects on alveolar macrophage phagocytosis and metabolism, *Arch. Environ. Health,* 26, 270, 1973.

71. **Huber, G. L., Mason, R. J., LaForce, M., Spencer, N. J., Gardner, D. E., and Coffin, D. V. M,** Alterations in the lung following the administration of ozone, *Arch. Int. Med. Symp.,* 9, 1971.

72. **Goldstein, E., Munson, E. S., Eagle, C., Martucci, R. W., and Hoeprich, P. D.,** Influence of anaesthetic agents on murine pulmonary bactericidal activity, *Antimicrob. Agents Chemother.,* 10, 231, 1971.

73. **Mustafa, M. G., Cross, C. E., and Tyler, W. S.,** Interference of cadmium ion with oxidative metabolism of alveolar macrophages, *Arch. Intern. Med. Symp.,* 9, 1971.

74. Bingham, E., Barkley, W., Zergas, M., Stemmer, K., and Taylor, P., Responses of alveolar macrophages to metals. I. Inhalation of lead and nickel, *Arch. Environ. Health*, 25, 406, 1972.

75. Waters, M. D., Gardner, D. E., Aranyi, C., and Coffin, D. L., Metal toxicity for rabbit alveolar macrophages *in vitro*, *Environ. Res.*, 9, 32, 1975.

76. Graham, J. A., Gardner, D. E., Waters, M. D., and Coffin, D. L., Effects of trace metals on phagocytosis by alveolar macrophages, *Infect. Immunol.*, 11, 1278, 1975.

77. Martin, R. R., and Warr, G. A., Cigarette smoking and human pulmonary macrophages, *Hosp. Pract.*, 12, 97, 1977.

78. Wynder, E. L. and Hoffmann, D., *Tobacco and Tobacco Smoke*, Academic press, New York, 1967.

79. Brody, A. R. and Craighhead, J. E., Cytoplasmic inclusions in pulmonary macrophages of cigarette smokers, *Lab. Invest.*, 32, 125, 1975.

80. Selikoff, J. J., Hammond, E. C., and Churg, J., Asbestos exposure, smoking, and neoplasia, *JAMA*, 203, 105, 1968.

81. Lundin, F. E., Lloyd, J. W., Smith, E. M., Archer, V. E., and Holaday, D. A., Mortality of uranium miners in relation to radiation, hard-rock mining, and cigarette smoking, *Health Phys*, 1950 through September 1967, 16, 571, 1969.

82. Feron, J. W., Emmelot, E., and Vossenaar, T., Lower respiratory tract tumors in Syrian golden hamsters after intratracheal installations of diethylnitrosamine alone and with ferric oxide, *Eur. J. Cancer*, 8, 445, 1972.

83. Pelfrene, A. F., Experimental evaluation of the clearance of 3,4-benzo(a)pyrene in association with talc from hamster lungs, *Am. Ind. Hyg. Assoc. J.*, 37, 706, 1976.

84. Niewoehner, D. E., Kleinerman, J., and Rice, D. B., Pathologic changes in the peripheral airways of young cigarette smokers, *N. Engl. J. Med.*, 291, 755, 1974.

85. Pratt, S. A., Finley, T. N., Morris, H. S., and Ladman, J., A comparison of alveolar macrophages and pulmonary surfactant obtained from the lungs of human smokers and non-smokers by endobronchial lavage, *Anat. Rec.*, 163, 497, 1969.

86. Harris, J. O., Swenson, E. W., and Johnson, J. E., Human alveolar macrophages: comparison of phagocytic ability, glucose utilization, and ultrastructure in smokers and nonsmokers, *J. Clin. Invest.*, 49, 2086, 1970.

87. Reynolds, H. Y. and Newball, H. H., Analysis of proteins and respiratory cells obtained from human lungs by bronchial lavage, *J. Lab. Clin. Med.*, 84, 559, 1974.

88. Low, R. B., Davis, G. S., and Giancola, M. S., Biochemical analysis of broncho-alveolar lavage fluids of healthy human volunteer smokers and nonsmokers, *Am. Rev. Respir. Dis.*, 118, 863, 1978.

89. Frasca, J. M., Auerbach, O., Parks, V. R., and Jamieson, J. D., Electron microscopic observations on pulmonary fibrosis and emphysema in smoking dogs, *Exp. Mol. Pathol.*, 15, 108, 1971.

90. Matulionis, D. H. and Traurig, H. H., *In situ* response of lung macrophages and hydrolase activities to cigarette smoke, *Lab. Invest.*, 37, 314, 1977.

91. Martin, R. R., Altered morphology and increased acid hydrolase content of pulmonary macrophages from cigarette smokers, *Am. Rev. Respir. Dis.*, 107, 596, 1973.

92. Harris J. O., Olsen, G. N., Castle, J. R., and Maloney, A. S., Comparison of proteolytic enzyme activity in pulmonary alveolar macrophages and blood leukocytes in smokers and nonsmokers, *Am. Rev. Respir. Dis.*, 111, 579, 1975.

93. Laurenzi, G. A., Guaneri, J. J., Endriga, R. B., and Carey, J. P., Clearance of bacteria by the lower respiratory tract, *Science*, 142, 1572, 1963.

94. Kass, E. H. and Green, G. M., Mechanisms of resistance to chronic pulmonary infection, in *Bronchitis: An International Symposium*, Grie, N. G. M. and Sluiter, H. J., Eds. Groningen, The Netherlands, 1964, 73.

95. Spurgash, A., Ehrich, R., and Petzold, R., Effects of cigarette smoke on resistance to respiratory infection, *Arch. Environ. Health*, 16, 385, 1968.

96. Green, G. M. and Carolin, D., The depressant effect of cigarette smoke on the *in vitro* antibacterial activity of alveolar macrophages, *N. Engl. J. Med.*, 276, 422, 1967.

97. Cutting, M., LaGuarda, R., Pereira, W., and Huber, G., The effect of *in vitro* exposure to cigar smoke on alveolar macrophage bactericidal function, *Clin. Res.*, 22, 716a, 1974.

98. Huber, G. L., Cutting, M. E., McCarthy, C. R., Simmons, G. A., LaGuarda, R., and Pereira, W., The depressant effect of marijuana smoke on the antibacterial activity of pulmonary alveolar macrophages, *Chest*, 68, 769, 1975.

99. Cutting, M., Watson, A., Goodenough, S., Simmons, G., LaGuarda, R., Huber, G., Impairment of alveolar macrophage bactericidal activity by synthetic tobacco substitutes, *Am. Rev. Respir. Dis.*, 109, 726, 1974.

100. Powell, G. M. and Green, G. M., Cigarette smoke — a proposed metabolic lesion in alveolar macrophages, *Biochem. Pharmacol.*, 21, 1785, 1972.

101. Jakab, G. J., Adverse effect of a cigarette smoke component, acrolein, on pulmonary antibacterial defenses and on viral-bacterial interactions in the lung, *Am. Rev. Respir. Dis.*, 115, 33, 1977.

102. **Green, G. M.,** Cigarette smoke: protection of alveolar macrophages by glutathione and cysteine, *Science,* 162, 810, 1968.
103. **Stuart, R. S., Higgins, W. H., and Brown, D. W.,** *In vitro* toxicity of tobacco smoke solutions to rabbit alveolar macrophages, *Arch. Environ. Health,* 33, 135, 1978.
104. **York, G. K., Arth, C., Stumbo, J. A., Cross, C, E., and Mustafa, M. G.,** Pulmonary macrophages respiration as affected by cigarette smoke and tobacco extract, *Arch. Environ. Health,* 27, 96, 1973.
105. **Holt, P. G. and Keast, D.,** Acute effects of cigarette smoke on murine macrophages, *Arch. Environ. Health,* 26, 300, 1973.
106. **Low, R. B. and Bulman, C. A.,** Stubstrate transport by the pulmonary alveolar macrophage, *Am. Rev. Respir. Dis.,* 116, 423, 1977.
107. **Kaltreider, H. B.,** State of the art: expressions of immune mechanisms in the lung, *Am. Rev. Respir. Dis.,* 113, 347, 1976.
108. **Schwartz, S. L. and Bellanti, J. A.,** The relationship of the alveolar macrophage to the immunologic responses of the lung, in *Respiratory Defense Mechanisms,* Vol. 2, Brain, J. D., Proctor, D. F., and Reid, L. M., Eds., Marcel Dekker, New York, 1977, 1053.
109. **Moore, V. L. and Myrvik, Q. N.,** The role of normal alveolar macrophages in cell-mediated immunity, *J. Reticuloendothel. Soc.,* 21, 131, 1977.
110. **Unanue, E. R.,** The regulatory role of macrophages in antigenic stimulation, *Adv. Immunol.,* 15, 95, 1972.
111. **Reynolds, H. Y., Kazmierowski, J. A., and Newball, H. H.,** Specificity of oposonic antibodies to exchange phagocytosis of *Pseudomonas aeruginosa* by human alveolar macrophages, *J. Clin. Invest.,* 56, 376, 1975.
112. **Reynolds, H. Y., Atkinson, J. P., Newball, H. H., and Frank, M. M.,** Receptors for immunoglobulin and complement on human alveolar macrophages, *J. Immunol.,* 114, 1813, 1975.
113. **Daughaday, C. C., and Douglas, S. D.,** Membrane receptors on rabbit and human pulmonary alveolar macrophages, *J. Reticuloendothel. Soc.,* 18, 37, 1976.
114. **Warr, G. A., and Martin, R. R.,** Immune receptors of human alevolar macrophages: comparison between cigarette smokers and nonsmokers, *J. Reticuloendothel. Soc.,* 22, 181, 1977.
115. **Mantovani, B. Rabinovitch, M., and Nussenweig, V.,** Phagocytosis of immune complexes by macrophages, *J. Exp. Med.,* 135, 780, 1972.
116. **Warr, G. A. and Martin, R. R.,** Chemotactic responsiveness of human alveolar macrophages: effects of cigarette smoking, *Infect. Immunity,* 9, 769, 1974.
117. **David, J. R.,** Macrophage activation by lymphocyte mediators, *Fed. Proc. Fed. Am. Soc. Exp. Biol.,* 34, 1730, 1975.
118. **Golde, D. W., Finley, T. N., and Cline, M. J.,** Production of colony stimulating factor by human macrophages, *Lancet,* 2, 1397, 1972.
119. **Kazmierowski, J. A., Gallin, J. I., and Reynolds, H. Y.,** Mechanism for the inflammatory response in primate lungs: demonstration and partial characterization of an alveolar macrophage-derived chemotactic factor with preferential activity for polymorphonuclear leukocytes, *J. Clin. Invest.,* 59, 273, 1977.
120. **Dauber, J. H. and Daniele, R. P.,** Chemotactic activity of guinea pig alveolar macrophages, *Am. Rev., Respir. Dis.,* 117, 673, 1978.
121. **Keast, D. and Holt, P.,** Smoking and the immune response, *New Sci.,* 28, 806, 1974.
122. **Finklea, J., Hasselblad, V., Riggan, W., Hammer, D., and Newill, V.,** Cigarette smoking and hemagglutination inhibition response to influenza after natural disease and immunization, *Am. Rev. Respir. Dis.,* 104, 368, 1971.
123. **Warr, G. A. and Martin, R. R.,** *In vitro* migration of human alveolar macrophages: effects of cigarette smoking, *Infect. Immun.,* 8, 222, 1973.
124. **Myrvik, Q. N., Leake, E. S., and Oshima, S.,** A study of macrophages and epitheloid-like cells from granulomatous (BCG-induced) lungs of rabbits, *J. Immunol.,* 89, 745, 1962.
125. **Saffioti, U., Montesano, R., Sellakumar, A. R., Cefis, F., and Kaufman, D. G.,** Respiratory tract carcinogensis in hamsters induced by different numbers of administrations of benzo[a]pyrene and ferric oxide, *Cancer Res,.* 32, 1073, 1972.
126. **Nebert, D. W. and Gelboin, H. V.,** The *in vivo* and *in vitro* induction of aryl hydrocarbon hydroxylase in mammalian cells of different species, tissues, strains, and developmental, and hormonal states, *Arch. Biochem. Biophys.,* 134, 76, 1969.
127. **Grover, P. L., Hewer, A., and Sims, P.,** Formation of K-region epoxides as microsomal metabolites of pyrene and benzo[a]pyrene, *Biochem. Pharmacol.,* 21, 2713, 1972.
128. **Cantrell, E. T., Warr, G. A., Busbee, D. L., and Martin, R. R.,** Induction of aryl hydrocarbon hydroxylase in human pulmonary alveolar macrophages by cigarette smoking, *J. Clin. Invest.,* 52, 1881, 1973.
129. **Carr, D. T. and Mountain, C. F.,** The staging of lung cancer, *Semin. Oncol.,* 1, 229, 1974.
130. **Davis, G.S.,** unpublished observations, 1978.

Chapter 2

RECRUITMENT OF INFLAMMATORY AND IMMUNOLOGICALLY COMPETENT CELLS

Marvin Lesser and Kaye H. Kilburn

TABLE OF CONTENTS

I. INTRODUCTION

Leukocytes begin to appear in the lung shortly after birth when the organ is thrown swiftly from a protected, sterile, wet environment into intimate contact with atmospheric gases and particles. Prior to birth neither neutrophils nor macrophages are found in airways or airspaces unless the fetus or its amniotic fluid have been disturbed by bacterial or viral infection, as by rupture of maternal membranes more than 24 hr before delivery.

After birth defenses against exogenous infectious particles become paramount and include isolation and detoxification by protective layers of mucus, surfactant, and immunoproteins, removal by the mucociliary escalator and lymphatics, and digestion and detoxification by scavenger cells. If these defenses are inadequate, or fail, the particles interact with the cells of the lung to stimulate, inhibit, or kill them. Although these last-ditch defenses by the epithelial and mesenchymal cells of the lung may be conservative and appropriate for the defense, they frequently encroach upon the airways or airspaces, further hampering defenses and reducing the lungs vital function of gas exchange.

The theme of this chapter is the mobilizing of the cellular defenses, i.e., the attraction of circulating leukocytes into the lung. That these cells play a vital part of the inflammatory process is well accepted. However, difficulties in sampling the mammalian lung in a precise manner have created grave problems in studies of the dynamics of cell recruitment. Furthermore, its complex organization constituting different zones, including a massive endothelial organ, a gossamer alveolar skin, and the interstitial space with its connective tissue and delivery systems for blood and air and removal of particles, add to the difficulties. Therefore, it calls for a certain trust in teleology, some reasoning from logical sequence, and extrapolation from in vitro and animal experiments to provide a coherent picture.

II. MECHANISMS OF NEUTROPHIL LOCOMOTION

The process of directed leukocyte movement in concentration gradients represents a series of complicated intracellular events that are initiated by interaction of specific cell receptors with chemoattractants. By using tritiated N-formylmethionyl-leucyl-phenylalanine (F-Met-Leu-[3H] Phe), a potent synthetic chemotactic peptide, Williams et al.[1] directly identified approximately 2000 binding sites per neutrophil. Of the 2000 potential receptors, only 100 to 200 needed to be occupied in order to obtain maximal chemotaxis. Showell et al.[2] synthesized 24 different tri- and tetrapeptides, mostly of the N-formylmethionyl group, and found that neutrophil chemotactic response was very specific in that small changes in the amino acid composition of the peptides, or even changes in amino acid position, altered activity markedly, suggesting that binding of the peptide with the receptor represents a stereospecific relationship.

In addition to stimulating chemotaxis, the interaction of small peptides with neutrophils has been found to induce coincidental lysosomal enzyme secretion.[2] Other agents, such as complement products and the chemotactic factor obtained from culture filtrates of *Escherichia coli*, also induce lysosomal enzyme release at the time of chemotaxis.[3] Such enzyme release may be mediated through cyclic nucleotides since cyclic adenosine monophosphate (cAMP), theophylline, prostaglandin E_1, and colchicine inhibit release, whereas cyclic guanosine monophosphate (cGMP) enhances it.[4] More recently, however, Spilberg et al.[5] found that the peptide Gly-His-Gly induced chemotaxis for human neutrophils without inducing lysosomal enzyme release, suggesting for the first time that chemotaxis and exocytosis may actually be mediated through separate receptors.

Besides causing chemotaxis and enzyme release, the interaction of chemoattractants with neutrophils also induces aggregation of cells and release of superoxide (O_2^-), both of which may contribute to acute injury of the lung endothelial cells. O'Flaherty et al.[5a] found that arachidonic acid stimulates human neutrophils to aggregate, but not to degranulate. On the basis of studies with three blockers of arachidonic acid metabolism, 5,8,11,14-eicosatetraynoic acid, indomethacin, and aspirin, the authors suggest that arachidonic acid may be a precursor of bioactive metabolites that mediate neutrophil function.[5a] Becker et al.[5b] found that N-formylmethionyl peptides stimulate O_2^- and H_2O_2 production in rabbit peritoneal neutrophils and suggest that the interaction of the peptides occurs at the same neutrophil receptor responsible for inducing chemokinesis, chemotaxis, granule enzyme secretion, and neutrophil aggregation.

Becker and Ward[6] have reported that neutrophils lose chemotactic responsiveness when incubated with phosphate esters, suggesting that an activated esterase in or on the neutrophil mediates cell response. Schiffman et al.[7] suggested a role for the esterase when they found that a chemotactic peptide, F-Met-Phe, was hydrolyzed to F-Met and Phe when incubated with neutrophils. This may be significant since further studies demonstrated that those formylated peptides that hydrolyze rapidly are better chemoattractants than those that hydrolyze slowly. Further support was provided by finding that reagents that inhibit hydrolysis also inhibit chemotaxis, suggesting that hydrolysis of peptides may be an obligatory step in the induction of directed cell movement.[7]

Once chemoattractants have interacted with the leukocyte surface to stimulate directed cell movement, changes occur in cellular K^+, Na^+, and Ca^{++}. Becker et al.[8] studied Na^+ and K^+ transmembrane fluxes of neutrophils with the chemotactic peptide N-formylmethionyl leucyl phenylalanine (f Met-Leu-Phe) and found that the peptide stimulated the Na^+-K^+ pump. It could not be decided, however, whether Na^+ efflux and K^+ influx played a direct role in cell movement towards the chemoattractant or served only to maintain equilibrium during movement. Boucek and Snyderman[9] measured calcium fluxes in neutrophils and found a marked influx of calcium when the cell was stimulated with a chemoattractant. On the basis of available information, Gallin et al.[10] proposed a hypothetical model of ionic control of leukocyte orientation during chemotaxis, suggesting that chemotactic factor interaction with the leukocyte membrane results initially in calcium influx and depolarization followed by hyperpolarization and finally calcium extrusion. These changes would provide an environment favorable for microtubule assembly, orientation, and pseudopod formation. More recently, Marasco et al.[10a] suggested that neither calcium nor magnesium is necessary for orientation in response to N-formylmethionyl-leucyl-phenylanine, but calcium is needed for maximum chemotactic response. In this scheme, the Na^+-K^+ pump would contribute to recovery.

As an alternate explanation, Lynn and Mukherjee[11] propose that hydroxy fatty acids, other lipids, and Ca^{++} ionophores stimulate cell movement by inducing accelerated Ca^{++} influx, whereas acidic peptides stimulate cells through monovalent cation influx, primarily Na^+. By whatever mechanism, the interaction of neutrophil and chemotactic factor quickly stimulates cell metabolism with an increase in both aerobic glycolysis and activity of the hexose monophosphate shunt.[12] Besides a need for energy, neutrophil locomotion requires a temperature between 25 and 40°C and a pH between 6.5 and 7.6.[13]

Flux changes in the leukocyte may involve only local areas of the cell membrane if a chemoattractant comes in contact with only that portion of the cell. Such a local process could lead to swelling and bulging of the cell membrane in that area into which cell contents could move as an early step in directed movement. In so doing, in contrast to the spherical shape in the circulation, migrating cells develop a forward, leading pseudopod, a mid-section containing the nucleus, and a trailing portion containing a few granules and mitochondria. Adherence is mainly in front. In moving through filters, the laminopodium is blunt, whereas in moving between endothelial or epithelial cells it is frequently pointed.[13] In neutrophil suspensions, the addition of chemotactic factors induces the development of elongated and bipolar cells within 10 min.[13a]

Cytochalasin B prevents neutrophil migration and decreases microfilaments, but allows normal orientation. Colchicine decreases centriole-associated microtubules and disturbs the orientation of nuclei and centrioles and pseudopod formation, thereby inhibiting directed movement, but not random migration.[14] Such studies suggest that although microfilaments are probably necessary for cell migration, intact microtubules are essential for normal pseudopod formation, orientation, and directed movement,[14] and that chemotaxis can be suppressed by conditions that inappropriately organize responsive microtubules in either a polymerized or depolymerized configuration.[14a]

III. IN VITRO CHEMOTAXIS

A. Neutrophils

Rapid advances in the understanding of leukocyte chemotaxis have occurred during the past 15 years with the use of the Boyden chamber.[15] The chamber consists of two compartments, separated by a micropore filter, in which cells are placed in the upper compartment and a soluble test substance is placed in the lower one. After incubation the filter is stained and examined under a microscope with chemotaxis being determined by several methods including

1. Counting the number of cells that have totally traversed the filter
2. Assessing the distance traversed by the advancing front of cells before they have moved completely through the filter[16]
3. Counting ^{51}Cr-labeled leukocytes that have migrated completely through the first filter and have fallen onto a second one.[17] Although the Boyden chamber has been primarily used to study chemotaxis of neutrophils, it can also be used to study eosinophils, basophils, lymphocytes, monocytes, fibroblasts, and neoplastic cells.

When tested in vitro, some substances attract neutrophils directly without the need for serum or other factors. Such substances have been classified as cytotaxins.[18] Substances that are not chemotactic alone but can act on substrate, usually serum, to generate a cytotaxin are classified as cytotaxigens (see Table 1 and Table 2).

Chemotactic components of complement activation have been the most extensively studied by in vitro methods. Complement components that have been found to act as cytotaxins include a trimolecular complex ($C\overline{567}$),[19] a split product of $C'3$ (C3a),[20] and a split product of $C'5$ (C5a).[21] More recent work using C6-deficient rabbit sera and purified human C3a and C5a suggests that C5a is the most active of the complement components.[22,23] It is now known that C5a is rapidly converted to C5a des Arg by a carboxypeptidase in serum, indicating that C5a des Arg may be the major active component in vivo under physiologic conditions.[23]

Any agent or substance that activates the classical or alternate complement pathway, or cleaves $C'5$ or $C'3$ directly, can function as a cytotaxigen. Of the numerous factors that can activate the classical pathway, antigen-antibody complexes appear to be the most important. Factors known to activate the alternate pathway include lipopolysaccharides,[24] asbestos fibers,[25] and many others. Substances acting directly on $C'3$ or $C'5$ to split off active factors include plasma[20] trypsin,[21] and a lysosomal enzyme from neutrophils.[26]

Bacterial products can function as cytotaxins or cytotaxigens. Many Gram-positive

Table 1

CYTOTAXINS FOR DIFFERENT LEUKOCYTES (INDICATED BY REFERENCE NUMBER)

Cytotaxin	Neutrophils	Lymphocytes	Mononuclears	Alveolar macrophages	Eosinophils	Fibroblasts
Complement products	19,20,21		86,96		121,122	
Bacterial products	18,27,30,48		30,86,96	96	121	
Low mol. wt. peptides	31		96	96		129
Virus-infected cell products	32		32			
Kallikrein	34		94			
Fibrinopeptide B	35					
Plasminogen activator	36		94			
Neutrophil fractions	37,38		86			
HETE	44					
Oxidized lipids	45					
Soluble collagen	46					129
Collagenolysis products	47					129
Lymphokines		84	90,91,92,96	96	123	128
Macrophage products	141	84				
ECF-A (mast cells + basophils)					108	
ECF (neutrophils)					114,115,116	
ECF (intermediate wt.)					117	
Histamine + metabolite					118,119	
Lung neoplasm components					124	
Anisakis larva extracts					125	

Table 2
CYTOTAXIGENS THAT INDUCE CHEMOTAXIS THROUGH
ACTIVATION OF COMPLEMENT PRODUCTS

Cytotaxigen	Neutrophils	Mononuclears	Eosinophils
Immune complexes	15	86	121
Lipopolysacchrides	24		
Asbestos fibers	25		
Plasma and trypsin	20,21	86	121
Lysosomal enzymes	26		
Bacterial proteinase	28		
Products of virus infected cells	33		
Neutrophil lysosomal fractions	26,37		
Tissue cell products	39		
Acid proteinase from lung + PAM's	88		
Heat killed *M. tuberculosis*	89		

and Gram-negative organisms release substances into the culture medium that directly attract neutrophils.[18,27] In addition, *Serratia marcescens* releases a proteinase that cleaves C3a from C3.[28]

In an attempt to identify specific bacterial components that induce chemotaxis, Schiffmann et al.[29] separated active peptides from *E. coli* culture filtrates and found that free carboxyl groups, but not free amino groups, are necessary for activity. Tainer et al.[30] isolated five lipid fractions from *E. coli* and found that one protein-free fraction attracted both neutrophils and macrophages. The other four fractions were found to be lipid-protein complexes that attracted macrophages only. However, when a peptide-free lipid extract of the four complexes was studied, it induced chemotaxis for neutrophils in a manner similar to arachiodonic acid (see below).

The observation that bacteria use N-formylmethionine in protein synthesis led investigators to study similar short-chained peptides for chemotactic activity.[31] It is now appreciated that a large number of peptides of the N-formylmethionyl group are chemoattractants (see Section II).

Viruses, like bacteria, can function as cytotaxins or cytotaxigens through their interaction with cells. Ward et al.[32] found that cells infected with mumps virus release a substance which attracts neutrophils directly. Brier et al.[33] found that rabbit kidney cells infected with *Herpes simplex* virus release a substance that interacts with serum to release C5a.

Several products of the kinin and coagulation systems also act as chemoattractants. Kaplan et al.[34] demonstrated that human plasma kallikrein attracts neutrophils in vitro, but Hageman factor fragments, prekallikrein, and bradykinin do not. In the coagulation system, fibrinopeptide B, but not fibrinopeptide A, AP, or AY,[35] and plasminogen activator[36] function as chemotactic factors.

Neutrophils have the ability to attract other neutrophils. This occurs through both cytotaxic activity which resides in postlysosomal supernatant fractions and cytotaxigenic activity which resides in lysosomal fractions.[37] Spilberg et al.[38] have also identified a heat-labile glycoprotein in the lysosomal fractions of human and rabbit neutrophils allowed to phagocytose monosodium urate crystals that acts as a cytotaxin.

Human alveolar macrophages release two substances into culture medium which attract blood polymorphonuclear granulocytes,[38a] with release being maximally stimulated by aggregated human immunoglobulin or zymosan particles. The larger substance had a mol wt of 10,000 daltons and was distinct from C5a. The smaller molecular weight substance was less well characterized.

Tissue cell products can also attract neutrophils, possibly explaining the appearance of neutrophils in areas of tissue damage. Hill and Ward[39] found that various rat tissues incubated in homologous serum cleaved C3 to its chemotactic fragment. The activity in rat heart tissue was due to a serine esterase with trypsin-like properties. The role of other intracellular components, namely cGMP and cAMP, in chemotaxis is unclear. It appears that agents that increase intracellular levels of cGMP, such as phenylephrine and prostaglandin F2a, tend to stimulate chemotaxis, whereas agents that increase cAMP, such as epinephrine, isoproterenol, and prostaglandin E_1 act to decrease chemotaxis.[40] However, cAMP alone in the Boyden chamber acts as a weak chemotaxin, whereas adenosine diphosphate (ADP) and adenosine triphosphate (ATP) act as inhibitors and adenosine monophosphate (AMP) is without effect.[41]

Higgins et al.[42] found that prostaglandin E_1 is chemotactic at concentrations as low as 10 ng/mℓ for rabbit neutrophils, whereas prostaglandins E_2 and F_{2a} had little or no chemotactic effect at concentrations up to 10 μg/mℓ. On the other hand, Till et al.[42a] found that in the absence of bovine serum albumin, prostaglandins of the F type (10^{-7} to 10^{-5} M) induced a chemokinetic and chemotactic response in rabbit peritoneal neutrophils, whereas prostaglandins of the E and A type had no significant effect. Human neutrophils, however, in vitro do not demonstrate chemotactic activity towards prostaglandins, prostaglandin precursors, or prostaglandin metabolites.[43] The difference in response between rabbit and human neutrophils may be due to species variation or to technical problems in handling lipids.[44]

Turner et al.[45] found that oxidized arachidonic acid, eicosapentaenoic acid, linolenic acid, docosahexaenoic acid, and arachidonyl acetate attracted human neutrophils in vitro, whereas none did so in the nonoxidized state. A metabolite of arachidonic acid, HETE (12-Hydroxy, 5,8,10,15 eicosatetraenoic acid), is also chemotactic in vitro for human neutrophils at concentrations between 10^{-4} and 10^{-7} M.[44] Since arachidonic acid is an important component of mammalian tissues, HETE may function as a physiologic chemoattractant through a process of

1. Disruption of plasma membranes with release of arachidonic acid through action of phospholipases,
2. Tissue conversion of arachidonic acid to HETE
3. Recruitment of cells by HETE

Products of collagenolysis produced by cutaneous collagenase, but not by bacterial collagenase, also attract neutrophils. These collagenolytic products consisted of at least 8 polypeptides between 1,000 and 30,000 daltons with 7 of them being leukotactic in vivo at a concentration of 10^{-10} M.[46,47] Stecher[48] found that bacterial collagenase was chemotactic for neutrophils in the Boyden chamber and confirmed that collagen degradation products following digestion with bacterial collagenase were not chemotactic. She also found that while fibrinogen, fibrin, and plasmin are not chemotactic in vitro, fibrin degradation products of human, bovine, sheep, and equine origin possess strong leukotactic activity.

1. Natural Inhibitors of Neutrophil Chemotaxis

Neutrophils can become irreversibly unresponsive to a chemoattractant (deactivated) if preincubated with the same chemoattractant before being placed in the Boyden chamber.[49] The process is very specific in that incubation with a dissimilar chemoattractant will not cause deactivation.[50] Deactivation is associated with a burst of activity of the hexose monophosphate shunt even though the cell remains immobile, indicating that deactivation is not due to inactivation.[12] The dicotomy may be explained by the recent suggestion that the apparent immobility is actually due to increased cell adhesiveness.[50a]

Normal serum contains two identified chemotactic factor inhibitors (CF-I) that inhibit the action of chemoattractants.[51] One, a β-globulin, inactivates C3a, and the other, an α-globulin, inactivates C5a.[52] Both appear to inactivate kallikrein, bacterial chemotactic factors, and a lymphokine chemotactic for monocytes.[52] The chemotactic factor inhibitors appear to function through aminopeptidase activity.[53]

Neutrophils produce several types of chemotactic inhibitors. One type, called neutrophil-immobilizing factor (NIF), inhibits passive motility and chemotaxis of neutrophils and eosinophils, but not monocytes.[17,54] It exists performed in neutrophils and monocytes and is released during phagocytosis. Another type, resembling CF-I, acts like a serum chemotactic inhibitor through inactivation of C5a, C3a, and a chemotactic factor derived from *E. coli*.[55] Elastase and cathepsin D appear to be the active factors released by the neutrophil that inactivate C5a.[55]

2. Clinical Disorders Associated with Abnormal Levels of Inhibitors

Abnormal neutrophil chemotaxis may occur in the presence of elevated levels of circulating or cell-directed inhibitors. Excess levels of serum CF-I have been detected in patients with cirrhosis,[56] uremia,[57] Hodgkin's disease,[58] sarcoidosis,[59] and cutaneous anergy.[60] Van Epps et al.[61] found that the presence of chemotactic inhibitor in serum directly paralleled skin test anergy and that the return of skin test reactivity coincided with a fall in chemotactic inhibitor activity. However, other factors are also involved since patients with anergy also demonstrate decreased lymphocyte-derived chemotactic factor production and poor response of neutrophils and monocytes to normal chemotactic factors.[62] Christou and Meakins[62a] suggest that decreased neutrophil chemotaxis observed in anergy is due to the *de novo* appearance of a circulating inhibitor with a mol wt of 310,000 daltons.

In contrast to the diseases associated with elevated levels of serum inhibitors, patients with a$_1$-antitrypsin deficiency and emphysema have a deficiency of chemotactic factor inactivator.[63] Such a deficiency may contribute to the pathogenesis of emphysema through excess neutrophil activity.

Excess levels of cell-directed inhibitors have been found infrequently. Smith et al.[64] described a patient with recurrent infections who had a neutrophil-directed inhibitor. Maderazo et al.[65] found an elevated level of a cell-directed inhibitor (CDI) in a patient with acute *Listeria* meningitis. They also found a normal antagonist of the inhibitor in normal serum, suggesting that CDI and its antagonist may function as normal regulators of chemotaxis. Patients with neoplasms involving lung and other organs also have elevated levels of inhibitors directed towards neutrophils and monocytes.[66,67]

Van Epps and Williams[68] found that serum from a patient with IgA myeloma suppressed neutrophil chemotaxis. The inhibitory factor was in the isolated IgA M component and acted on neutrophils. Davis et al.[69] described a child with recurrent pyogenic infections and elevated IgA who had neutrophil inhibition due to an IgM-IgA cryoglobulin complex.

3. Clinical Disorders Associated with Abnormal In Vitro Neutrophil Chemotaxis

A number of patients have been described whose leukocytes demonstrated abnormal chemotaxis in vitro. In most cases, the abnormality was attributed to a basic neutrophil defect, although in most situations a search for chemotactic inhibitory factors was not made. Such patients experience recurrent infections frequently involving the upper and lower respiratory tract. Some of these reported cases of abnormal in vitro chemotaxis and other clinical and laboratory abnormalities include 2 children with associated impaired random mobility,[70] 2 kindred with associated congenital ichthyosis,[71] a patient with associated congenital agammaglobulinema and abnormal phagocytosis,[72] 1 girl with associated decreased cellular immunity,[73] 3 children with associated elevated IgE levels and eczema,[74] 2 patients with elevated IgE and mucocutaneous candidiasis,[75] and 11 people with elevated IgE levels, eosinophilia, recurrent infections, and eczematous dermatitis.[76] Additional cases include 5 family members with asthma, eczema, and the histocompatibility antigen HLA-B12,[77] 14 patients with recurrent episodes of otitis media and diarrhea,[78] 10 patients with Wegener's granulomatosis,[79] several patients with Chediak-Higashi syndrome,[80] and patients with rheumatoid arthritis.[81] In rheumatoid arthritis, the defect may be due to neutrophil phagocytosis of immune complexes since normal human neutrophils incubated with purified rheumatoid factor complexes demonstrate abnormal chemotaxis.[81]

B. Lymphocytes

Although lymphocytes are motile cells and migrate through tissue, in a 1953 review Harris[82] found no evidence that they exhibit chemotaxis. Subsequent studies by other investigators have revealed that many of the substances that attract neutrophils and macrophages in vitro, such as C5a and bacterial products, have no detectable effect on lymphocytes. Ward et al.,[83] however, found in 1971 that rat lymphocytes were chemotactic to a product found in culture fluids of antigen-stimulated guinea pig lymphocytes. Recently Ward et al.[84] found that rat lymphocytes also show chemotaxis towards mixed lymphocyte culture fluids, fluid from concanavalin A-stimulated cells, fluids from phagocytizing macrophages, and antirat IgG. Upon separating the test lymphocytes, spleen T cells responded to the mixed lymphocyte cultures, whereas B cells responded poorly. Only B cells responded to anti-IgG.

Houck and Chang[85] isolated a protein from thymus extracts of vaccinated calves that attracted lymphocytes both in vitro and in vivo. It was found to have a mol wt of 10,500 daltons and appeared to be a sialoprotein.

C. Monocytes and Macrophages

Most in vitro studies of mononuclear cells have been done with peritoneal macrophages and peripheral blood monocytes. Few studies have been done with alveolar macrophages (see below). Ward[86] found that peritoneal mononuclear cells from rabbits responded to rabbit serum treated with immune complexes or streptokinase and plasminogen, to soluble factors produced by bacteria, and to lysates obtained from rabbit neutrophils. The active component in the lysates, which did not attract neutrophils, appeared related to cationic peptides of lysosomal granules. In addition, peritoneal mononuclear cells respond to a number of other factors that activate C5a, including endotoxin, cobra venom factor, and an acid proteinase from macrophages and lung.[87,88] Symon et al.[89] found that heat killed *Mycobacterium tuberculosis*-activated plasma to generate a factor chemotactic for guinea pig peritoneal mononuclear cells. Although not fully characterized, the factor differed from that generated by *Shigella flexneri* endotoxin, but was inactivated with several complement inhibitors. Activity was found in several protein fractions of *M. tuberculosis*, in culture filtrates, and was still present after lipid had been extracted.

Some lymphocyte products released from sensitized cells after stimulation attract mononuclear cells. Ward et al.[90] identified such a lymphokine from guinea pigs that attracted peritoneal mononuclear cells and differed from migration inhibition factor (MIF). Wahl et al.[91] also identified a lymphokine in guinea pigs that attracted mononuclear cells, but it differed by elution patterns from the one described by Ward. Altman et al.[92] found that stimulated peripheral human blood leukocytes and purified lymphocytes released a substance that attracted homologous monocytes. It was heat stable, nondialyzable, had a mol wt of around 12,500, was not a complement product, and seemed to differ from other described lymphokines. Wahl et al.[93] studied the interrelationship of macrophages in the production of two lymphokines, monocyte chemotactic factor and macrophage activating factor, and found that T cells required viable macrophage cooperation to produce the lymphokines.

As discussed previously, Hageman factor-dependent activation of the fibrinolytic and kinin pathways generates plasminogen activator and kallikrein which are chemotactic for neutrophils. Gallin and Kaplan[94] found that both enzymes also attract human mononuclear cells isolated from heparinized peripheral blood by Hypaque-Ficoll separation. Alpha-macroglobulin inhibited the chemotactic activity of kallikrein.

Virus-infected cells release substances that attract neutrophils and mononuclear cells and also substances which interact with human C3 or C5 to generate activity (cytotaxigens).

In a study of peripheral human blood monocytes, Gallin et al.[95] found that ionophore A23187 and PGE_1 increased intracellular cAMP and inhibited cell locomotion. Ascorbic acid and serotonin increased cGMP and enhanced chemotactic responsiveness, but this effect could be inhibited when cAMP was increased. The results suggest that a fine balance may exist in intracellular cyclic nucleotides in modulating locomotion and chemotaxis.

In studies with alveolar macrophages, Ward[86] found that rabbit alveolar macrophages responded poorly to all agents that attracted peritoneal mononuclear cells. In a recent detailed study, Dauber and Daniele[96] compared the responsiveness of guinea pig alveolar and peritoneal macrophages and found that peritoneal macrophages responded to endotoxin-activated guinea pig serum, lymphocyte-derived chemotactic factor, bacterial chemotactic factor and the peptides N-formylmethionyl-alanine (F-Met-Ala), and N-formylmethionyl-phenylalanine (F-Met-Phe), whereas alveolar macrophages migrated equally well only toward the peptides. The response to endotoxin-activated guinea pig serum was minimal, whereas the response to lymphocyte derived chemotactic factor and bacterial chemotactic factor was intermediate. Alveolar macrophages from smokers demonstrate higher random migration and greater chemotactic responsiveness to casein than do those from nonsmokers.[97] Alveolar macrophages obtained by lavage from patients with acute smoke inhalation reveal decreased chemotaxis.[97a]

Lynn and Mukherjee[97b] have demonstrated that alveolar macrophages are also activated by unsaturated fatty acids. In addition, they showed that rabbit alveolar macrophages, when incubated, release unsaturated fatty acids, primarily linoleic acid, that stimulate motility of other macrophages, but have no effect on neutrophils. Anionic phospholipids, e.g., phosphatidylglycerol, which is secreted in large amounts in mammalian airways, also activate migration of macrophages, but do not activate migration of neutrophils. On the basis of these and additional studies, they suggest that the elaboration of unsaturated fatty acids, as well as of nonspecific proteins, is responsible for accumulation of macrophages in injured body spaces such as alveoli or pleura.[97b]

Both chemotactic and nonchemotactic factors can stimulate macrophages to release lysosomal enzymes which include lactate dehydrogenase, β-glucoronidase, acid phosphatase,[98] elastase,[99] collagenase,[100] and plasminogen activator.[101] The release of some of these by recruited macrophages may function in inflammation, tissue destruction, and collagen turnover.

Inhibition of monocyte and macrophage chemotaxis — has been found in association with infections and neoplasms. Human blood monocytes exposed to *Herpes simplex* or influenza virus showed reduced in vitro chemotaxis, whereas those exposed to vaccina, polio, and reovirus did not.[102] The reduced chemotaxis was not due to virus-induced cytotoxicity. Monocyte chemotaxis has been found to be reduced in patients with active breast cancer,[103] with Stage III melanoma,[104] or with metastatic bronchial carcinoma.[105] The role of monocyte inhibitors in neoplasms is unclear. Normann and Sorkin[106] found that culture supernatants from several tumor cells lines inhibited rat peritoneal mononuclear cell chemotaxis in vitro, whereas Meltzer et al.[107] found that the culture fluids from five murine sarcomas attracted peritoneal mononuclear cells from mice infected with *Mycobacterium bovis*.

D. Eosinophils

Kay et al.[108] were the first to isolate a substance from lung that selectively recruited eosinophils in vitro. Named eosinophilic chemotactic factor of anaphylaxis (ECF-A), it exits in a preformed state in mast cells and basophils and is released through antigen-IgE interaction.[109] Release involves five sequential stages including

1. A calcium-requiring activation of a diisopropylphosphofluoridate-sensitive serine esterase
2. The further autocatalytic activation of the esterase
3. A 2-DG-inhibitable energy requiring step
4. A second calcium-requiring, EDTA-inhibitable stage
5. A cyclic AMP-inhibitable step[110]

Goetzl and Austen[111] purified ECF-A and identified two tetrapeptides with the amino acid sequence of Val-Gly-Ser-Glu and Ala-Gly-Ser-Glu. Both, along with an analogue Val-Gly-Asp-Glu, promote eosinophil chemotaxis in vitro.[112] Reduction of the tetrapeptides to tripeptides by deleting glycine decreases in vitro activity tenfold, suggesting that spatial distance between NH_2 and COOH is critical for activity.[113]

In addition to mast cells, neutrophils also release an eosinophil chemotactic factor (ECF). Release occurs following stimulation by calcium ionophore A23187 or as the result of phagocytosis of zymosan particles, zymosan coated with complement, or zymosan in the presence of serum.[114,115] Neutrophils also release ECF following incubation with larvae of *Nippostrongylus brasiliensis*.[116] By elution patterns ECF appears to be very similar to ECF-A.[115]

Recently, Boswell et al.[117] identified several intermediate molecular weight eosinophil chemotactic factors in rat peritoneal mast cells. The factors were in the 1500- to 2500-mol wt. range, as contrasted to 300 to 1000 for ECF-A, and induced both eosinophil chemotaxis and deactivation. It is presumed that these newly identified factors function similarly to ECF-A in vivo following mast cell release.

Histamine in vitro attracts eosinophils at critical concentrations. Clark et al.[118] found that histamine attracts eosinophils in a concentration between 3×10^{-7} M and 1.25×10^{-6} M/ℓ, but is inhibitory at higher concentrations. Imidazole acetic acid, a major metabolite of histamine, also attracts eosinophils, but other histamine catabolites do not.[119] The inhibitory effect of histamine at higher concentrations is modulated through the H-2 receptor with an increase in intracellular cyclic AMP.[120]

Eosinophils will respond chemotactically to many of the substances that attract neutrophils, including bacterial products, serum treated with immune complexes, and a mixture of plasminogen and streptokinase.[121] Since such a response, with the exception of that to bacterial products, is mediated through complement activation, it is clear that eosinophils respond to C3a and C5a.[121,122]

Eosinophils are also attracted to lymphocyte products. Sensitized lymphocytes cultured in the presence of specific antigen release a number of lymphokines into the surrounding medium. Some of these react with immune complexes in vitro to generate a chemotactic factor for eosinophils.[123] Generation is dependent on the presence of the same antigen in the immune complexes as was used to sensitize and stimulate the lymphocytes.[123]

In addition, two other substances have been identified that attract eosinophils in the Boyden chamber. Goetzl et al.[124] isolated a peptide, eosinophil chemotactic factor of lung squamous cell carcinoma (ECF-LSC), from extracts of lung carcinomas from three patients who also had eosinophilia. It was comparable to ECF-A, but eluted from Dowex-1 at a more alkaline pH. Tanaka and Torisu[125] found that soluble extracts from *Anisakis* larva strongly attract eosinophils without serum or additional factors, offering evidence that eosinophils can be recruited by parasites directly.

E. Basophils

As stated previously, basophils, like mast cells, release mediators of immediate hypersensitivity. In addition, however, Kay and Austen[126] found that basophils from two patients with high basophil counts responded chemotactically in vitro to a number of different chemotactic agents, including diffusates from lung fragments challenged with pollen antigen, kallikrein, and C5a. This suggests that basophils may play several roles in immediate hypersensitivity reactions by responding to chemotaxins, releasing mediators, and attracting eosinophils. Of possible clinical importance, Hirsch[127] found elevated levels of blood basophils in symptomatic hay fever subjects that decreased when the symptoms decreased and that these patients had a basophil chemotactic factor in the serum and circulating basophils with a receptor for that factor.

F. Fibroblasts

An application of modified Boyden chambers has demonstrated chemotaxis of human dermal fibroblasts to factors derived from stimulated lymphocytes incubated in the presence of macrophages. The factors were found to be heat stable, trypsin sensitive, and neuraminidase resistant.[128] Using this same system, it was shown that human dermal fibroblasts in culture are attracted to Type I, II, and III human collagens and α-chains. Collagenase digestion of the three types of collagen produced peptides which were also chemotactic as were synthetic di- and tripeptides and hydroxyproline.[129] These findings support the hypothesis that remodeling of connective tissue and response to injury and inflammation may, at times, be independent of leukocytes and macrophages and depend upon fibroblasts alone. Fibroblasts themselves elaborate substances chemotactic for neutrophils and monocytes which are distinct from collagen and products of complement activation.[129a] Fibroblasts also secret a factor that activates complement to generate C5a from human serum.[129a]

G. Effects of Drugs and Lipids on In Vitro Chemotaxis

Various antibiotics, steroids, or lipids have been added to neutrophils in the Boyden chamber to note their modifying effects on in vitro chemotaxis. Chloramphenicol, rifampin, clindamycin, erythromycin, tetracycline, and gentamicin suppress the neutrophil response to chemoattractants.[130-132a] Penicillin G-Na, sulfapyridine, and dapsone are without effect,[132] while gramicidin S, tyrocidin, and bacitracin attract neutrophils.[133] The mechanisms by which antibiotics alter in vitro chemotaxis is not known, but tetracycline may bind with the chemoattractant.[131]

Hydrocortisone sodium succinate at concentrations from 5 to 125 μg/mℓ induces a progressive inhibition of neutrophil chemotaxis that cannot be reversed by washing the cells.[134] High doses of methylprednisolone sodium succinate also inhibit chemotaxis, whereas medroxyprogesterone acetate and cortisone acetate produce mild stimulation.[135]

Oleic acid, an unsaturated fatty acid, moderately inhibits chemotaxis only at very high concentrations.[136] Palmitic acid, a saturated fatty acid, also inhibits chemotaxis at high concentrations, but, in addition, inhibits at low concentrations that are within the range found in serum in various diseases including Gram-negative sepsis. Electron microscopic studies of neutrophils incubated with palmitic acid reveal that the cells contain cleft-like dilatations of the endoplasmic reticulum resembling crystals. The crystals may act to inhibit chemotaxis through interference with intracellular processes.[136]

IV. IN VIVO CHEMOTAXIS — ANIMALS

Despite an impressive array of information concerning chemotaxis of neutrophils, macrophages, and eosinophils in vitro, a well-accepted system for studying chemotaxis in vivo has not emerged. The Rebuck window and a modification using a filter and pad containing a chemoattractant serve well for studies of cutaneous reactions.[46] Perhaps the most satisfactory model that allows study of the time course of leukocyte recruitment is that of the rat peritoneum following injection of glycogen or endotoxin.[137] The disadvantages include inability to visualize the process and confusion from other inflammatory events that cannot be controlled. The airway has been infrequently used as a method of assessing chemotaxis even though a number of materials including endotoxin, bacteria, cotton bract, bagasse (sugarcane), moldy hay, and cigarette smoke can be given as aerosols or intratracheal injections.

A. Complement Products and Leukocyte Recruitment

Ward et al.[138] were the first to demonstrate that chemotactic complement products could be generated in vivo following i.v. injection of complement fixing agents. Further support was obtained when extracts of tissue lesions from rats with reversed passive Arthus reactions were found to be rich in leukotactic activity as measured in vitro.[139] On further analysis, the leukotactic activity was found to be associated with $C\overline{567}$ and C5 cleavage products. Also, C5a appears in the peritoneal fluid of guinea pigs following injection of glycogen or endotoxin and occurs before the accumulation of neutrophils. The peritoneal fluid of mice that are C5 deficient does not generate C5a, and such mice do not accumulate neutrophils in the abdomen following injection.[137] Jones et al.[140] found that complement products can function in vivo when they demonstrated that ^{51}Cr-labeled homologous neutrophils will accumulate at guinea pig skin sites following intradermal injection of factors derived from complement-activated serum.

In a study of rhesus monkeys, Kazmierowski et al.[141] noted that approximately 4 hr after initial bronchoalveolar lavage with 0.9% saline an increase in numbers of neutrophils were found when lavage was repeated. Such bronchoalveolar lavage fluid was studied in vitro and found to recruit human neutrophils and mononuclear cells. Gel filtration chromatography of the lavage fluid disclosed two peaks of chemotactic activity. One had an estimated mol wt of 15,000 daltons and was analogous to C5a. The other had a mol wt of about 5,000 daltons and was released from alveolar macrophages. This study shows that complement activation can occur in the lung and that alveolar macrophages can release a chemotactic material into the airways.

Henson et al.[141a] have reported on an extensive study of complement fragments, alveolar macrophages, and alveolitis in the rabbit. They found that the i.v. injection of substances that activate complement leads to neutrophil accumulation in the pulmonary vasculature, but that airway instillation of complement activating substances is necessary for induction of pneumonitis. They determined that the active complement-derived chemotactic factor generated in the airway was C5a des Arg, rather than C5a, and that C5 is normally available in the lung at levels that would allow generation of both C5a and C5a des Arg. They propose a schema by which complement fragments can induce inflammatory responses in the lung through:

1. Cleavage of C5 in airspaces or interstitium by macrophage- or neutrophil-derived proteases or by activation of complement pathways
2. Removal of the C-terminal arginine from the C5a to yield C5a des Arg
3. Attraction of neutrophils from the capillary directly and/or by inductive release of chemotactic factors from the resident macrophages

These cells are also stimulated to secrete proteases, which cleave C5 and further enhance the reaction.[141a]

Desai et al.[141b] have found that the intratracheal administration of purified human

C5 into the lungs of hamsters led to accumulation of leukocytes within lung parenchyma when observed at 4 hr. They propose that this response may be due to the action of lung-associated proteases, possibly elastase, resulting in the *in situ* production of chemotactic factors.

Johnson et al.[142] demonstrated that chemotactic factor inhibitor also has a role in vivo. In a reversed passive Arthus rat model the intrabronchial administration of anti-BSA antibody followed by BSA intravenously resulted in an intense pneumonic reaction consisting of neutrophil infiltrates and hemorrhage. Animals receiving 150 μl CFI mixed with the antibody before intrabronchial injection had only a minimal reaction. The results suggest that CFI may be important in the control of inflammation.

B. Endotoxin and Bacteria

Pernis et al.[143] noted that rabbits given aerosols of *Salmonella* endotoxin developed fever and labored breathing, whereas those given crude cotton dust extracts did not. Snell[144] studied the microscopic changes associated with the acute reaction to *E. coli* endotoxin and noted alveolar edema and cellular infiltration of neutrophils, eosinophils, and macrophages at 24 hr and obliteration of many alveolar spaces with macrophages at 48 hr. Some neutrophils were also recruited to the bronchi and bronchioles. Cavagna et al.[145] studied the long-term effects of *E. coli* endotoxin given over a 5-month period and observed exfoliation of bronchial cells and peribronchial lymphocyte infiltrates.

Studies have involved quantitating neutrophils in bronchopulmonary lavage and assessing recruitment into bronchi and bronchioles by *in situ* fixation following administration of *Salmonella typhosa* or *E. coli* endotoxin to guinea pigs or hamsters by a Collison nebulizer.[146] After 4 hr, an average of 28 million leukocytes were lavaged from guinea pigs exposed to endotoxin compared to 5 million from animals exposed to a water aerosol. Sections of airways and lung which had been fixed *in situ* with 2% osmium tetroxide in fluorocarbon embedded in plastic and cut at 1 μm showed peaks of 53.9 neutrophils per 100 epithelial cells at 4 hr for guinea pigs and 99.7 neutrophils per 100 epithelial cells at 6 hr for hamsters. The airway neutrophil counts of controls were 0.1 to 0.2 per 100 epithelial cells.

Pierce et al.[147] used similar techniques in mice to show that recruitment of neutrophils to bronchi and alveoli occurs within 4 hr following aerosol exposure to *Klebsiella pneumoniae* or *E. coli*, but not *Staphylococcus aureus*. In a study of guinea pigs given *Listeria monocytogenes,* naive animals exposed to microorganisms developed an acute illness with neutrophil infiltrates which were gradually replaced by macrophages whereas animals immunized to the organism did not develop acute illness and had an initial cellular response consisting of macrophages rather than neutrophils.[148,149]

C. Cotton Dust

In studies designed to determine the pathogenesis of byssinosis, Prausnitz[150] exposed guinea pigs to sieved cotton dust in a chamber for 3 to 4 hr/day, 5 days/week, for 1 to 6 months. After 1 month, edema and infiltration consisting of neutrophils and macrophages were seen in alveoli near aiways. Controls, exposed to chalk, were normal, while those given chalk plus histamine showed slight alveolar changes. Similar experiments with rabbits by Cavagna et al.,[145] done in parallel with their endotoxin studies referred to previously, showed that cotton extracts prepared by grinding and freeze-drying had about 1/100 the pyogenic activity of endotoxin from *E. coli*. Rabbits exposed to 2 mg of the cotton extract in 2 ml saline 5 days/week for 20 weeks developed peribronchial lymphocytes, alveolar thickening, goblet cell hyperplasia, and neutrophil infiltrations of bronchi and bronchioles.

Recent studies have involved efforts to appraise the nature of cotton factors that might be responsible for byssinosis. Cotton mill trash or cotton bracts were extracted with warm water or ethyl acetate and sterilized by filtration through 0.22 µm millipore filters. Aerosol exposure to hamsters recruited neutrophils to airway walls and lumens within 2 hr. Neutrophil numbers peaked at 6 hr, but persisted for 24 hr. Repeated exposure continued to recruit only neutrophils. Quercetin and related flavonoids from cotton gave similar reactions, but required high doses. Other cotton extract fractions obtained by high pressure liquid chromatography including lacinilene-C7 methyl ether have been tested and found to recruit neutrophils.[151,152] Possible pathways for generation of mediators in the airway include

1. Direct effect of the chemical
2. Stimulation of macrophages which serve as sentinels
3. Stimulation of an epithelial cell
4. A combined macrophage to epithelial mediation (see Figure 1)

Another way to obtain quantitative data is to do repeated bronchopulmonary lavages with saline following cotton dust exposure. Such methods have also demonstrated striking increase in neutrophils, but not macrophages, following exposure,[153] although, as stated previously, interpretation may be difficult because saline lavage alone activates complement and induces neutrophil accumulation in some animals.

D. Chemical Agents and Carrier Molecules

In a series of experiments, the hamster airway was used to measure and time the sequence of responses to simple chemicals administered alone and in combination or adsorbed on carbon particles. Sulfur dioxide, formaldehyde, acrolein, and the vapor phase of cigarette smoke were given at doses producing microscopic abnormalities extending from slight changes of cytoplasmic vacuolation and pallor to severe cytotoxic changes of nuclear extrusion and exfoliation of cells. Sulfur dioxide at 200 to 400 ppm for 6 weeks caused loss of cilia, vacuolation, pyknotic nuclei, extrusion of cells, and mild recruitment of neutrophils. A lower dose, 40 ppm, for 6 weeks had no effect, but when combined with 0.74 g/m³ of carbon, it recruited neutrophils to the airways and induced cytoxic changes.[154] Formaldehyde at 600 ppm was highly cytotoxic, but at 6 ppm with carbon, it recruited neutrophils at 24 to 48 hr. Acrolein at 6 ppm was cytotoxic, but when combined with carbon, it induced neutrophil recruitment.[155] The vapor phase of cigarette smoke obtained by drawing smoke through dual Cambridge filters was similarly cytotoxic alone (20 cigarettes in 4 hr), but when combined with 283 mg/mℓ of carbon, it recruited neutrophils.[156] Whole cigarette smoke and particle phase alone (charcoal filtered) recruited neutrophils, but was not cytotoxic.

A number of other agents, including paraquat,[157] chlorogenic acid, catechols, tannins, gossypol, phenol, and polyhydroxyl phenols are also cytotoxic if given as aerosols, but in the same or lower doses combined with carbon or silica flour, they recruit neutrophils.

Thus, as demonstrated by these experiments, it appears that in most instances the combination of a bland particle and a toxic molecule is required for neutrophil recruitment to airways. Particles can be so small as to avoid sedimentation at 30,000 to 60,000 ×g for an hour as is the case for *E. coli* endotoxin, cotton, and tobacco extracts which are active even after centrifugation, suggesting that the supernatant may still contain submicron particles. The possible mechanisms for the airways' cellular responses to environmental messages (mediators) are shown in Figure 1.

The in vivo and in vitro effects of cigarette smoke differ. Guinea pigs exposed to 7 cigarettes developed a reduction in macrophages and neutrophils obtained by lavage at 2 hr, but a slight rise at 6 hr.[158] No observations were made at 12 or 24 hr, so

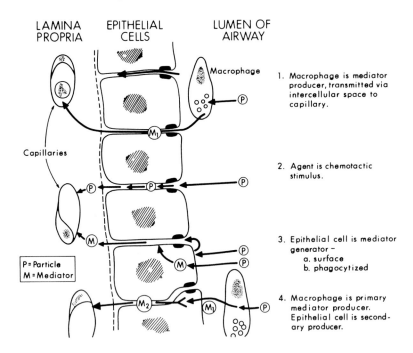

FIGURE 1.   Possible pathways for generation of mediators to recruit neutrophils in the airway.

increases in neutrophils at that time may have been overlooked. A total of 4 cigarettes per day for 4 and 8 weeks raised macrophage numbers about 20% and neutrophil numbers about 50%.[159] In vitro experiments have shown that whole tobacco smoke and components of cigarette smoke, particularly acrolein and crotonaldehyde and to a lesser extent cyanide, acetaldehyde, furfural, and nicotine, inhibit human neutrophil chemotaxis to serum activated by endotoxin without altering neutrophil viability.[160] Thus, the findings that whole cigarette smoke or the vapor phase plus carbon recruits neutrophils in the airway contrasts with the in vitro effects of whole smoke and suggests that care must be exercised in extrapolating from in vitro to in vivo effects of agents on cell behavior.

E. Foreign Proteins (Fungi and Organic Materials)

A number of different animal models have been developed to investigate the pathogenesis of hypersensitivity pneumonitis. One model that closely resembles human disease involves giving an antigen repeatedly via the respiratory route without otherwise sensitizing the animals. Following three intratracheal injections of *Micropolyspora faeni* in rabbits, Salvaggio et al.[161] noted sequential microscopic changes consisting of

1. Day 3 — a mixed cellular infiltrate in the terminal and respiratory bronchioles and alveoli
2. Day 9 — bronchiolocentric and interstitial infiltration with macrophages and lymphocytes
3. Day 14 — interstitial histiocytes and multinucleated giant cells surrounded by lymphocytes
4. Day 21 — giant cells and histiocytes in well-developed granulomas

The animals also developed specific serum precipitating antibodies, Arthus-type skin reactions, and delayed skin reactivity, suggesting Type III (immune complex) and Type

IV (cell-mediated) reactions. In the same model, alveolar macrophage migration was significantly inhibited in the presence of *M. faeni* antigen, suggesting that specifically sensitized lymphocytes were present in the free bronchoalveolar cell population.[162] With a different antigen, dinitrophenylated human immunoglobulin G, Henney and Waldman[163] found sensitized lymphocytes in the respiratory tract of guinea pigs given the antigen in the form of nose drops, but not in those animals immunized parenterally.

Other animal models have been developed to further explore immunologic mechanisms. Santives et al.[164] challenged guinea pigs by aerosol with ovalbumin or pigeon serum after s.c. sensitization and noted that those given ovalbumin developed severe pneumonitis, but those given pigeon serum did not. The total antibody activity and specific IgG and and IgG_2 responses were similar in the groups, but the IgE-like antibody response was markedly higher in the group given ovalbumin, suggesting that IgE antibody may function in initial injury. The pneumonitis induced in the animals, however, was hemorrhagic and therefore atypical for hypersensitivity pneumonitis.

Richerson[165] immunized guinea pigs in various ways to stimulate antibody- or cell-mediated hypersensitivity and challenged them with appropriate aerosolized antigens. Those animals with an induced Type I reaction developed anaphylaxis and peribronchial eosinophilia, while those with an induced Type III reaction developed a severe hemorrhagic pneumonia with neutrophil infiltration in 4 to 6 hr. Those with an induced Type IV reaction developed alveolitis at 24 hr of predominately mononuclear cells. The same results were obtained in monkeys given either specific precipitating antibody or sensitized lymphocytes passively and challenged by pigeon serum aerosols.[166] The pathologic changes in humans with hypersensitivity pneumonias, to be discussed later, more closely resemble the animal Type IV reactions.

Clearly none of the animal models totally explain the immunologic events in hypersensitivity pneumonitis. Most of the evidence suggests a Type III and/or a Type IV reaction, but it is possible that neither of these reactions is a primary event.

Olenchock and Burrell[167] exposed unimmunized rabbits to aerosols of *Aspergillus* spores and noted that postchallenge depressions in arterial oxygen tension could be prevented by prior complement depletion, suggesting that nonspecific complement activation was related to the hypoxia. These results were supported by Edwards et al.,[168] who found that unsensitized rabbits exposed to zymosan, a substance known to activate the alternate pathway of complement, developed the same pathologic changes as those exposed to moldy hay dust. Further support of possible clinical significance comes from studies showing that respirable fractions of moldy hay and grain dust activate the alternate pathway of complement when incubated with fresh human serum.[169]

Animal studies also suggest that cofactor agents of inflammation, once called adjuvants in the lung, may potentiate the effects of the organic antigens associated with hypersensitivity pneumonitis. Rabbits exposed to pigeon antigens and immunized with carrageenan or bacillus Calmette-Guerin (BCG) develop a more severe pneumonitis than with carrageenan or BCG alone and develop cell-mediated hypersensitivity to the inhaled antigen in bronchoalveolar cells.[170,171]

An animal model has also been developed for study of purified protein derivative (PPD).[172] Guinea pigs immunized by an injection of dry-killed tubercle bacilli and then challenged by inhaled PPD developed an exudative pneumonic process.[172] The infiltrative process consisted of neutrophils initially, but maximal infiltrative changes occurred at 24 to 48 hr and consisted of large collections of mononuclear cells, mostly lymphocytes. The process gradually subsided within 7 to 20 days. This model shows that a delayed hypersensitivity reaction can be produced in the lung.

F. Parasitic Infections

Eosinophil response in animals secondary to induced parasitic infections is a useful way of studying eosinophil recruitment and function. Although most studies have not focused on pulmonary aspects, in one model animals inoculated with *Trichinella* larvae fail to develop an eosophilia unless organisms are given in such a manner that they lodge in the lung.[173]

Results from several studies indicate that the immunologic response of the host is complex. Animals develop high levels of specific IgE following immunization with a number of different parasites,[174] suggesting that immediate hypersensitivity and release of mediators could contribute to the eosinophilia. Such a mechanism was partially supported by the work of Archer et al.,[175] who found that phospholipid preparations from *Ascaris suum* or cysts of *Echinococcus granulosis* (hydatid cysts) induced eosinophilia, mast cell hyperplasia, and mast cell granule lysis following i.p. injection in rats. However, they also found that the active material in the phospholipid preparations, lecithin and lecithin plasmalogen, stimulated complement breakdown via the alternative complement pathway and therefore released other factors chemotactic for eosinophils.

Lymphocytes also play a role in parasite-induced eosinophilia. Procedures which deplete lymphocytes, such as neonatal thymectomy or prolonged thoracic duct drainage, result in a marked reduction in eosinophil response in rats immunized with *Trichinella*.[176] In addition, eosinophilia could be induced in nonimmunized animals by transfer of large lymphocytes, but not by plasma or cell-free lymph, from infected animals. The transferred lymphocytes induced eosinophilia even if implanted in cell-tight diffusion chambers. Although the active lymphocyte product was not identified, Colley,[177] in a later study with *Schistosoma mansoni*-infected mice did isolate an active factor and called it eosinophil stiulation promoter (ESP). More recently Green and Colley[178] found that ESP is produced by T lymphocytes and that possible interaction with macrophages is necessary for its production.

Although the specific function of eosinophils in parasitic infections is not known, they may play a direct role in combating parasitic infections. Mahmoud et al.[179] found that mice infected with 10 cercariae of *S. mansoni* 16 and 36 weeks before challenge with 500 cercariae showed a 40% reduction in *Schistosomula* recovered from the lung as compared to a group that were not immunized. Treatment of the animals with antilymphocyte, antimacrophage, or antineutrophil serum did not alter the numbers of *Schistosomula* recovered from the lungs of immune animals, but in those treated with antieosinophil serum, the numbers of *Schistosomula* increased to the levels seen in nonimmune animals. In the *S. mansoni* models, eosinophils appear to kill parasites through IgG antibody-dependent damage following adherence via the Fc receptors[180] and through activation of complement at the parasite surface by the alternative pathway with C-3 mediated adherence.[181]

V. IN VIVO CHEMOTAXIS — HUMANS

A. Acute and Chronic Bronchitis

Evidence for recruitment of neutrophils in airways from the nose to the trachea to the terminal bronchioles may be inferred from the massive outpouring of neutrophils into the sputum during exacerbations of bronchitis[182] and from the histology of these airways as seen in biopsy[183] and autopsy material.[153] Moreover, as efforts have been made to correlate functional impairment of bronchioles with structural changes in cigarette smokers, inflammatory infiltrates in bronchioles have been frequently observed.[185] Patients with airway failure have a significant increase in neutrophils, particularly in mucus in lumens of small airways and in the epithelium of bronchi that may contribute to the stickiness of mucus and plugging of lumens, and to peribronchiolar fibrosis with distortion of obliterative airways obstruction.[186] Finally, when neutrophils are carefully looked for between epithelial cells in bronchial biopsies of patients with chronic bronchitis, especially those hospitalized for exacerbations, they are almost invariably found and appear to be roughly proportional to the purulence of the sputum.[187-189] Counts of cells in sputum show that chronic bronchitic patients expel as many as 254×10^6 neutrophils and 30.6×10^6 macrophages per day during exacerbations.[182]

Inhalations of a variety of inorganic and organic materials causes an acute syndrome within a few hours consisting of fever, chills, malaise, nausea, cough, and shortness of breath. A number of different metals have been associated with the syndrome, including copper, magnesium, aluminum, iron, and, more importantly, zinc. Tungsten carbide or hard metal, which is made by fusing tungsten and carbon with cobalt, causes a purulent bronchitis, suggesting that cobalt recruits neutrophils.[190] Copper and its salts have been shown to cause leukocyte recruitment in the lung.[191]

Some of the environmental or occupational settings where the acute syndrome has been related to the inhalation of organic materials include

1.   Sewage workers exposed to aerosols or dusts of bacteria[192]
2.   Individuals exposed to humidifiers contaminated with bacteria, fungi, and protozoa[193,194]
3.   Workers who developed mill fever, cotton fever, or cardroom fever after exposure to cotton,[195,196] flax, hemp, or kapok dusts[197]
4.   Individuals exposed to a vast array of materials associated with hypersensitivity pneumonitis (to be discussed later in this section)

In cotton workers, fever, peripheral blood leukocytes, airway leukocytosis, and airway narrowing occur together following exposure[198] (see Figure 2). When dust is higher, the sequence occurs earlier. The time sequence is similar in guinea pigs following exposure to cotton dust or endotoxin.[146] Thus, fever, chills, malaise, and shortness of breath may be due to recruitment of neutrophils into capillaries and their margination (adherence) and degranulation with release of enzymes and possibly pyrogens, following stimulation.[199]

There is little evidence that macrophages pass through airway walls, although they are found in clear sputum and tracheobroncial secretions obtained from normal subjects. The site of entry for macrophages onto the mucociliary escalator in mammalian lungs appears to be in the distal airways — i.e., the respiratory bronchioles or the junction between these and the terminal bronchioles.[200] Macklin[201] described these as the "sumps" or entry points to macrophages, and Green[202] suggested that macrophages lacking a means of access to ciliated airways from alveoli could move onto the terminal bronchioles from lymphatics which drain alveolar ducts to this site. There has been no direct demonstration of this postulated mechanism nor is there a precedent.

B. Alveolitis and Pneumonitis

A most obvious example of neutrophil recruitment in the lung is the third stage or grey hepatization of pneumococcal pneumonia. It follows the first stage which is outpouring of edema fluid triggered by the pneumococci and by bacterial cell products demonstrated in culture fluid[203] and the second stage which is red hepatization with alveolar filling by erythrocytes, fibrin and some neutrophils. In the inflammatory response to Streptococci of group A, the organisms need not be alive.[204]

Pneumonias as a general term for recruitment of inflammatory cells to alveoli due

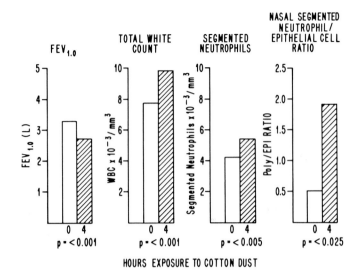

FIGURE 2.   Responses of a panel of 11 textile workers to heavy cotton dust exposure.

to viruses, bacteria, fungi, and foreign particles such as silica all have a stage of leukocytic infiltration. For example, in influenza initial alveolar damage produces edema containing erythrocytes, plasma, proteins, and fibrin-forming hyaline membranes. After further damage, and in fatal cases, alveolar walls are destroyed and neutrophils are conspicuous. Epithelium of small airways is severely damaged and is exfoliated, denuding the basal lamina. As discussed in the in vitro section, both virus-infected cells and damaged cells release substances that attract neutrophils. With lesser damage to alveoli and survival of the host, monocytic infiltration follows, and unless bacteria are secondary invaders, resolution with removal of cell products and cellular debris is complete with restoration of alveoli.

We can assume from animal experiments[205] that the initial response of human lung to quartz particles repeats this stepwise cascade of first, edema (water and protein), second, erythrocytes and fibrin, third, neutrophil infiltration, and fourth, macrophage infiltration. The cascade continues to a fifth stage consisting of an outpouring of phospholipid and protein into alveoli which exceeds the removal capacity, producing lipoproteinosis.[206] In the fifth stage, alveolar Type II cells, which synthesize surfactant, are active in contrast to alveolar lining cells (Type I) which do not seem involved. The sixth phase is fibrosis which may reflect direct effects upon fibroblasts or more probably the results of interaction with other cells, particularly macrophages and lymphocytes.

Tuberculosis represents an example of the cascading stages recounted above, but the order and the time course of transmutation are disturbed so that the problem focuses upon macrophages which apparently have difficulty digesting mycobacteria and their products.[207] With the prolonged macrophage stage, giant cells form and fibroblasts are stimulated to encapsulate and sequester these slow and incomplete reactions with development of granulomas and necrotic (caseous) foci.[208] The same modifications of the cascade apply to the fungus diseases, such as histoplasmosis and coccidiodomycosis, although the sequence time is shorter than tuberculosis and approximates that of carrageenin granuloma in guinea pigs.

The granuloma of beryllium, resembling in most particulars the entire sarcoidosis class of granulomas, is another recapitulation of the theme outlined above, but emphasizes the fibrotic rather than the necrotic end stage. Thus, caseation does not occur. A consistent feature of the granulomatous disease cascade is recruitment of lymphocytes which surround the macrophages granulomas. They are noteworthy in farmer's lung, alveolitis, but the role of these cells and the mechanisms remain obscure.

C. Hypersensitivity Pneumonias

Hypersensitivity pneumonias develop as the result of repeated inhalation of vegetable or animal products in a vast array of occupational settings. The clinical and pathologic changes, however, are very similar. Clinically the patients experience episodes of shortness of breath, fever, and pulmonary infiltrates by chest roentgenograms, all developing 4 to 6 hr after exposure to the antigen.

The major pathologic findings during the acute stage consist of obstructive bronchiolitis and centrilobular bronchopneumonia, characterized by a mixture of neutrophils, eosinophils, monocytes, lymphocytes, and plasma cells.[209] Additional findings include interstitial infiltrates, proliferation of alveolar epithelium, and vasculitis involving the alveolar capillaries.

During the subacute stage, bronchitis and bronchiolitis are still prominent features, but more of the cells in the alveoli and interstitium are lymphocytes and macrophages.[210] Other findings in this stage include foamy macrophages, lymphoid follicles, and peribronchiolar granulomas containing giant cells.

The major pathologic changes during the chronic stage consist of peribronchial and interstitial fibrosis, cystic changes, and few distinct granulomas. A small number of lymphocytes, plasma cells, macrophages, and giant cells are also present.[210]

The microscopic changes in the acute stage are related to antigen deposition in the distal lung. Wenzel et al.[211] studied two patients with acute farmer's lung and found that the walls of the bronchioles stained with fluorescein-labeled gamma globulins obtained from the serum of patients with farmer's lung, suggesting that high concentrations of *M. faeni* antigens were present. Similar staining of lung samples from two patients with chronic disease failed to reveal fluorescence. Histiocytic cells from all four patients stained for C3 complement, suggesting the antecedent presence of antigen-antibody complexes.

The actual mechanisms of leukocyte recruitment into the lung is unclear, but probably complex. Patients with hypersensitivity pneumonia demonstrate several features and characteristics of Type III reactions including:

1. Specific serum precipitins to the inciting antigen
2. Positive "Arthus" skin reactions
3. The onset of symptoms 4 to 6 hr after exposure

However, such findings are difficult to integrate with the observations that asymptomatic exposed individuals also have specific serum precipitins, and even sensitive solid-phase radioimmunoassay methods fail to separate the two groups on the basis of antibody titers.[212] Both groups also have precipitins to trichloroacetic acid (TCA) — extractable antigens which represent the polysaccharide component of *M. faeni*.[213] Boyd, however, has described a radioimmunoassay method that demonstrates higher circulating humoral antibody responses in symptomatic farmers and symptomatic pigeon breeders as compared to those who are asymptomatic.[213a]

The role of complement is unclear. Moore et al.[214] found that serum CH_{50} levels were actually lower in asymptomatic pigeon breeders than symptomatic breeders and that the levels fell significantly following inhalational challenge with aerosolized pigeon serum only in the asymptomatic group. This suggests that antigen-antibody formation and complement activation may serve a protective role in clearing inhaled antigen.

Berrens et al.,[215] on the other hand, found that serum hemolytic complement from symptomatic pigeon fanciers underwent rapid decomposition when exposed in vitro to substances found in pigeon excreta. The authors postulated that the serum of symptomatic pigeon breeders contains an unusually labile variant of C3PA which, once activated, can initiate the rapid decomposition of C3. Marx and Flaherty[216] offered support when they found that *M. faeni*, three species of *Aspergillus*, and two strains of *Thermoactinomyces vulgaris* consume complement and convert C3PA to C3A in the absence of detectable antibodies.

Patients with hypersensitivity pneumonias also develop circulating stimulated lymphocytes.[217] A greater number of symptomatic pigeon breeders have sensitized lymphocytes as compared to an asymptomatic group, but, as with serum precipitins, the test is not of diagnostic value because of overlap.[218] Bronchial lavage of patients with chronic hypersensitivity pneumonias yields a high percentage of T lymphocytes,[219] indicating that lymphocytes are recruited during the chronic stages and suggesting that cellular immunity is involved in the disease process.

Clearly several immunologic processes occur in asymptomatic and symptomatic exposed individuals, but no current immunologic tests separate the two groups or explain why the one group develops pathologic changes.

Therefore, recent work has focused on attempting to define the various antigenic components of *M. faeni* and pigeon products. *M. faeni* contains major antigenic components in a polysaccharide fraction and a protein fraction. Enzymes make up a portion of the protein fraction and are of potential significance because of their ability to activate complement. Roberts[220] studied proteolytic enzymes from 20 to 30 different protein bands and found that diisopropylflurophosphate (DFP) inhibited all major enzymes, indicating that nearly all of the enzymes belonged to a serine-protease group. Inhibition with DFP had little or no effect on complement activation by the antigen mixtures, indicating that proteolytic enzymes may not be responsible for such activity. Some, but not all of the enzymes were inhibited with α_1-antitrypsin, suggesting that some could act uninhibited in the lung. Nicolet et al.[211] studied a "Chymotrypsin-like enzyme", Enzyme 1, and found that both asymptomatic and symptomatic farmers had serum precipitins to the enzyme fraction.

Pigeon excreta antigens have been separated into a major fraction A which consists of a mixture of heteropolysaccharides and a fraction B which consists of glycoproteins.[222] Several components of the glycoprotein fractions have been identified by immunoelectrophoresis and labeled PDE$_1$, PDE$_3$, and PDE$_B$.[223] No information is available as to the significance of these glycoproteins in human subjects.

D. Eosinophil Recruitment
1. Allergic Bronchopulmonary Aspergillosis

Patients with allergic bronchopulmonary aspergillosis experience asthmatic symptoms, fever, and productive cough. Laboratory studies frequently reveal pulmonary infiltrates, blood eosinophilia, serum precipitins, and positive sputum cultures for *Aspergillus fumigatus, Aspergillus flavus,* or *Aspergillus niger.*[224] Skin testing reveals a dual response of an immediate, Type I, response and an Arthus, Type III, reaction. Because of the combination of abnormal immunologic findings, eosinophilia could be the result of a Type I or a Type III reaction in such patients.

The immunologic mechanisms cannot be understood until more information is available regarding the chemistry and antigenic components of *Aspergillus* organisms. Bardana[225] studied a labeled trichloroacetic acid supernatant fraction from *A. fumigatus* and found that all individuals tested had antibodies to the fraction, but those with allergic bronchopulmonary aspergillosis and aspergilloma had much higher titers. The antigen fraction was not further separated. Other investigators[226,227] have also separated *Aspergillus* antigen groups, but, in general, work in the field has not progressed to the stage where distinct antigens are available for specific immunologic studies.

2. Atopic Diseases

Increased numbers of eosinophils are found in the blood, lungs, airways and bronchial secretions of patients with extrinsic asthma and allergic rhinitis. Current theory is that such patients have an inherited predisposition to producing specific IgE antibody to inhaled allergens. The IgE antibodies fix to mast cells and with further allergenic challenge cause the release of mediators. Two of the mediators, histamine and slow reactive substance of anaphylaxis (SRS-A), induce edema and bronchoconstriction, while a third, platelet-activating factor (PAF), causes secretion of amines from platelets. A fourth, eosinophil chemotactic factor of anaphylaxis (ECF-A), acts to recruit eosinophils.

The in vivo significance of in vitro chemoattractants of eosinophils other than ECF-A, such as C5a and mast cell intermediate weight chemotactic factors, is unknown. Although histamine attracts eosinophils in vitro, it does not appear to do so in vivo.[228] Histamine in tissues may appear to recruit eosinophils, but probably only retains eosinophils in the area for a longer period of time than neutrophils.[228]

The function of eosinophils in the lung in atopic disorders is diverse. Once attracted by ECF-A, eosinophils appear to serve a regulatory function in controlling mediator activity through the enzymes arylsulfatase, phospholipase D, and histaminase which inactivate SRS-A,[229] PAF,[230] and histamine,[231] respectively. Eosinophils also actively phagocytize mast cell granules[232] and appear to delay or inhibit the restoration of histamine levels following anaphylaxis.[233]

Eosinophils also release a soluble factor (EDI) which acts to inhibit the release of histamine from sensitized cells by increasing intracellular levels of cyclic AMP.[234] The factor has been found to consist of prostaglandins E_1 and E_2,[235] suggesting a possible dual role for these prostaglandins in not only inhibiting histamine release, but also acting directly as bronchodilators.

3. Parasitic Infections

Eosinophil infiltration and peripheral eosinophilia are found in association with many parasitic diseases. Frequently larvae migrate through the lungs in the early stages of the diseases, and in one, tropical eosinophilia, pulmonary symptoms are associated with sequestration of filiaria in the pulmonary parenchyma. Four male students, who ingested massive numbers of *A. suum* ova, developed extensive pulmonary infiltrates, asthma, eosinophilia reaching a peak during the recovery phase, and elevated IgE levels.[236] The IgG and IgA levels remained normal, but two patients developed elevated levels of IgM and precipitating antibodies to *Ascaris* antigen.

The findings of asthmatic symptoms, elevated serum levels of IgE, and occasional anaphylactic reactions (hydatid cyst rupture) in patients with parasitic infections suggest that eosinophil recruitment and eosinophilia is part of a hypersensitivity reaction. In animal studies, eosinophils also accumulate after complement activation, lymphocyte sensitization, or direct attraction by parasite products (see Sections III D and IV F). The significance of these findings in humans is unknown.

4. Pulmonary Infiltrates with Eosinophilia (PIE)

The syndrome of pulmonary infiltrates with blood eosinophilia (Loeffler's syndrome) is characterized by fever, sore throat, cough, dyspnea, wheezing, cyanosis, and rigors or muscle pains plus finely nodular pulmonary infiltrates. Histology shows alveolar infiltration with eosinophils, neutrophils, and some lymphocytes often near terminal bronchioles. Large mononuclear cells are plentiful, and there may be accompanying vasculitis or granuloma formation.[237] Chemotherapeutic agents and antibiotics frequently associated with this syndrome include nitrofurantoin, paraaminosalicyclic acid, methotrexate, penicillin, and sulfonamides.[238-240] Occasional instances due to other agents have been reported including lymphangiogram media in oils.[241]

In addition to *Aspergillus*, parasitic infections, and drugs discussed above, bacterial infections (tuberculosis, brucellosis, coccidiomycosis, and histoplasmosis), sarcoidosis, and Hodgkin's disease have been associated with PIE with a continuum from the transient to the sustained.[242] Allergic subjects are especially prone, and infiltrates with asthma are not uncommon.[237] Chronic eosinophilic pneumonia was designated as a distinct syndrome after studies of nine women revealed characteristic abnormalities of high fevers, night sweats, severe dyspnea, and progressively dense patchy peripheral infiltrates in chest roentgenograms. Six of the group developed asthma. Lung biopsies were distinctive and showed dense interstitial infiltrates of histiocytes, lymphocytes, eosinophils, and occasional plasma cells, while alveolar spaces were filled with macrophages, histiocytic giant cells, and many eosinophils.[243,244] Systemic periarteritis nodosa has been an infrequent end stage in some patients with chronic PIE or cryptogenic pulmonary eosinophilia.[245]

VI. SUMMARY

The basic mechanisms of recruitment of inflammatory and immunologically competent cells into the human lung are poorly understood with studies of such movement and recruitment still at the descriptive stage. For this reason, it is necessary to extrapolate from data provided by in vitro experiments. The list of agents that attract leukocytes in the Boyden chamber continues to expand with recent interest in lipids and N-formylmethionyl peptides. Likewise, the number of different cells that demonstrate directed movement in vitro has expanded to include fibroblasts and alveolar macrophages. The findings that soluble collagens and collagen digestion products attract fibroblasts suggests a direct interrelationship in modeling and remodeling of the lung framework. The observation that alveolar macrophages are more chemotactic towards small peptides than other agents tested may reflect the importance of such cells in defense against bacterial organisms.

In vitro studies have also provided important information regarding the basic events of attractant-receptor interaction, ion fluxes, microtubule formation and directed movement. Of probable equal importance in vivo, in vitro methods have allowed study of enzyme release which generally occurs at the time of chemotaxis. An understanding of both processes may allow insight into the intricate aspects of inflammation and tissue destruction. In vitro methods have also revealed interdependence of leukocytes in chemotaxis as shown, for example, by the release of a substance from alveolar macrophages into the airways that attracts neutrophils or the dependence of lymphocytes on macrophage interaction for release of some lymphokines.

Animal studies have revealed that neutrophils are recruited to the airway by a variety of substances, including endotoxin, cotton trash products, and many chemical agents absorbed on carbon particles. Studies with organic materials and fungi have been generally concerned with exploring the immunological events in hypersensitivity pneumonias, but recent work suggests that many inhaled organic materials are capable of activating complement by the alternate pathway without prior immunization of the host. Animal models with parasitic infections are now providing information regarding the mechanisms of eosinophilia and eosinophil recruitment and the combative role of the eosinophil.

Human studies have described the neutrophil recruitment in the airways of patients with chronic bronchitis and byssinosis and various combinations of all inflammatory cells in different pneumonic diseases. Numerous studies have been applied to asymptomatic and symptomatic individuals exposed to foreign organic materials, and although the sequence of leukocyte recruitment in the lung is known, immunologic studies have not successfully explained individual susceptibility. Some information is available regarding eosinophil recruitment and function in the lung in atopic diseases and parasitic infections, but the mechanisms of eosinophil recruitment in the clinical disorders of PIE is essentially unknown.

REFERENCES

1. Williams, L. T., Synderman, R., Pike, M. C., et al., Specific receptor sites for chemotactic peptides on human polymorphonuclear leukocytes, *Proc. Natl. Acad. Sci. U.S.A.,* 74, 1204, 1977.
2. Showell, H. J., Freer, R. J., Zigmond, S. H., et al,. The structure-activity relations of synthetic peptides as chemotactic factors and inducers of lysosomal enzyme secretion for neutrophils, *J. Exp. Med.,* 143, 1154, 1976.
3. Becker, E. L., Showell, H. J., Henson, P. M., et al., The ability of chemotactic factors to induce lysosomal enzyme release. I. The characteristics of the release, the importance of surfaces and the relation of enzyme release to chemotatctic responsiveness, *J. Immunol.,* 112, 2047, 1974.
4. Goldstein, I., Hoffstein, S., Gallin, J., et al., Mechanisms of lysosomal enzyme release from human leukocytes: microtubule assembly and membrane fusion induced by a component of complement, *Proc. Natl. Acad. Sci. U.S.A.,* 70, 2916, 1973.
5. Spilberg, I., Mandell, B., Mehta, J., et al., Dissociation of the neutrophil functions of exocytosis and chemotaxis, *J. Lab. Clin. Med.,* 92, 297, 1978.
5a. O'Flaherty, J. T., Showell, H. J., Ward, P. A., et al., A possible role of arachidonic acid in human neutrophil aggregation and degranulation, *Am. J. Pathol.,* 96, 799, 1979.
5b. Becker, E. L., Sigman, M., Oliver, J. M., Superoxide production induced in rabbit polymorphonuclear leukocytes by synthetic chemotactic peptides and A23187, *Am. J. Pathol.,* 95, 81, 1979.
6. Becker, E. L. and Ward, P. A., Partial biochemical characterization of the activated esterase required in the complement-dependent chemotaxis of rabbit polymorphonuclear leukocytes, *J. Exp. Med.,* 125, 1021, 1967.
7. Schiffman, E., Corcoran, B. A., and Aswanikumar, S., Molecular events in the response of neutrophils to synthetic N-fMET chemotatctic peptides: demonstration of a specific receptor, in *Leukocyte Chemotaxis,* 1st ed., Gallin, J. and Quie, P. G., Eds., Raven Press, New York, 1978, 97.
8. Becker, E. L., Showell, H. J., Naccache, P. H., et al., Enzymes in granulocyte movement: preliminary evidence for the involvement of Na +, k + ATPase, in *Leukocyte Chemotaxis,* 1st ed., Gallin, J. and Quie, P. G., Eds., Raven Press, New York, 1978, 113.
9. Boucek, M. M. and Synderman, R., Calcium influex requirement for human neutrophil chemotaxis: inhibition by lanthanum chloride, *Science,* 193, 905, 1976.
10. Gallin, J. I., Gallin, E. K., Malech, H. L., et al., *Structural and Ionic Events During Leukocyte Chemotaxis,* 1st ed., Gallin, J. and Quie, P. G., Eds., Raven Press, New York, 1978, 123.
10a. Marasco, W. A., Becker, E. L., and Oliver, J. M., The ionic basis of chemotaxis, *Am. J. Pathol.,* 98, 749, 1980.
11. Lynn, W. S. and Mukherjee, C., Motility of human polymorphonuclear leukocytes, *Am. J. Pathol.,* 91, 581, 1978.
12. Goetzl, E. J. and Austen, K. F., Stimulation of human neutrophil leukocyte aerobic glucose metabolism by purified chemotactic factors, *J. Clin. Invest.,* 53, 591, 1974.
13. Zigmond, S., Chemotaxis by polymorphonuclear leukocytes, *J. Cell. Biol.,* 77, 269, 1978.
13a. Smith, C. W., Hollers, J. C., Patrick, R. A., et al., Motility and adhesiveness in human neutrophils, *J. Clin. Invest.,* 63, 221, 1979.
14. Malech, H. L., Root, R. K., and Gallin, J. I., Structural analysis of human neutrophil migration, *J. Cell Biol.,* 75, 666, 1977.
14a. Spilberg, I., Mandell, B., and Hoffstein, S., A proposed model for chemotactic deactivation, *J. Lab. Clin. Med.,* 94, 361, 1979.
15. Boyden, S., The chemotactic effect of mixtures of antibody and antigen on polymorphonuclear leucocytes, *J. Exp. Med.,* 115, 453, 1962.
16. Zigmond, S. H. and Hirsch, J. G., Leukocyte locomotion and chemotaxis, *J. Exp. Med.,* 137, 387, 1973.

17. Gallin, J. I. and Wolff, S. M., Leukocyte chemotaxis: physiological considerations and abnormalities, *Clin. Haematol.*, 4, 567, 1967.
18. Keller, H. U. and Sorkin, E., Studies on chematoxis, *Int. Arch. Alergy*, 31, 505, 1957.
19. Ward, P. A., Cochrane, C. G., and Muller-Eberhard, H. J., The role of serum complement in chemotaxis of leukocytes *in vitro*, *J. Exp. Med.*, 122, 327, 1965.
20. Ward, P. A., A plasmin-split fragment of C′3 as a new chemotactic factor, *J. Exp. Med.*, 126, 189, 1967.
21. Ward, P. A. and Newman, L. J., A neutrophil chemotactic factor from human C′5, *J. Immunol.*, 102, 93, 1969.
22. Snyderman, R., Phillips, J., and Mergenhagen, S. E., Polymorphonuclear leukocyte chemotactic activity in rabbit serum and guinea pig serum treated with immune complexes; evidence for C5a as the major chemotactic factor, *Infect. Immunol.*, 1, 521, 1970.
23. Fernandez, H. N., Henson, P. M., Otani, A., et al., Chemotactic response to human C3a and C5a anaphylatoxins. I. Evaluation of C3a and C5a leukotaxis in vitro and under simulated *in vivo* conditions, *J. Immunol.*, 120, 109, 1978.
24. Bitter-Suermann, D., Hadding, U., Schorlemmer, H. U., et al., Activation by some T-independent antigens and B cell mitogens of the alternative pathway of the complement system, *J. Immunol.*, 115, 425, 1975.
25. Wilson, M. R., Gaumer, H. R., and Salvaggio, J. E., Activation of the alternative complement pathway and generation of chemotactic factors by asbestos, *J. Allergy Clin. Immunol.*, 60, 218, 1977.
26. Ward, P. A. and Hill, J. H., C5 chemotactic fragments produced by an enzyme in lysosomal granules of neutrophils, *J. Immunol.*, 104, 535, 1970.
27. Ward, P. A., Lepow, I. H., and Newman, L. J., Bacterial factors chemotactic for polymorphonuclear leukocytes, *Am. J. Pathol.*, 52, 725, 1968.
28. Chapitis, J., Ward, P. A., and Lepow, I. H., Generation of chemotactic activity from human serum and purified components of complement by Serratia proteinase, *J. Immunol.*, 107, 317, 1971.
29. Schiffman, E., Showell, H. V., Corcoran, B. A., et al., The isolation and partial characterization of neutrophil chemotactic factors from *Escherichia coli*, *J. Immunol.*, 114, 1831, 1975.
30. Tainer, J. A., Turner, S. R., and Lynn, W. S., New aspects of chemotaxis, *Am. J. Pathol.*, 81, 401, 1975.
31. Schiffmann, E., Corcoran, B. A., and Wahl, S. M., N-formylmethionyl peptides as chemoattractants for leucocytes, *Proc. Natl. Acad. Sci. U.S.A.*, 72, 1059.
32. Ward, P. A., Cohen, S., and Flanagen, T. D., Leukotactic factors elaborated by virus-infected tissues, *J. Exp. Med.*, 135, 1095, 1972.
33. Brier, A. M., Snyderman, R., Mergenhagen, S. E., et al., Inflammation and *Herpes simplex* virus: release of a chemotaxis-generating factor from infected cells, *Science*, 170, 1104, 1970.
34. Kaplan, A. P., Kay, A. B., and Austen, K. F., A prealbumin activator of prekallikrein. III. Appearance of chemotactic activity for human neutrophils by the conversion of human prekallikrein to kallikrein, *J. Exp. Med.*, 135, 81, 1972.
35. Kay, A. B., Pepper, D. S., and McKenzie, R., The identification of fibrinopeptide B as a chemotactic agent derived from human fibrinogen, *Br. J. Haematol.*, 27, 669, 1974.
36. Kaplan, A. P., Goetzl, E. J., and Austen, K. F., The fibrinolytic pathway of human plasma. III. The generation of chemotactic activity by activation of plasminogen proactivation, *J. Clin. Invest.*, 52, 2591, 1973.
37. Borel, J. F., Keller, H. U., and Sorkin, E., Studies on chemotaxis. XI. Effect on neutrophils of lysosomal and other subcellular fractions from leukocytes, *Int. Arch. Allergy*, 35, 194, 1969.
38. Spilberg, I., Gallacher, A., Mehta, J. M., et al., Urate Crystal-induced chemotactic factor: isolation and partial characterization, *J. Clin. Invest.*, 58, 815, 1976.
38a. Merrill, W. W., Naegel, G. P., Matthay, R. A., et al., Alveolar macrophage-derived chemotactic factor, *J. Clin. Invest.*, 65, 268, 1980.
39. Hill, J. H. and Ward, P. A., C3 leukotactic factors produced by a tissue protease, *J. Exp. Med.*, 130, 505, 1969.
40. Hill, H. R., Cyclic nucleotides as modulators of leukocyte chemotaxis, in *Leukocyte Chemotaxis*, 1st ed., Gallin, J. I. and Quie, P. G., Eds., Raven Press, New York, 1978.
41. Rivkin, I. and Becker, E. L., Effect of exogenous cyclic AMP and other adenine nucleotides on neutrophil chemotaxis and motility, *Int. Arch. Allergy Appl. Immunol.*, 50, 95, 1976.
42. Higgs, G. A., McCall, E., and Youlten, L. J. F., A chemotactic role of prostaglandins released from polymorphonuclear leukocytes during phagocytosis, *Br. J. Pharmacol.*, 53, 539, 1975.
42a. Till, G., Kownatzki, E., Seitz, M., et al., Chemokinetic and chemotactic activity of various prostaglandins for neutrophil granulocytes, *Clin. Immunol. Immunopathol.*, 12, 111, 1979.
43. Pazzaglia, A., Barker, A., Warin, A. P., et Al., Failure of prostaglandins, prostaglandin metabolites and arachidonic acid to elicit chemotaxis of human polymorphonuclear leukocytes, *Br. J. Dermatol.*, 96, 533, 1977.

44. Turner, S. R. and Lynn, W. S., Lipid molecules as chemotactic factors, in *Leukocyte Chemotaxis*, 1st ed., Gallin, J. I. and Quie, P. G., Eds., Raven Press, New York, 1978, 289.

45. Turner, R. S., Campbell, J. A., and Lynn, W. S., Polymorphonuclear leukocyte chemotaxis toward oxidized lipid components of cell membranes, *J. Exp. Med.*, 141, 1437, 1975.

46. Chang, C. and Houck, J. C., Demonstration of the chemotactic properties of collagen, *Proc. Soc. Exp. Biol. Med.*, 134, 22, 1970.

47. Houck, J. C. and Chang, C., The chemotactic properties of the products of collagenolysis (35834), *Proc. Soc. Exp. Biol. Med.*, 138, 69, 1971.

48. Stecher, V. J., The chemotaxis of selected cell types to connective tissue degradation products, *Ann. N.Y. Acad. Sci.*, 257, 177, 1975.

49. Ward, P. A. and Becker, E. L., The deactivation of rabbit neutrophils by chemotactic factor and the nature of the activatable esterase, *J. Exp. Med.*, 127, 693, 1968.

50. Goetzl, E. J., Plasma and cell-derived inhibitors of human neutrophil chemotaxis, *Ann. N.Y. Acad. Sci.*, 256, 210, 1975.

50a. Fehr, J. and Dahinden, C., Modulating influences of chemotactic factor-induced cell adhesiveness on granulocyte function, *J. Clin. Invest.*, 64, 8, 1979.

51. Berenberg, J. L. and Ward, P. A., Chemotactic factor inactivator in normal human serum, *J. Clin. Invest.*, 52, 1200, 1973.

52. Till, G. and Ward, P. A., Two distinct chemotactic factor inactivators in human serum, *J. Immunol.*, 114, 843, 1975.

53. Ward, P. A. and Ozols, J., Characterization of the protease activity in the chemotactic factor inactivator, *J. Clin. Invest.*, 58, 123, 1976.

54. Goetzl, E. J. and Austen, K. F., A neutrophil-immobilizing factor derived from human leukocytes. I. Generation and partial characterization, *J. Exp. Med.*, 136, 1564, 1972.

55. Bronza, J. P., Senior, R. M., and Kreutzer, D. L., Chemotactic factor inactivators of human granulocytes, *J. Clin. Invest.*, 60, 1280, 1977.

56. Maderazo, E. G., Ward, P. A., and Quintiliani, R., Defective regulation of chemotaxis in cirrhosis, *J. Lab. Clin. Med.*, 85, 621, 1975.

57. Siriwatratananonta, P., Sinsakul, V., Stern, K., et al., Defective chemotaxis in uremia, *J. Lab. Clin. Med.*, 92, 402, 1978

58. Ward, P. A., and Berenberg, J. L., Defective regulation of inflammatory mediators in Hodgkin's disease: supernormal levels of chemotactic factor inactivator, *N. Engl. J. Med.*, 290, 76, 1974.

59. Maderazo, E. G., Ward, P. A., Woronick, C. L., et al., Leukotactic dysfunction in sarcoidosis, *Ann. Intern. Med.*, 84, 414, 1976.

60. Van Epps, D. E., Palmer, D. L., and Williams, R. C., Characterization of serum inhibitors of neutrophil chemotaxis associated with energy, *J. Immunol.*, 113, 189, 1974.

61. Van Epps, D. E. and Williams, R. C., Serum inhibitors of leukocyte chemotaxis and their relationship to skin test energy, in *Leukocyte Chemotaxis*, 1st ed., Gallin, J. I. and Quie, P. G., Eds., Raven Press, New York, 1978, 237.

62. Wilson, W. R., Ritts, R. E., and and Hermans, P. E., Abnormal chemotaxis in patients with cutaneous anergy, *Mayo Clin. Proc.*, 52, 1976, 1977.

62a. Christou, N. V. and Meakins, J. L., Neutrophil function in surgical patients: two inhibitors of granulocyte chemotaxis associated with sepsis, *J. Surg. Res.*, 26, 355, 1979.

63. Ward, P. A. and Talamo, R. C., Deficiency of the chemotactic factor inactivator in human sera with α_1-antitrypsin deficiency, *J. Clin. Invest.*, 52, 516, 1973

64. Smith, C. W., Hollers, J. C., Dupree, E., et al., A serum inhibitor of leukotaxis in a child with recurrent infections, *J. Lab. Clin. Med.*, 79, 878, 1972.

65. Maderazo, E. G., Ward, P. A., Woronick, C. L., et al., Partial characterization of a cell-directed inhibitor of leukotaxis in human serum, *J. Lab. Clin. Med.*, 89, 190, 1977.

66. Maderazo, E. G., Anton, T. F., and Ward, P. A., Serum-associated inhibition of leukotaxis in humans with cancer, *Clin. Immunol. Immunopathol.*, 9, 166, 1978.

67. Ward, P. A., Anton, T., and Maderazo, E., Defective leukotaxis in cancer patients, *Clin. Res.*, 24, 463a, 1976.

68. Van Epps, D. E. and Williams, R. C., Suppression of leukocyte chemotaxis by human IgA myeloma components, *J. Exp. Med.*, 144, 1227, 1976.

69. Davis, A. T., Grady, P. G., Shapira, E., et al., PMN chemotactic inhibition associated with a Cryoglobulin, *J. Pediatr.*, 90, 229, 1977.

70. Miller, M. E., Oski, F. A., and Harris, M. B., Lazy-leucocyte syndrome: a new disorder of neutrophil function, *Lancet*, I, 665, 1971.

71. Miller, M. E., Norman, M. E., Koblernzer, P. J., et. al., A new familial defect of neutrophil movement, *J. Lab. Clin. Med.*, 82, 1, 1975.

72. Steerman, R. L., Snyderman, R., Leikin, S. L., et al., Intrinisic defect of the polymorphonuclear leucocyte resulting in impaired chemotaxis and phagocytosis, *Clin. Exp. Immunol.*, 9, 939, 1971.

73. Clark, R. A., Root, R. K., Kimball, H. R., et al., Defective neutrophil chemotaxis and cellular immunity in a child with recurrent infecttions, *Ann. Intern. Med.*, 78, 515, 1973.

74. Hill, H. R. and Quie, P. G., Raised serum-IgE levels and defective neutrophil chemotaxis in three children with eczema and recurrent bacterial infections, *Lancet*, 1, 183, 1974.

75. Van Scoy, R. E., Hill, H. R., Ritts, R. E., et al., Familial neutrophil chemotaxis defect, recurrent bacterial infections, mucocutaneous candidiasis, and hyperimmunoglobulinemia E, *Ann. Intern. Med.*, 82, 766, 1975.

76. Dahl, M. V., Greene, W. H., and Quie, P. G., Infection, dermatitis, increased IgE, and impaired neutrophil chemotaxis, *Arch. Dermatol.*, 112, 1387, 1976.

77. Jacobs, J. C. and Norman, M. E., A familial defect of neutrophil chemotaxis with asthma, eczema, and recurrent skin infections, *Pediatr. Res.*, 11, 732, 1977.

78. Hill, H. R., Book, L. S., Hemming, V. G., et al., Defective neutrophil chemotactic responses in patients with recurrent episodes of otitis media and chronic diarrhea,, *Am. J. Dis. Child.*, 131, 433, 1977.

79. Niinaka, T., Okochi, T., Watanabe, Y., et al., Chemotactic defect in Wegener's granulomatosis, *J. Med.*, 8, 161, 1977.

80. Clark, R. A. and Kimball, H. R., Defective granulocyte chemotaxis in the Chediak-Higashi syndrome, *J. Clin. Invest.*, 50, 2645, 1971.

81. Mowat, A. G. and Baum, J., Chemotaxis of polymorphonuclear leukocytes from patients with rheumatoid arthritis, *J. Clin. Invest.*, 50, 2541, 1971.

82. Harris, H., The movement of lymphocytes, *Br. J. Exp. Pathol.*, 34, 599, 1953.

83. Ward, P. A., Offen, C. D., and Montogomery, J. R., Chemoattractants of leukocytes, with special reference to lymphocytes, *Fed. Proc. Fed. Am. Soc. Exp. Biol.*, 30, 1721, 1971.

84. Ward, P. A., Unanue, E. R., Goralnick, S. J., et al., Chemotaxis of rat lymphocytes, *J. Immunol.*, 119, 416, 1977.

85. Houck, J. C. and Chang, C. M., The purification and characterization of a lymphokine chemotactic for lymphocytes-lymphotactin, *Inflammation*, 2, 105, 1977.

86. Ward, P. A., Chemotaxis of mononuclear cells, *J. Exp. Med.*, 128, 1201, 1968.

87. Snyderman, R. and Mergenhagen, S. E., *Immunobiology of the Macrophage, Chemotaxis of Macrophages*, Nelson, D. S., Ed., Academic Press, New York, 1976, 323.

88. Snyderman, R., Shin, H. S., and Dannenberg, A. M., Macrophage proteinase and inflammation: the production of chemotactic activity from the fifth component of complement by macrophage proteinase, *J. Immunol.*, 109, 896, 1972.

89. Symon, D. N. K., McKay, J. C., and Wilkinson, P. C., Plasma-dependent chemotaxis of macrophages towards *Mycobacterium tuberculosis* and other organisms, *Immunology.*, 22, 267, 1972.

90. Ward, P. A., Remold, H. G., and David, H. R., The production by antigen-stimulated lymphocytes of leukotactic factor distinct from migration inhibitory factor, *Cell. Immunol.*, 1, 162, 1970.

91. Wahl, S. M., Altman, L. C., Oppenheim, J. J., In Vitro studies of a chemotactic lymphokine in the guinea pig, *Int. Arch. Allergy*, 46, 768, 1974.

92. Altman, L. C., Snyderman, R., Oppenheim, J. J., et al., A human mononuclear leukocyte chemotactic factor: characterization, specificity and kinetics of production by homologous leukocytes, *J. Immunol.*, 110, 801, 1973.

93. Wahl, M. S., Wilton, J. M., Rosenstreich, D. L., et al., The role of macrophages in the production of lymphokines by T and B lymphocytes, *J. Immunol.*, 114, 1296, 1975.

94. Gallin, J. I. and Kaplan, A. P., Mononuclear cell chemotactic activity of kallikrein and plasminogen activator and its inhibition by Cl inhibitor and α_2-macroglobulin, *J. Immunol.*, 113, 1928, 1975.

95. Gallin, J. E., Sandler, J. A., Clyman, R. I., et al., Agents that increase cyclic AMP and inhibit accumulation of cGMP and depress human monocyte locomotion, *J. Immunol.*, 120, 492, 1978.

96. Dauber, J. H. and Daniele, R. P., Chemotactic activity of guinea pig alveolar macrophages, *Am. Rev. Respir. Dis.*, 117, 673, 1978.

97. Warr, G. A. and Martin, R. R. Chemotactic responsiveness of human alveolar macrophages: effects of cigarette smoking, *Infect. Immunol.*, 9, 769, 1974.

97a. Demarest, G. B., Hudson, L. D., and Altman, L. C., Impaired alveolar macrophage chemotaxis in patients with actue smoke inhalation, *Am. Rev. Respir. Dis.*, 119, 279, 1979.

97b. Lynn, W. S., Mukherjee, C., Motility of rabbit alveolar cells, *Am. J. Pathol.*, 96, 663, 1979.

98. Pantalone, R. M. and Page, R. C., Lymphokine-induced production and release of lysosomal enzymes by macrophages, *Proc. Natl. Acad. Sci. U.S.A.*, 72, 2091, 1975.

99. Werb, Z. and Gordon, S., Elastase secretion by stimulated macrophages, *J. Exp. Med.*, 142, 361, 1975.

100. Wahl, L. M., Wahl, S. M., Mergenhagen, S. E., et al., Collagenase production by endotoxin-activated macrophages, *Proc. Natl. Acad. Sci. U.S.A.*, 71, 3598, 1974.

101. Unkeless, J. C., Gordon, S., and Reich, E., Secretion of plasminogen activator by stimulated macrophages, *J. Exp. Med.*, 139, 834, 1974.

102. Kleinerman, E. S., Snyderman, R., and Daniels, C., Depression of human monocyte chemotaxis by *Herpes simplex* and influenza viruses, *J. Immunol.*, 113, 1562, 1974.

103. Snyderman, R., Meadows, L., Holder, W., et al., Abnormal monocyte chemotaxis in patients with breast cancer: evidence for a tumor-mediated effect, *J. Natl. Cancer Inst.*, 60, 737, 1978.

104. Rubin, R. H., Cosimi, B. A., and Goetzl, E. J., Defective human mononuclear leukocyte, chemotaxis as an index of host resistance to malignant melanoma, *Clin. Immunol. Immunopathol.*, 6, 376, 1976.

105. Kay, A. B. and McVie, J. G., Monocyte chemotaxis in bronchial carcinoma and cigarette smokers, *Br. J. Cancer*, 36, 461, 1977.

106. Normann, S. J. and Sorkin, E., Inhibition of macrophage chemotaxis by neoplastic and other rapidly proliferating cells *in vitro, Cancer Res.*, 37, 705, 1977.

107. Meltzer, M. S., Stevenson, M. M., and Leonard, E. J., Characterization of macrophage chemotaxins in tumor cell cultures and comparison with lymphocyte-derived chemotactic factors, *Cancer Res.*, 37, 721, 1977.

108. Kay, A. B., Stechschulte, D. J., and Austen, K. F., An eosinophil leukocyte chemotactic factor of anaphylaxis, *J. Exp. Med.*, 133, 602, 1971.

109. Parish, W. E., Eosinophilia. III. The anaphylactic release from isolated human basophils of a substance that selectively attracts eosinophils, *Clin. Allergy*, 2, 381, 1972.

110. Kaliner, M. and Austen, K. F., A sequence of biochemical events in the antigen-induced release of chemical mediators from sensitized human lung tissue, *J. Exp. Med.*, 138, 1077, 1973.

111. Goetzl, E. J. and Austen, K. F., Purification and synthesis of eosinophilotactic tetrapeptides of human lung tissue: identification as eosinophil chemotactic factor of anaphylaxis, *Proc. Natl. Acad. Sci. U.S.A.*, 72, 4123, 1975.

112. Turnbull, L. W., Evans, D. P., and Kay, A. B., Human eosinophils, acidic tetrapeptides (ECF-A) and histamine, *Immunology*, 32, 57, 1977.

113. Goetzl, E. J. and Austen, K. F., Structural determinants of the eosinophil chemotactic activity of the acidic tetrapeptides of eosinophil chemotactic factor of anaphylaxis, *J. Exp. Med.*, 144, 1424, 1976.

114. Czarnetzki, B. M., Konig, W., and Lichtenstein, L. M., Eosinophil chemotactic factor (ECF). I. Release from polymorphonuclear leukocytes by the calcium ionophore A23187, *J. Immunol.*, 117, 229, 1976.

115. Konig, W., Czarnetzki, B. M., and Lichtenstein, L. M., Eosinophil chemotactic factor (ECF). II. Release from human polymorphonuclear leukocytes during phagocytosis, *J. Immunol.*, 117, 235, 1976.

116. Czarnetzki, B. M., Eosinophil chemotactic factor release from neutrophils by *Nippostrongylus brasiliensis* larvae, *Nature (London)*, 271, 553, 1978.

117. Boswell, R. N., Austen, K. F., and Goetzl, E. J., Intermediate moleculear weight eosinophil chemotactic factors in rat peritoneal mast cells: immunologic release, granule association, and demonstration of structural heterogeneity, *J. Immunol.*, 120, 15, 1978.

118. Clark, R. A. F., Gallin, J. I., and Kaplan, A. P., The selective eosinophil chemotactic activity of histamine, *J. Exp. Med.*, 142, 1462, 1975.

119. Turnbull, L. W. and Kay, A. B., Histamine and imidazole acetic acid as chemotactic agents for human eosinophil leukocytes, *Immunology*, 31, 797, 1976.

120. Clark, R. A. F., Sandler, J. A., Gallin, J. I., Histamine modulation of eosinophil migration, *J. Immunol.*, 118, 137, 1977.

121. Ward, P. A., Chemotaxis of human eosinophils, *Am. J. Pathol.*, 54, 121, 1969.

122. Kay, A. B., Studies on eosinophil leucocyte migration. II. Factors specifically chemotactic for eosinophils and neutrophils generated from guinea-pig serum by antigen-antibody complexes, *Clin. Exp. Med.*, 7, 732, 1970.

123. Cohen, S., Ward, P. A., *In vitro* and *in vivo* activity of a lymphocyte and immune complex-dependent chemotactic factor for eosinophils, *J. Exp. Med.*, 133, 133, 1971.

124. Goetzl, E. J., Tashjian, A. H., Ruben, R. H., et al., Production of a low molecular weight eosinophil polymorphonuclear leukocyte chemotactic factor by anaplastic squamous cell carcinomas of human lung, *J. Clin. Invest.*, 61, 770, 1978.

125. Tanaka, J. and Torisu, M., Anisakis and eosinophil. I. Detection of a soluble factor selectively chemotactic for eosinophils in the extract from anisakis larvae, *J. Immunol.*, 120, 745, 1978.

126. Kay, A. B. and Austen, K. F., Chemotaxis of human basophil leukocytes, *Clin. Exp. Immunol.*, 11, 557, 1972.

127. Hirsch, S. R., Serum basophil chemotactic factor, *J. Allergy Clin. Immunol.*, 57, 193, 1976.

128. Postlethwaite, A. E., Synderman, R., and Kang, A. H., The chemotactic attraction of human fibroblasts to a lymphocyte-derived factor, *J. Exp. Med.*, 144, 1188, 1976.

129. Postlethwaite, A. E., Seyer, J. M., and Kang, A. H., Chemotactic attraction of human fibroblasts to Type I, II and III collagens and collagen-derived peptides, *Proc. Natl. Acad. Sci. U.S.A.*, 75, 871, 1978.

129a. Sobel, J. D. and Gallin, J. I., Polymorphonuclear leukocyte and monocyte chemoattractants produced by human fibroblasts, *J. Clin. Invest.*, 63, 609, 1979.

130. Forsgren, A. and Schmeling, D., Effects of antibiotics on chemotaxis of human leukocytes, *Antimicro. Agents Chemother.*, 11, 580, 1977.

131. Majeski, J. A. and Alexander, J. W., Evaluation of tetracycline in the neutrophil chemotactic response, *J. Lab. Clin. Med.*, 90, 259, 1977.

132. Esterly, N. B., Furey, N. L., and Flanagan, L. E., The effect of antimicrobial agents on leukocyte chemotaxis, *J. Invest. Dermatol.*, 70, 51, 1978.

132a. Khan, A. J., Evans, H. E., Glass, L., et al., Abnormal neutrophil chemotaxis and random migration induced by aminoglycoside antibiotics, *J. Lab. Clin. Med.*, 93, 295, 1979.

133. Aswanikumar, S., Schiffman, E., Corcoran, B. A., et al., Antibiotics and peptides with agonist and atagonist chemotactic activity. *Biochem. Res. Commun.*, 80, 464, 1978.

134. Shea, C. and Morse, E. D., Inhibition of human neutrophil chemotaxis by corticosteroids, *Ann. Clin. Lab. Sci.*, 8, 30, 1978.

135. Majeski, J. A. and Alexander, J. W., The steroid effect on the in vitro human neutrophil chemotactic response, *J. Surg. Res.*, 21, 265, 1976.

136. Hawley, H. P. and Gordon, G. B., The effects of long chain free fatty acids on human neutrophil function and structure, *Lab. Invest.*, 34, 216, 1976.

137. Snyderman, R., Phillips, J. K., and Mergenhagen, S. E., Biological activity of complement, *in vivo*, *J. Exp. Med.*, 134, 1131, 1971.

138. Ward, P. A., Cochrane, C. G., and Muller-Eberhard, H. J., Further studies on the chemotactic factor of complement and its formation *in vivo*, *Immunology*, 11, 141, 1966.

139. Ward, P. A. and Hill, J. H., Biologic role of complement products, *J. Immunol.*, 108, 1137, 1972.

140. Jones, D. G., Richardson, D. L., and Kay, A. B., Neutrophil accumulation in vitro following the administration of chemotactic factors, *Br. J. Haematol.*, 35, 19, 1977.

141. Kazmierowski, J. A., Gallin, J. I., and Reynolds, H. Y., Mechanism for the inflammatory response in primate lungs, *J. Clin. Invest.*, 59, 273, 1977.

141a. Henson, P. M., McCarthy, K., Larsen, G. L., et al., Complement fragments, alveolar macrophages, and alveolitis, *Am. J. Pathol.*, 97, 93, 1979.

141b. Desai, U., Kreutzer, D. L., Showell, H., et al., Acute inflammatory pulmonary reactions induced by chemotactic factors, *Am. J. Pathol.*, 96, 71, 1979.

142. Johnson, K. J., Anderson, T. P., and Ward, P. A., Suppression of immune complex-induced inflammation by the chemotactic factor inactivator, *J. Clin. Invest.*, 59, 951, 1977.

143. Pernis, B., Vigliani, E. C., Cavagna, C., et al., The role of bacterial endotoxins in occupational diseases caused by inhaling vegetable dusts, *Br. J. Indust. Med.*, 18, 120, 1961.

144. Snell, J. D., Effects of inhaled endotoxin, *J. Lab. Clin. Med.*, 67, 624, 1966.

145. Cavagna, G., Foa, F., and Vigliani, E. C., et al., Effects in man and rabbits of inhalation of cotton dust or extracts and purified endotoxins, *Br. J. Industr. Med.*, 26, 314, 1969.

146. Hudson, A. R., Kilburn, K. H., Halprin, G. M., et al., Granulocyte recruitment to airways exposed to endotoxin aerosols, *Am. Rev. Respir. Dis.*, 115, 89, 1977.

147. Pierce, A. K., Reynolds, R. C., and Harris, G. D., Leukocyte response to inhaled bacteria, *Am. Rev. Repir. Dis.*, 116, 679, 1977.

148. Blanden, R. V., Lefford, M. J., and Mackaness, G. B., The host response to calmette-guerin bacillus infection in mice, *J. Exp. Med.*, 129, 1079, 1969.

149. McGregor, D. D., Koster, F. T., and Mackaness, G. B., The mediator of cellular immunity. I. The life-span and circulation dynamics of the immunologically committed lymphocyte, *J. Exp. Med.*, 133, 389, 1971.

150. Prausnitz, C., Investigations on Respiratory Dust Disease in Operations in the Cotton Industry, Medical Research Council, His Majesty's Stationery Office, London, 1936.

151. Kilburn, K. H., Leukocyte recruitment and histamine release by Lacinilene-C7-Methylether: isolated from cotton dust and synthesized, in press.

152. Kilburn, K. H., Lynn, W. D., Tres, L. L., et al., Leukocyte recruitment through airway walls by condensed vegetable tannins and quercetin, *Lab. Invest.*, 28, 55, 1973.

153. Thurlbeck, W. M., Henderson, J. A. M., Fraser, R. G., et al., Chronic obstructive lung disease: a comparison between clinical, roentgenologic, functional, and morphologic criteria in chronic bronchitis, emphysema, asthma, and bronchiectasis, *Medicine*, 49, 81, 1970.

154. Asmundsson, T., Kilburn, K. H., and McKenzie, W. N., Injury and metaplasia of airway cells due to SO_2, *Lab. Invest.*, 29, 41, 1973.

155. Kilburn, K. H. and McKenzie, W. N., Leukocyte recruitment to airways by aldehyde-carbon combinations that mimic cigarette smoke, *Lab. Invest.*, 38, 134, 1978.

156. Kilburn, K. H. and McKenzie, W. N., Leukocyte recruitment to airways by cigarette smoke and particle phase in contract to cytotoxicity of vapor, *Science*, 189, 634, 1975.

157. Kilburn, K. H. and McKenzie, W. N., in press,

158. Rylander, R., Free lung cell studies in cigarette smoke inhalation experiments, *Scand. J. Respir. Dis.,* 52, 121, 1971.

159. Rylander, R., Pulmonary cell responses to inhaled cigarette smoke, *Arch. Environ. Health,* 29, 329, 1974.

160. Bridges, R. B., Kraal, J. H., Haung, L. J. T., et al., Effect of cigarette smoke components on *in vitro* chemotaxis of human polymorphonuclear leukocytes, *Infect. Immun.,* 16, 240, 1977.

161. Salvaggio, J., Phanuphak, P., Stanford, R., et al., Experimental production of granulomatous pneumonitis, *J. Allergy Clin. Immunol.,* 56, 346, 1975.

162. Harris, J. O., Bice, D., and Salvaggio, J. E., Cellular and humoral bronchopulmonary immune resonse of rabbits immunized with thermophilic actinomyces antigen, *Am. Rev. Respir. Dis.,* 114, 29, 1976.

163. Henney, C. S., Waldman, R. H., Cell-mediated immunity shown by lymphocytes from the respiratory tract, *Science,* 169, 696, 1970.

164. Santives, T., Roska, A. K., Hensley, G. T., et al., Immunologically induced lung disease in guinea pigs, *J. Allergy Clin. Immunol.,* 57, 582, 1976.

165. Richerson, H. B., Acute experimental hypersensitivity pneumonitis in the guinea pig, *J. Lab. Clin. Med.,* 79, 745, 1972.

166. Hensley, G. T., Fink, J. N., Barboriak, J. J., et al., Hypersensitivity pneumonitis in the monkey, *Arch. Pathol.,* 97, 33, 1974.

167. Olenchock, S. A. and Burrell, R., The role of precipitins and complement activation in the etiology of allergic lung disease, *J. Allergy Clin. Immunol.,* 58, 76, 1976.

168. Edwards, J. H., Wagner, J. C., and Seal, R. M. E., Pulmonary responses to particulate materials capable of activating the alternative pathway of complement, *Clin. Allergy,* 6, 155, 1976.

169. Edwards, J. H., Baker, J. T., and Davies, B. H., Precipitin test negative farmer's lung-activation of the alternative pathway of complement by moldy hay dusts. *Clin. Allergy,* 4, 379, 1974.

170. Moore, V. I., Hensley, G. T., and Fink, J. N., An animal model of hypersensitivity pneumonitis in the rabbit, *J. Clin. Invest.,* 56, 937, 1975.

171. Peterson, L. B., Thrall, R. S., Moore, V. L., et al., An animal model of hypersensitivity pneumonitis in the rabbit. Induction of cellular hypersensitivity to inhaled antigens using carrageenan and BCG, *Am. Rev. Respir. Dis.,* 116, 1007, 1977.

172. Miyamoto, T., Kabe, J., Noda, M., et al., Physiologic and pathologic respiratory changes in delayed type hypersensitivity reaction in guinea pigs, *Am. Rev. Respir. Dis.,* 103, 509, 1971.

173. Basten, A., Boyer, M. H., and Beeson, P. B., Mechanism of eosinophilia. I. Factors affecting the eosinophil response of rats to *Trichinella spiralis, J. Exp. Med.,* 131, 1271, 1970.

174. Bazin, H., Elevation of total serum IgE in rats showing helminth parasite infection, *Nature (London),* 251, 613, 1974.

175. Archer, G. T., Robson, J. E., and Thompson, A. R., Eosinophilia and mast cell hyperplasia induced by parasite phospholipid, *Pathology,* 9, 137, 1977.

176. Basten, A. and Beeson, P. B., Mechanism of eosinophilia. II. Role of the lymphocyte, *J. Exp. Med.,* 131, 1288, 1970.

177. Colley, D. G., Eosinophils and immune mechanisms. I. Eosinophil stimulation promoter (ESP): a lymphokine induced by specific antigen or phytohemagglutinin, *J. Immunol.,* 110, 1419, 1973.

178. Greene, B. M. and Colley, D. G., Eosinophils and immune mechanisms. III. Production of the lympokine eosinophil stimulation promoter by mouse T lymphocytes, *J. Immunol.,* 116, 1078, 1976.

179. Mahoumoud, A. A. F., Warren, K. S., and Peters, P. A., A role for the eosinophil in acquired resistance to *Schistoma mansoni* infection as determined by antieosinophil serum, *J. Exp. Med.,* 142, 805, 1975.

180. Butterworth, A. E., David, J. R., and Frants, D., Antibody-dependent eosinophil-mediated damage to ^{51}Cr-labeled schistosomula of *Schistosoma mansoni, J. Exp. Med.,* 145, 136, 1977.

181. Ramalho-Finto, F. J., McLaren, D. J., and Smithers, S. R., Complement-mediated killing of schistosomula of *Schistosoma mansoni* by rat eosinophils, *in vitro, J. Exp. Med.,* 147, 147, 1978.

182. Chodosh, S., Zaccheo, C. W., and Segal, M. S., The cytology and histochemistry of sputum cells. I. Preliminary differential counts in chronic bronchitis, *Am. Rev. Respir. Dis.,* 85, 635, 1962.

183. Glynn, A. A. and Muchaels, L., Bronchial biopsy in chronic bronchitis and asthma, *Thorax,* 15, 142, 1960.

184. Ottensen, E. A., *Eosinophilia and the Lung-In Immunologic and Infectious Reactions in the Lung,* Kirkpatrick, C. H. and Reynolds, H. Y., Eds., Marcel Dekker, New York, 1976, 289.

185. Cosio, M., Ghezzo, H., Hogg, J. C., et al., The relations between structural changes in small airways and pulmonary function tests, *N. Engl. J. Med.,* 298, 1277, 1978.

186. Karpick, R. J., Pratt, P. C., Asmundsson, T., et al., Pathological findings in respiratory failure, *Ann. Intern. Med.,* 72, 189, 1970.

187. McLean, K. H., The pathology of acute bronchiolitis — a study of its evolution. I. The exudative phase, *Aust. Ann. Med.,* 5, 254, 1956.

188. **Engel, S.,** Bronchiolitis, *Br. J. Dis. Chest.,* 53, 125, 1959.
189. **Spencer, H.,** *Pathology of the Lung (Excluding Pulmonary Tuberculosis),* Pergamon press, New York, 1977, chap. 1.
190. **Coates, E. O. and Watson, J. H. L.,** Diffuse interstitial lung disease in tungsten carbide workers, *Ann. Intern. Med.,* 75, 709, 1971.
191. **Pimentel, J. C. and Marques, F.,** Vineyard sprayer's lung: a new occupational disease, *Thorax,* 24, 678, 1969.
192. **Rylander, R.,** Studies on humans exposed to airborne sewage sludge, *Schweiz. Med. Wochenschr.,* 107, 182, 1977.
193. **Edwards, J. H., Griggiths, A. J., and Mullens, J.,** Protozoa as sources of antigen in "humidifier fever", *Nature (London),* 264, 438, 1976.
194. **Friend, J. A. R., Palmer, K. N. V., Gaddie, J., et al.,** Extrinsic allergic alveolitis and contaminated cooling-water in factory machine, *Lancet,* 1, 297, 1977.
195. **Trice, M. F.,** Card-room fever, *Textile World,* 90, 68, 1940.
196. **Ritter, W. L. and Nussbaum, M. A.,** Occupational illnesses in cotton industries, *Miss. Doctor,* 22, 96, 1944.
197. **Uragoda, C. G.,** An investigation into the health of kapok workers, *Br. J. Industr. Med.,* 34, 181, 1977.
198. **Merchant, J. A., Halprin, G. M., Hudson, A. R., et al.,** Responses to cotton dust, *Arch. Environ. Health,* 30, 222, 1975.
199. **Ratcliff, N. B., Wilson, J. W., Mikat, E., et al.,** The lung in hemorragic shock. IV. The role of neutrophilic polymorphonuclear leukocytes, *Am. J. Pathol.,* 65, 325, 1971.
200. **Kilburn, K. H.,** Clearance zones in the distal lung, *Ann. N. Y. Acad. Sci.,* 221, 276, 1974.
201. **Macklin, C. C.,** Pulmonary sumps, dust accmulations, alveolar fluid, and lymph vessels, *Acta Anat.,* 23, 1, 1955.
202. **Green, G. M., Jakab, G. J., Low, R. B., et al.,** Defense mechanisms of the respiratory membrane, *Am. Rev. Respir. Dis.,* 115, 479, 1977.
203. **Sutliff, W. D. and Friedmann, T. E.,** A soluble edema-producing substance from the pneumococcus, *J. Immunol.,* 34, 455, 1938.
204. **Davies, P., Page, R. C., and Allison, A. C.,** Changes in cellular enzyme levels and extracellular release of lysosomal acid hydrolases in macrophages exposed to group A streptococcal cell wall substance, *J. Exp. Med.,* 139, 1262, 1974.
205. **Zaidi, S. H., Shanker, R., and Dogra, R. K. S.,** Experimental studies on early stages of the development of pulmonary silicosis in pups, *Environ. Res.,* 4, 243, 1971.
206. **Heppleston, A. G., Wright, N. A., and Stewart, J. A.,** Experimental alveolar lipo-proteinosis following the inhalation of silica, *J. Pathol.,* 101, 293, 1970.
207. **Spector, W. G., Reichold, N., and Ryan, G. B.,** Degradation of granuloma-inducing micro-organisms by macrophages, *J. Pathol.,* 101, 339, 1970.
208. **Forbus, W. D.,** *Granulomatous Inflammation,* Charles C Thomas, Springfield, Ill., 1949, 3.
209. **Barrowcliff, D. F. and Arblaster, P. G.,** Farmer's lung: a study of an acute fetal case, *Thorax,* 23, 490, 1968.
210. **Seal, R. M. E., Hapke, E. J., Thomas, G. O.,** The pathology of the acute and chronic stages of farmer's lung, *Thorax,* 23, 469, 1968.
211. **Wenzel, F. J., Emanuel, D. A., and Gray, R. L.,** Immunofluorescent studies in patients with farmer's lung, *J. Allergy Clin. Immunol.,* 48, 224, 1971.
212. **Patterson, R., Roberts, M., Roberts, R. C.,** Antibodies of different immunoglobulin classes against antigens causing farmer's lung, *Am. Rev. Respir. Dis.,* 114, 315, 1976.
213. **Roberts, R. C., Zais, D. P., and Emanuel, D. A.,** The frequency of precipitins to trichloracetic acid-extractable antigens from thermophilic actinomycetes in farmer's lung patients and asymptomatic farmers, *Am. Rev. Respir. Dis.,* 114, 23, 1976.
213a. **Boyd, G.,** Clinical and immunological studies in pulmonary extrinsic allergic alveolitis, *Scot. Med. J.,* 23, 267, 1978.
214. **Moore, V. L., Fink, J. N., Barboriak, J. J., et al.,** Immunologic events in pigeon breeder's disease, *J. Allergy Clin. Immunol.,* 53, 319, 1974.
215. **Berrens, L., Guikers, C. L. H., and Van Dijk, A.,** The antigens in pigeon-breeder's disease and their interaction with human complement, *Ann. N.Y. Acad. Sci.,* 221, 153, 1974.
216. **Marx, J. J. and Flaherty, D. K.,** Activation of the complement sequence by extracts of bacteria and fungi associated with hypersensitivity pneumonitis, *J. Allergy Clin. Immunol.,* 57, 328, 1976.
217. **Caldwell, J. R., Pearce, D. E., Spencer, C.,** Immunologic mechanisms in hypersensitivity pneumonitis. I. Evidence for cell-mediated immunity and complement fixation in pigeon breeder's disease, *J. Allergy Clin. Immunol.,* 52, 225, 1973.
218. **Fink, J. N., Moore, V. L., and Barboriak, J. J.,** Cell-mediated hypersensitivity in pigeon breeders, *Int. Arch. Allergy Appl. Immunol.,* 49, 831, 1975.

219. Reynolds, H. Y., Fulmer, J. D., Kazmierowski, J. A., et al., Analysis of cellular and protein content of broncho-alveolar lavage fluid from patients with idiopathic pulmonary fibrosis and chronic hypersensitivity pneumonitis, *J. Clin. Invest.*, 59, 165, 1977.

220. Roberts, R., Fractionation and characterization of thermophilic actinomycetes, *J. Allergy Clin. Immunol.*, 61, 234, 1978.

221. Nicolet, J., Bannerman, E. N., De Haller, R., Farmer's lung: immunological response to a group of extracellular enzymes of *Micropolyspora faeni*, *Clin. Exp. Immunol.*, 27, 401, 1977.

222. Berrens, L., Antigen diversity in pigeon breeder's disease, *J. Allergy Clin. Immunol.*, 61, 219, 1978.

223. Fredericks, W., Antigen in pigeon dropping extracts, *J. Allergy Clin. Immunol.*, 61, 221, 1978.

224. Khan, Z. U., Sandu, R. S., Randhawa, H. S., et al., Allergic broncho-pulmonary aspergillosis: a study of 46 cases with special reference to laboratory aspects, *Scand. J. Respir. Dis.*, 57, 73, 1976.

225. Bardana, E. J., Culture and antigen variants of *Aspergillus*, *J. Allergy Clin. Immunol.*, 61, 225, 1978.

226. Reed, C., Variability of antigenicity of *Aspergillus fumigatus*, *J. Allergy Clin. Immunol.*, 61, 227, 1978.

227. Kobayashi, G., Fractionation of *Aspergillus* antigens, *J. Allergy Clin. Immunol.*, 61, 230, 1978.

228. Parish, W. E., Substances that attract eosinophils *in vitro* and *in vivo*, and that elicit blood eosinophilia, *Antibiot. Chemother.*, 19, 233, 1974.

229. Wasserman, S. I., Goetzl, E. J., and Austen, K. F., Inactivation of slow reacting substance of anaphylaxis by human eosinophil arylsulfatase, *J. Immunol.*, 114, 645, 1975.

230. Kater, L. A., Goetzl, E. J., and Austen, K. F., Isolation of human eosinophil phospholipase D, *J. Clin. Invest.*, 57, 1173, 1976.

231. Zeiger, R. S., Yurdin, D. L., and Colten, H. R., Histamine metabolism. II. Cellular and subcellular localization of the catabolic enzymes, histaminase and histamine methyl transferase in human leukocytes, *J. Allergy Clin. Immunol.*, 58, 172, 1976.

232. Welsh, R. A. and Geer, J. C., Phagocytosis of mast cell granules by the eosinophilic leukocyte in the rat, *Am. J. Pathol.*, 35, 103, 1959.

233. Jones, D. G. and Kay, A. B., Eosinophils as regulators of repair following anaphylaxis, *Fed. Proc. Fed. Am. Soc. Exp. Biol.*, 35, 515, 1976.

234. Hubscher, T., Role of the eosinophil in the allergic reactions. I. EDI — an eosinophil-derived inhibitor of histamine release, *J. Immunol.*, 114, 1379, 1975.

235. Hubscher, T., Role of the eosinophil in the allergic reactions. II. Release of prostaglandins from human eosinophilic leukocytes, *J. Immunol.*, 114, 1389, 1975.

236. Phills, J. A., Harrold, A. J., Whiteman, G. V., et al., Pulmonary infiltrates, asthma, and eosinophilia due to *Ascaris suum* infestation in man, *N. Engl. J. Med.*, 286, 965, 1972.

237. Croften, J. W., Livingstone, J. L., Oswald, N. C., et al., Pulmonary eosinophilia, *Thorax*, 7, 1, 1952.

238. Nicklaus, T. M. and Snyder, A. B., Nitrofurantoin pulmonary reaction, *Arch. Int. Med.*, 121, 151, 1968.

239. Everts, C. S., Westcott, J. L., and Bragg, D. G., Methotrexate therapy and pulmonary disease, *Radiology*, 107, 539, 1973.

240. DeWeck, A. L., The formation of penicillin antigens, *Proc. R. Soc. Med.*, 61, 894, 1968.

241. Kilburn, K. H., Pulmonary diseases induced by drugs, in press.

242. Patterson, R., Irons, J. S., Kelly, J. F., et al., Pulmonary infiltrates with eosinophilia, *J. Allergy Clin. Immunol.*, 53, 245, 1974.

243. Carrington, C. B., Addington, W. W., and Goff, A. M., Chronic eosinophilic pneumonia, *N. Engl. J. Med.*, 280, 787, 1969.

244. Liebow, A. A. and Carrington, C. B., The eosinophilic pneumonias, *Medicine*, 48, 251, 1969.

245. McCarthy, D. S. and Pepys, J., Cryptogenic pulmonary eosinophilias, *Clin. Allergy*, 3, 339, 1973.

246. Ottensen, E. A., *Eosinophilia and the Lung-In Immunologic and Infectious Reactions in the Lung*, Kirkpatrick, C. H. and Reynolds, H. Y., Eds., Marcel Dekker, New York, 1976, 289.

Chapter 3

RELEASE OF PHARMACOLOGICAL AGENTS AND MEDIATORS FROM THE LUNGS

Sami I. Said

TABLE OF CONTENTS

I. INTRODUCTION

The release of pharmacologically active mediators from the lung has been considered for some time as an important factor in relation to anaphylaxis and extrinsic asthma.[1] It has only recently been recognized, however, that the lung is capable of synthesizing and releasing a variety of biologically active substances.[2-4] The possible importance of this phenomenon in the regulation of pulmonary function and in the mediation of pulmonary injury is now coming under increasing investigation.

Much of the evidence for the release of biologically active compounds from the lung has been derived from experiments on animals, isolated lungs, or on fragments of lung tissue and has been based on bioassay or on the use of pharmacologic antagonists and metabolic inhibitors. In many instances therefore the identities and concentrations of released agents remain to be established by more specific and precise techniques. Moreover, confirmation of this release and assessment of its importance in humans are still lacking.

It must be noted, further, that the pulmonary release of active substances often represents a balance between (1) *de novo* synthesis followed by discharge of these substances and (2) their removal or inactivation by the lung.

II. METHODS FOR DETECTION AND ASSAY OF RELEASED SUBSTANCES

Much of the data on the pulmonary release of biologically active substances has been acquired through bioassay techniques. In one such technique which has proved especially valuable, a series of sensitive smooth muscle organs, attached to transducers, are superfused with physiologic salt soltuions (see Figure 1).[5-6] The addition of biologically active substances to the superfusing solution is detected by the responses of assay organs, and the nature and approximate concentration of a given humoral agent may be deduced by comparing these responses with those elicited by standard reference solutions of known concentrations. Selection of assay organs depends on the substance or substances suspected of being released (see Table 1; see also References 6 and 7). The specificity of the responses of the assay organs is enhanced by pretreating them with specific pharmacologic antagonists or inhibitors. This technique is applicable for the analysis of "spot" samples and for the continuous assay of a perfusate from an isolated lung or of a stream of blood from a living animal.[6,7] This method has the advantages of relative simplicity and sensitivity and of providing rapid, on-line results. Its main drawback is that it can permit only a tentative identification of the active agent based on one type of biological action, usually the contraction or relaxation of certain smooth muscles. Other limitations of this method are that it is semiquantitative and may be insensitive to certain released substances, if these are inactive on the smooth muscle organs selected for the assay or if mediators are released only locally as "tissue hormones", without reaching the perfusate or other external medium.

Another important approach to investigating the release of certain humoral agents from the lung has been the use of inhibitors of their biosynthesis. This approach is useful when the release of these agents, e.g., the prostaglandins, follows stimulation of their biosynthesis and is not the result of their discharge from preexisting stores.[8] Thus, if the biosynthesis of prostaglandins is prevented, none could be released. The discovery that aspirin and indomethacin can inhibit the biosynthesis of prostaglandins in many systems has therefore provided a valuable tool in exploring the occurrence, magnitude, and impact of prostaglandin synthesis and release.[9]

Specific, quantitative, and often more sensitive assays of released mediators depend on their identification and measurement by chemical anaylses, including special extrac-

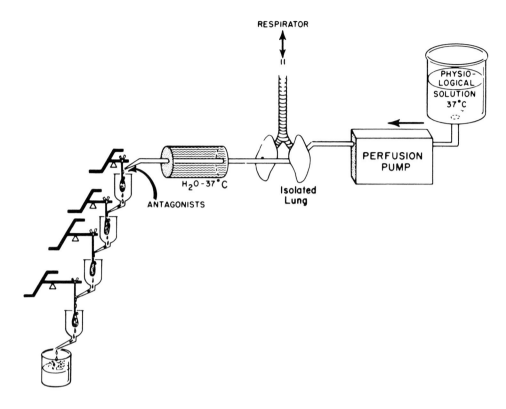

FIGURE 1. Schema for bioassay of lung perfusate, using the superfusion technique. The lung is isolated and perfused *in situ*, at constant flow, with physiologic solution at 37°C. Perfusate is rewarmed and pumped onto isolated smooth muscle organs, placed in series. Lung may be ventilated mechanically at different tidal volumes, using different gas mixtures. (Reprinted from Said, S. I., *Metabolic Functions of the Lung*, Vol. 4, Bakhle, Y. S. and Vane, J. R., Eds., by courtesy of Marcel Dekker, Inc., New York, 1977, chap. 10.)

tion and purification, thin-layer chromatography, gas-liquid chromatography, and mass spectrometry.[10] These methods, however, require specialized skills, expertise, longer time, and more elaborate equipment. Specific radioimmunoassays are available for at least some of the mediators and offer the advantages of relative simplicity, precision, and sensitivity.

III. CRITERIA FOR ESTABLISHING A MEDIATOR ROLE FOR A GIVEN SUBSTANCE

For the purpose of this discussion, mediators are defined as compounds that are either locally released or carried in blood or tissue fluids and that may participate in initiating, perpetuating, or aggravating a pathologic process.

The mere finding of a particular biologically active substance in pulmonary perfusate, blood, or other biological fluid does not necessarily mean that that substance is causally related to an associated response. However, such a relationship is likely if certain criteria are satisfied. For example:

1. The substance in question must be capable of producing, alone or with other compounds that also are released, the effects it is suspected of mediating.
2. The substance must be released in "sufficient" concentrations at the scene of its postulated actions.

Table 1

BIOLOGICALLY ACTIVE SUBSTANCES THAT MAY BE DETECTED AND MEASURED BY BIOASSAY

Compound	Basis for bioassay[a]
Amines	
Histamine	Contraction of GPI, GPGB
Serotonin	Contraction of RSS
Peptides	
Bradykinin	Contraction of GPGB, RU; relaxation of RC
Angiotensin II	Contraction of RC, GPGB
Vasoactive intestinal peptide	Relaxation of RSS, GPT, GPL, GPGB, CR; vasodilation
Spasmogenic lung peptide	Contraction of RSS, GPT, GPL, GPPA, GPI, GPGB, CR
Substance P	Contraction of GPT, GPI; vasodilation
Lipids	
PGE$_2$	Contraction of RSS, GPGB; CR; weaker contraction of RC and relaxation of GPT, GPL
PGF$_{2\alpha}$	Contraction of RC, GPT; weaker contraction of GPGB, CR
PG endoperoxides	Contraction of airway and pulmonary vascular smooth muscle
Thromboxane A$_2$	Contraction of airway, pulmonary vascular and aortic smooth muscle; platelet aggregation
Prostacyclin	Relaxation of coronary (bovine) and pulmonary vascular smooth muscle; platelet disaggregation
Slow-reacting substance of anaphylaxis	Contraction of GPI, GPT, in presence of atropine and mepyramine

[a] Abbreviations: CR, chick rectum; GPGB, guinea pig gallbladder; GPI, guinea pig ileum; GPL, guinea pig lung; GPPA, guinea pig pulmonary artery; GPT, guinea pig trachea; RSS, rat stomach strip; RC, rat colon; RU, rat uterus (estrus).

3. Inhibition of the release of this substance, or of its actions, should reduce or abolish the suspected effect.

IV. BIOLOGICALLY ACTIVE SUBSTANCES THAT MAY BE RELEASED FROM THE LUNG

Any substance that the lung is capable of storing or synthesizing may, under certain conditions, be released into the bloodstream. Active substances whose release from the lung has been demonstrated or is considered likely or at least possible include biogenic amines, polypeptides, proteins, lipids, and other compounds that remain incompletely identified (see Tables 2 to 6).

A. Biogenic Amines
1. Histamine
Histamine is probably the best known mediator substance. Its release has often been used as a yardstick for measuring "mediator release" as a whole, especially in immediate hypersensitivity reactions.

The mast cell is the principal target cell in immediate hypersensitivity. A series of intracellular reactions, triggered by antigen-IgE interaction, culminate in the degranulation of the mast cell. In the lung, mast cells are located in the bronchi, around smaller blood vessels, in alveolar walls, and in the pleura. The release of histamine, and other mediators, from mast cells is a noncytotoxic process in which the cell granules are discharged while the cell remains basically intact. This mediator release is actually an example of secretion and therefore is energy dependent, requires the presence of calcium ion, involves the contractile elements of the cell, and is influenced by the levels of the cyclic nucleotides (cyclic AMP and GMP).[11]

Table 2
ESTABLISHED AND POTENTIAL HUMORAL MEDIATORS IN LUNG AND THEIR PRINCIPAL BIOLOGICAL ACTIONS — BIOGENIC AMINES

Mediator	Action
Histamine	Constriction of bronchial and alveolar duct smooth muscle, decreased lung compliance and increased resistance; pulmonary vasoconstriction; increased fluid transudation from bronchial and (?) pulmonary vessels; systemic hypotension
Serotonin	Bronchoconstriction; vasoconstriction (systemic and pulmonary vessels)

Table 3
ESTABLISHED AND POTENTIAL HUMORAL MEDIATORS IN LUNG AND THEIR PRINCIPAL BIOLOGICAL ACTIONS — POLYPEPTIDES

Mediator	Action
Bradykinin	Contraction of bronchial smooth muscle [(?) through release of PGs]; increased capillary permeability [systemic and (?) pulmonary vessels]; systemic hypotension
Angiotensin II	Vasoconstriction, raised blood pressure, aldosterone release
VIP or VIP-like peptide	Systemic vasodilation; relaxation of tracheobronchial and other smooth muscle; stimulation of cyclic AMP production in many tissues
Spasmogenic lung peptide	Bronchoconstriction, contraction of other smooth muscle
RCS - releasing factor	Release of "Rabbit-Aorta-Contracting Substance" (see below)
Eosinophil chemotactic factor of anaphylaxis	Chemotaxis of eosinophils in immediate hypersensitivity
Substance P	Contraction of tracheobronchial and other smooth muscle
Bombesin	Contraction of tracheobronchial and other smooth muscle
ACTH and other hormones	Specific endocrine syndromes

The main actions of histamine include constriction of bronchial and alveolar duct smooth muscle, leading to a fall in pulmonary compliance and an increase in resistance to breathing. Histamine also constricts pulmonary vessels, raising pulmonary vascular resistance, but dilates systemic vessels and lowers systemic arterial blood pressure. There is ample proof that histamine increases systemic vascular permeability, but whether it has a similar effect on pulmonary vessels is doubtful and, in any case, probably minor.

2. Serotonin

Serotonin (5-Hydroxytryptamine) in the lung may be released from platelets which tend to accumulate in the pulmonary circulation in certain pathologic conditions, such

Table 4
ESTABLISHED AND POTENTIAL HUMORAL MEDIATORS IN LUNG AND THEIR PRINCIPAL BIOLOGICAL ACTIONS — PROTEINS

Mediator	Action
Complement	Immunologic injury
Lymphokines	"Cell-mediated" hypersensitivity
Proteolytic enzymes	
Elastase	Inflammation, hemorrhage, tissue destruction (acute); emphysema (more delayed)
Kallikrein	Release of bradykinin
Other enzymes	
Angiotensin converting enzyme	Activation of angiotensin; inactivation of bradykinin
Superoxide dismutase	Protection against oxygen toxicity
Mixed function oxidases	Metabolism of xenobiotics
Thromboplastin	Activation of extrinsic clotting mechanism

Table 5
ESTABLISHED AND POTENTIAL HUMORAL MEDIATORS IN LUNG AND THEIR PRINCIPAL BIOLOGICAL ACTIONS — LIPIDS

Mediator	Action
Prostaglandins	
$PGF_{2\alpha}$	Constriction of bronchi, alveolar ducts and pulmonary vessels
PGE_2	Bronchial relaxation (in vitro and in animals, but not consistently in humans); increased cAMP production; systemic vasodilation
PG endoperoxides	Contraction of airways (8 to 10 times more potent than $PGF_{2\alpha}$); contraction of other smooth muscle
Thromboxane A_2	Platelet aggregation, bronchoconstriction (10 times more potent than endoperoxides)
Prostacyclin (PGI_2)	Platelet disaggregation, systemic and pulmonary vasodilator
Slow-reacting substance of anaphylaxis (Leukotriene D)	Bronchoconstriction (more prolonged than with histamine), bronchial edema
RCS	Mixture of thromboxane A_2 and PG endoperoxide

Table 6
INHIBITORS OF BIOSYNTHETIC PATHWAYS FROM ARACHIDONIC ACID

Site of action	Examples[a]
Lipoxygenase	ETYA, phenidone
Cyclo-oxygenase	Aspirin, indomethacin, ETYA, phenidone
Prostacyclin synthetase	15-HPAA, tranylcypromine
Thromboxane synthetase	Imidazole
Phospholipase A_2	Corticosteroids

[a]   ETYA, 5,8,11-eicosatriynoic acid; phenidone, 1-phenyl-3-pyrazolidone; 15-HPAA, 15-hydroperoxy-arachidonic acid.

as pulmonary embolism and endotoxin shock. Another possible source of serotonin within the lung are the "neuroepithelial bodies", located in bronchial and alveolar walls. Lauweryns et al. showed these bodies to have fluorescent granules containing serotonin.[12] The amounts of serotonin in neuroepithelial bodies may be small, but owing to their strategic location, the serotonin they release may have important physiological and pharmacological effects[13](see Table 2).

B. Polypeptides

Among the biologically active peptides that may be produced by the lung (see Table 3) are

1. *Bradykinin* is generated through the action of activated kallikrein on a protein substrate (kininogen) in plasma or in lung tissue. Normal lung, it should be recalled, is capable of effectively removing bradykinin from the circulation.
2. *Angiotensin II* is the potent vasopressor resulting from the action of angiotensin-converting enzyme (kininase II) on angiotensin I. This is the same enzyme that catalyzes the inactivation of bradykinin and is concentrated in pulmonary endothelium.[14]
3. *Vasoactive intestinal peptide (VIP)* was originally isolated from porcine small intestine and this peptide is now known to occur widely in the GI tract, brain, peripheral nerves, and ganglia of mammalian and nonmammalian species.[15] Immunoreactive VIP is also present in the lung,[16] in locations that include mast cells[17] and nerves in the bronchial wall, especially near blood vessels and glandular structures.[18] VIP effects on lung include relaxation of tracheobronchial smooth muscle, protection against the bronchoconstrictor action of histamine and $PGE_{2\alpha}$, and stimulation of adenylate cyclase activity.
4. *A spasmogenic lung peptide,* with smooth muscle effects opposite to those of VIP, is extractable from normal porcine lung.[16] Although this peptide has yet to be chemically identified, it is apparently distinct from known peptides with similar biological activity.[16]
5. *The eosinophil chemotactic factor of anaphylaxis (ECF-A)* attracts eosinophils to the site of the anaphylactic reaction. ECF-A extracted from human lung appears to be composed of at least two tetrapeptides which have been prepared by synthesis.[11]
6. *Substance P,* a vasodilator of systemic vessels that contracts bronchial and other smooth muscle, was first discovered in extracts of intestine and of brain. Substance P immunoreactivity has recently been identified in lung tissue.[19]
7. *Bombesin,* was isolated from amphibian skin; a bombesin-like peptide has been found to occur in intestine, and has also been demonstrated in fetal lung by immunofluorescence.[20] Bombesin induces constriction of tracheobronchial and other smooth muscle.
8. A variety of peptide hormones, including *adrenocorticotrophic hormone (ACTH), antidiuretic hormone,* and *parathyroid hormone* may be released by the lung. This release is most commonly associated with pulmonary neoplasms, but may occur with inflammatory lesions (see later section in this chapter). The secretion of these hormones may result in specific endocrine syndromes (ectopic, paraneoplastic syndromes) or may remain clinically silent, being detectable only by sensitive, specific assays.

C. Proteins

A number of biologically active proteins occur, or may be generated, in the lung and may participate in important metabolic, inflammatory, and other reactions (Table 4). These proteins include

1. Complement, a major mediator of immunologic injury[21]
2. Lymphokines, a group of compounds that mediate "cell-mediated" (delayed) hypersensitivity[22]

3. Proteases, such as (a) elastase, which can produce acute lesions of inflammation, necrosis, and hemorrhage[23] or delayed injury simulating emphysema,[24] and (b) kallikrein which, upon activation, produces the release of bradykinin

4. Superoxide dismutase, an enzyme that destroys the superoxide radical,[25] believed to mediate the toxic effects of oxygen and other forms of lung injury, thus serving a protective function

5. Angiotensin-converting enzyme (kininase II, peptidyl dipeptidase), the enzyme responsible for converting angiotensin I to angiotensin II and for inactivating bradykinin.[14] Pulmonary endothelium is rich in this enzyme, but it also occurs in extrapulmonary sites, including glomeruli and intestinal epithelium.

6. The lung is rich in thromboplastin, an enzyme that can set off the activation of the extrinsic clotting mechanism, and in plasminogen activator, catalyzing the formation of plasmin, the key enzyme in fibrinolysis.[26]

7. Mixed-function oxidases and other drug-metabolizing enzymes present in lung microsomes may also be responsible for metabolizing polycyclic aromatic hydrocarbons, e.g., benzo(a)pyrene, into carcinogenic and mutagenic compounds.[27]

D. Lipids (see Table 5)

Most of the active lipid compounds that may be synthesized by the lung originate from one common precursor, arachidonic acid.[10] The two main synthetic pathways, the resulting compounds and their metabolites, are shown schematically in Figure 2. The principal products in the lung are prostacyclin (PGI_2)[27] and the thromboxanes. The former compound predominates in vascular endothelium and the latter in platelets.[10]

The activities of these compounds are summarized in Table 5. (Relatively little is known the biological actions of HETE and HPETE, two of the products catalyzed by lipoxygenase.) The potent endoperoxides have a short half-life of about 5 min, and the more potent thromboxane A_2 has an even shorter half-life of 30 sec. The slow-reacting substance of anaphylaxis (SRS-A) is now known to be derived from arachidonic acid,[28] through the action of the lipoxygenase enzyme.[28a]

These biosynthetic transformations can be blocked by inhibitors acting at different sites (see Figure 3); some of these inhibitors are listed in Table 6.[10]

V. PREFORMED VS. NEWLY SYNTHESIZED OR ACTIVATED MEDIATORS

Some of the active agents discussed above are preformed, e.g., histamine and ECF-A, contained within mast cell granules, and proteases, are normally confined within lysosomal membranes. Other active compounds, e.g., the prostaglandins and related lipids, must be generated by new synthesis before they can be released. This new synthesis may be stimulated by a variety of physical, chemical, neurogenic, and other stimuli (see later section). Activation is required for the kallikrein-kinin system and for complement to play a mediator role.

VI. MECHANISMS OF RELEASE OF MEDIATORS

Intracellular mediators may be released by either of two distinct mechanisms:[29]

1. *Cytotoxic release.* The cell membrane is disrupted and cytoplasmic enzymes and other contents are liberated. Examples of this mechanism are (a) the complement dependent reaction of antibody directed against the cell, (b) the involvement of platelets as ''innocent bystanders'' in the presence of immune complexes and

SOME ARACHIDONIC ACID
TRANSFORMATIONS IN LUNG

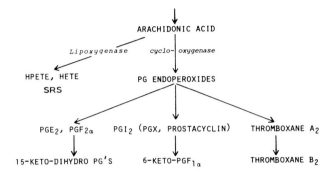

FIGURE 2.   Schema of biosynthetic pathways from arachidonic acid in lung. Major metabolites are shown on last line.

INHIBITION OF ARACHIDONIC ACID
TRANSFORMATIONS IN LUNG

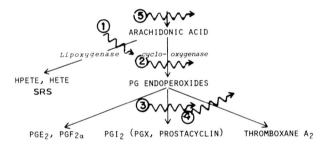

FIGURE 3.   Sites of possible inhibition (wavy arrows) of biosynthetic transformations from arachidonic acid. Examples of compounds acting at these different sites are given in Table 6.

complement, and (c) the lysis of macrophages by particles they phagocytize, e.g., silica.

2.   *Noncytotoxic release.* The granules to be discharged are thought to migrate toward the plasma membrane; the granule membrane fuses with the plasma membrane and the granules are extruded by a process of exocytosis.

Stimuli for this release appear to act at the cell surface and include (a) immunoglobulins interacting with specific receptors by the Fc portion of the molecule, (b) small proteins or peptides, e.g., complement -derived anaphylatoxins, (c) certain proteolytic enzymes, e.g., thrombin acting on platelets, and (d) cell-cell (e.g., basophil-platelet) interactions.

The noncytotoxic release reaction bears many similarities to the secretory process by which hormones, enzymes, and neurotransmitters are secreted. Both processes require energy (ATP), Ca^{++} in the external medium, and the participation of microtubules and microfilaments. Both processes are also influenced by the cyclic nucleotides, though in opposite fashion; whereas increased cyclic AMP concentration stimulates or enhances glandular and endocrine secretion, it inhibits the release of mediators.

Table 7
CONTRIBUTION OF CELLS TO MEDIATOR RELEASE

Cell	Associated mediators
Mast cell, basophil	Histamine, other mediators of anaphylaxis
Polymorphonuclear leukocyte	Lysosomal enzymes, superoxide
Macrophage	
Lymphocyte (stimulated)	Lymphokines
Plasma cell	Immunoglobulins
Platelet	Amines, PGs, PG endoperoxides, thromboxanes
Endothelium	PGs, bradykinin, angiotension converting enzyme
Neuroendocrine (APUD cell, neuroepithelial body)	Serotonin and other amines, peptide hormones

VII. CELLULAR ORIGIN OF MEDIATORS

As mentioned above, mediators normally occur as inactive precursors or are contained within intracellular sites from which they are discharged only following appropriate stimulation. A discussion of mediators should therefore include reference to the cells from which they originate and with which they may interact.

Table 7 summarizes the cellular origin of the major humoral mediators. Mast cells and basophils probably contribute most of the mediators of immediate hypersensitivity. Polymorphonuclear leukocytes and, to a smaller degree, alveolar macrophages, contain many proteolytic and other hydrolytic enzymes within their lysosomes. Lymphocytes, upon stimulation, release lymphokines. Plasma cells synthesize immunoglobulins. Platelets are a storehouse of biogenic amines, especially serotonin, but are also rich in prostaglandins and even richer in PG endoperoxides and thromboxanes. The latter two groups of compounds are also formed in lung tissue. Endothelial cells are the main sites of uptake and metabolism of serotonin, bradykinin, angiotensin I, and possibly other compounds. Finally, neuroendocrine cells, also known as Feyrter, Kultschitzky, or "APUD" (amine precursor uptake and decarboxylation) cells, may be the major serotonin- and peptide-containing cells in the lung (see Figure 4). The latter cells may occur in clusters of innervated cells and are then referred to as "neuroepithelial bodies".

VIII. CONDITIONS ASSOCIATED WITH PULMONARY RELEASE OF BIOLOGICALLY ACTIVE AGENTS

A. Anaphylaxis[1,11,30,31]

This is probably the condition that has been most extensively studied in relation to mediator release. As mentioned earlier, histamine is the prototype mediator in this condition, but by no means the only one, nor is it likely to be the most important. Other mediators include ECF-A, neutrophil chemotactic factors, bradykinin, SRS-A, prostaglandins, thromboxane A_2 (the major component of "RCS"), and platelet-activating factors. Evidence for the release of these substances is derived mainly from experiments on guinea pig lungs. With the exception of "RCS", the same agents are released from sensitized human lungs upon challenge with antigen.

The immunologic release of histamine and SRS-A from guinea pig lung occurs within 30 sec of antigen challenge; histamine release is maximal at 2 min and complete within 30 min, while that of SRS-A is maximal at 4 min (20 min in human lung) and continues after 30 min. Because of their rapid appearance, histamine and SRS-A are spoken of as "primary" mediators, while the release of other agents, including the prostaglandins, is thought to be "secondary" to that of the former compounds. This

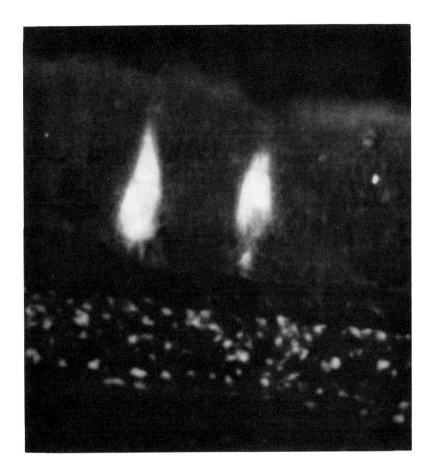

FIGURE 4. Formaldehyde-induced fluorescence in two serotonin-containing cells in the tracheal epithelium of an adult rabbit. The apexes of the cells taper toward the lumen, the wider bases are near the autofluorescent elastic lamina. Most of the fluorescent material is located above the nucleus toward the lumen. The cells measure 30 to 40 μm tall and 10 to 15 μm at the widest point. (Magnification $\times$ 715.) (Courtesy of Richard D. Dey, Ph.D., Dallas, Tex.).

distinction refers more to the chronology of release than to the biological importance of the respective compounds.

The released substances (especially histamine, SRS-A, $PGF_{2\alpha}$, endoperoxides, and thromboxanes A_2) cause constriction of airway smooth muscle, contractile elements in the lung, and pulmonary vessels (see Tables 2 to 5); attract eosinophils and polymorphs (ECF-A, neutrophil chemotaxins); and induce platelet aggregation (thromboxane A_2, platelet activating factors). Other substances are released, however, which tend to oppose the actions of these mediators or the process of mediator release itself. Such substances include:

1. PGE_2, released from unknown sites in the lung
2. VIP, released from the lung on immunologic challenge, and from mast cells, concomitantly with histamine, by compound 48/80 and by Ca^{2+} ionophore
3. Catecholamines, released through the action of histamine on the adrenal medulla

These three compounds induce relaxation of airway smooth muscle and promote cyclic AMP accumulation in the lung, thus opposing the IgE-mediated degranulation of mast cells. Another example of "negative feedback" in anaphylactic release is the inactivation of ECF-A through the action of the enzyme arylsulfatase, contained within the chemically attracted eosinophils.

B. Mechanical Stimulation

1. Stimulation of the External Surface of the Lung

The first indication that mechanical stimulation of the lung could provoke the release of active agents came with the discovery that gentle stroking or massaging of the external surface of isolated, perfused guinea pig lungs caused the appearance in the perfusate of substances with PG-like activity, "rabbit aorta contracting substance (RCS)", and histamine.[32]

The possible release of active substances from the lung with mechanical stimulation of the external surface of the lung in vivo, such as occurs in the course of thoracic surgery, has not been investigated.

The stirring of suspensions of chopped lung (from sensitized or unsensitized guinea pigs), as with a nylon rod for 5 to 6 min, was also found to release from the lung a mixture of smooth muscle-contracting substances.[33] This release could be demonstrated when stirring was repeated, although the concentration of released materials gradually decreased. A similar release of spasmogens was detected on mechanical agitation of chopped human lung.

2. Stimulation of the Alveolar Surface: Hyperinflation

The possibility that other, possibly more physiological forms of physical stimulation, e.g., hyperinflation, may also provoke the release of mediators was tested in the isolated lung of dogs and later in intact dogs.[34-36] In the former preparation the lungs were mechanically ventilated with 5% CO_2 in O_2, and perfused at constant flow with Krebs solution. The perfusate continually superfused strips of rat stomach and rat colon (chosen for the detection and assay of PGE and PGF compounds, see Table 1) which had been rendered insensitive to catecholamines, histamine, serotonin (5-hydroxytryptamine), and acetylcholine. During control ventilation (at predicted normal tidal volume), there was no evidence of spasmogenic activity in the perfusate. On increasing tidal volume by 50 to 100% while maintaining the same minute ventilation and perfusate pH, both smooth muscle strips contracted (see Figure 3). The contractions, signaling the appearance of spasmogens with PG-like activity, began within 2 min of the stepped-up ventilation and correlated with breath size. The concentrations of PGs in the perfusate were estimated by bioassay to be 150 ng/min (using PGE_1 as reference). Concomitantly with the apparent release of PGs, the perfusion pressure of the lung required to maintain the same flow decreased, reflecting pulmonary vasodilation. After infusion of aspirin (1 mg) into the pulmonary circulation, hyperinflation no longer resulted in contraction of the smooth muscle assay organs or decrease in pulmonary perfusion pressure. These findings suggested that stretching of the lung was capable of provoking increased pulmonary synthesis of vasodilator PG-like compounds (and possibly other substances with similar activity), and their subsequent release into the circulation. Similar results were obtained in isolated guinea pig and rat lungs.[37] More recent work by Gryglewski et al. has demonstrated the release of prostacyclin during hyperinflation.

3. Hyperventilation and Respiratory Alkalosis

If a similar release of vasodilator PGs could occur in the whole animal during hyperinflation, it could contribute to the systemic hypotension that frequently complicates mechanical ventilation at large tidal volumes. This possibility was investigated in anesthetized, paralyzed, and mechanically ventilated dogs.[36] Following a control pe-

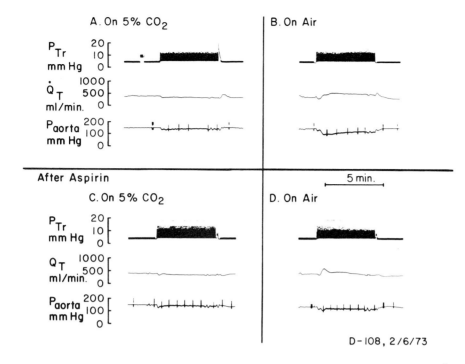

FIGURE 5. Upper panels: changes in mean aortic blood pressure (P aorta), cardiac output ($\dot{Q}_r$) and tracheal pressure (P_{Tr}) in anesthetized, paralyzed dog ventilated with 5% CO_2 in air (Panel A) or with room air (Panel B). Period of increased P_{Tr} (5 min) marks hyperventilation, achieved by increasing tidal volume fivefold. After administration of aspirin (30 mg/kg, i.v.), fall in blood pressure, previously seen during hyperventilation on air, was markedly attenuated.

riod of normal ventilation, tidal volume was increased fivefold and maintained at that level for 5 min, then returned to the normal level. The increased ventilation was carried out either with air alone or with 5% CO_2 added to air (see Figure 5). Hyperventilation with air was characterized by severe hypocapnia (arterial blood P_{CO_2} fell from 41 to 15 mmHg) and respiratory alkalosis (pH increased from 7.32 to 7.52). In these experiments, mean arterial blood pressure decreased by 32 (± 18)%. Increased ventilation with 5% CO_2 added to the inspired air, however, did not cause a change in arterial P_{CO_2} or pH. Under those circumstances, the fall in blood pressure in the same animals was 13(± 12)% of control value (significantly less than in the first group, $p < 0.001$). If both animal groups were pretreated with aspirin (30 mg/kg in saline, infused i.v.), the fall in blood pressure was reduced to 18 (± 10)% in the presence of respiratory alkalosis and to 8 (± 5)% without respiratory alkalosis. These experiments provided evidence that:

1. The systemic hypotension complicating mechanical hyperventilation is greater in the presence of respiratory alkalosis than if arterial blood pH remained normal.
2. This hypotension is mediated to a large extent by the release of vasodilator agents.
3. The responsible mediators probably include PGs (possibly PGEs) or compounds with PG-like activity, including prostacyclin.

C. Pulmonary Thromboembolism

For years it has been considered likely that pulmonary embolism leads to the release of humoral mediators from the lung. This impression has been gained largely from circumstantial indirect evidence, including the following:

1. Vascular obstruction alone, or with superimposed vagal reflexes, often fails to explain all the pulmonary (e.g., wheezing, pulmonary hypertension) and systemic (e.g., hypotension) manifestations of pulmonary embolism.
2. Certain humoral agents, such as histamine and serotonin, can mimic some of the pathophysiologic changes occurring in this condition[38] (see Table 2).
3. Pharmacologic agents that inhibit the actions of histamine and serotonin or deplete their stores can attenuate the vascular and pulmonary effects of experimental pulmonary embolism.[39]
4. In cross-circulation experiments, at least some of the cardiorespiratory effects of pulmonary embolism in one dog may be transmitted to another.[40]

The serotonin released in pulmonary embolism is probably derived largely from platelets which tend to accumulate within the pulmonary circulation, may aggregate and release their contents, and may form microemboli. An additional source of serotonin is lung tissue itself which, in certain species, e.g., rat, rabbit, and mouse, contains relatively high concentrations of this biogenic amine.[41] Neuroepithelial bodies, as mentioned earlier, contain serotonin-rich granules that can be discharged by appropriate stimuli.

In recent years, the superfusion technique for bioassay has made it possible to obtain more direct evidence for the release of biologically active substances after embolization of pulmonary vessels. On embolization of isolated lungs of guinea pigs and rats with fat emulsions, microspheres, and colloidal substances, ranging in size from 1 to 120 μm in diameter, there was evidence for the release of PGE_2, even when the lungs were perfused with platelet-free solutions.[42] In the same experimental preparation, there was release also of RCS and, in some instances, histamine. The magnitude of the release of these humoral agents with pulmonary embolism is generally less intense than with IgE-mediated release.

Additional, though indirect, evidence that PGs or related compounds mediate some of the effects of pulmonary embolism is derived from the use of inhibitors of PG synthesis. Pretreatment of anesthetized dogs with aspirin was found to prevent the rise in pulmonary vascular and airway pressures that otherwise follows thrombin- or protamine-induced platelet aggregation in pulmonary vessels, without preventing the platelets from aggregating.[43] Similarly, aspirin abolished the pulmonary hypertension caused by endotoxin-induced microembolization and the increase in airway pressure following barium sulfate microembolism.[44]

D. Pulmonary Microembolism: Intravascular Platelet Aggregation[45-47]

An important condition, related to pulmonary embolism, is now recognized, where platelets aggregate and become trapped in the pulmonary vascular bed, causing pulmonary microembolism.

Platelet reactions include first, adhesion (adherence) to particles or surfaces, followed by a release reaction, in which their contents are liberated, leading to aggregation (platelets binding to platelets) and usually further release of mediators.[29] It is this chain of reactions that is at the basis of pulmonary microembolism, which is thought to be an important factor in the pathogenesis of the respiratory distress syndrome.

A variety of stimuli may provoke the release reaction and aggregation of platelets. These stimuli include thrombin, collagen, thromboxanes, PG endoperoxides, ADP, platelet-activating factors (PAF) from basophils or mast cells, antibody, and complement.[29]

Platelet aggregation (and pulmonary microembolism) leads to intense constriction of all smooth-muscle structures in the lung: tracheobronchial tree, alveolar ducts, and pulmonary vessels. These effects are attributable in large measure to the release of the many potent vasoactive compounds normally confined within the platelets (see above).

E. Pulmonary Edema

Pulmonary edema is a serious, life-threatening condition that occurs as a reaction to a variety of drugs, toxins, and irritants and as a complication of cardiac failure or other disease states. Several pharmacologically active agents (e.g., histamine, brady-kinin, and epinephrine) are capable of causing pulmonary edema, but the release of mediators from the lung during pulmonary edema and its pathophysiologic importance has been inadequately examined.

Following the induction of edema in isolated, perfused cat lungs, perfusates and foam exhibited biological activity consistent with the presence of PGE_2 and $PGF_{2\alpha}$ and other unidentified spasmogens. When airway fluid and foam were extracted for PGs, thin layer chromatography of these extracts and bioassay of eluted portions corresponding to PGE_2 and $PGF_{2\alpha}$ confirmed the presence of these compounds in foam.[48] Radioimmunoassay of $PGF_{2\alpha}$ metabolite showed it to be present in elevated concentrations in arterial blood of dogs after induction of pulmonary edema with alloxan.[49] More recently, elevated levels of thromboxane B_2, the stable metabolite of thromboxane A_2, were measured in pulmonary lymph and in foam, during alloxan-induced pulmonary edema.[492] Immunoreactive VIP also has been measured in foam and in perfusates from edematous cat and rat lungs.

F. Hypoxic Pulmonary Hypertension

It is well known that alveolar hypoxia produces pulmonary vasoconstriction and hypertension, but the mechanism of this response remains poorly understood. Several lines of evidence suggest mediation by metabolic events, probably including the release of vasoactive substances. Efforts to identify these mediators have not been totally successful, but prostaglandin-like or prostaglandin-related compounds, as well as the spasmogenic lung peptide, may be involved.[50-52]

G. Conditions Associated with Respiratory Distress

A syndrome of respiratory distress, progressive hypoxia, decreasing lung compliance, and spreading infiltrations on chest X-ray, may afflict individuals with previously normal lungs, as a complication of numerous acute medical and surgical conditions.[53] The lungs in this adult respiratory distress syndrome (ARDS), show large-scale atelectasis, edema, and hemorrhage, much like the lungs of the neonatal respiratory distress syndrome ("hyaline membrane disease").

The conditions predisposing to the adult syndrome are multiple and seemingly unrelated. One common thread between them is the likely participation of humoral mediators in the pathogenesis of the pulmonary complications. Some of the therapeutic measures often used, especially oxygen administration or mechanical ventilation, may aggravate lung injury and the release of biologically active substances. Two conditions relevant to this syndrome, pulmonary microembolism and pulmonary edema, have been discussed earlier. A few others follow.

1. Endotoxin (Septic) Shock

Shock from any cause, but especially septic shock, frequently precedes the onset of the respiratory distress.

Some understanding of the pathogenicity of endotoxin to the lung and other organs has been gained from investigations in animals. Thus, i.v. administration of endotoxin induces systemic hypotension in all species, often accompanied by pulmonary hypertension. One mechanism of these responses is the release of prostaglandin-like compounds, since both reactions can be reduced or abolished by pretreating the animals with prostaglandin synthetase-inhibitors, such as aspirin or indomethacin.[54-55] This conclusion has recently been confirmed by bioassay.[56]

If the lungs are examined after one i.v. injection of endotoxin, fibrin thrombi are found in small pulmonary vessels (also in liver and spleen sinusoids). If a second sublethal dose of endotoxin is given i.v. (24 hr later), new fibrin thrombi are found in the lungs, but now also in the glomeruli of the kidney, leading to bilateral renal cortical necrosis. This pathologic picture is known as the generalized Schwartzmann reaction.[57-58] It is now believed that this process of intravascular coagulation is mediated by the granular leukocytes, since the reaction can be prevented by depletion of these cells with nitrogen mustard[59] and leucocyte granules can substitute for the first (preparing) injection of endotoxin.[60] The leukocytes apparently acquire enough procoagulant (thromboplastic) activity in the presence of endotoxin to trigger intravascular clotting, via the extrinsic pathway.[61]

2. Disseminated Intravascular Coagulation

This clinical syndrome is the result of pathologic activation of blood coagulation and fibrinolysis. When fully expressed, it is manifested by bleeding (due to depletion of coagulation factors and platelets), organ ischemia (due to deposition of fibrin in small vessels), and hemolytic anemia (due to fibrin-induced red cell destruction).[61-63] Intravascular coagulation may either precede or follow the development of the respiratory distress syndrome. In cases where the coagulopathy occurs first, the lung pathology may be partly related to the small-vessel occlusion and leukocytic enzymes. Conversely, lung injury may itself "trigger" intravascular coagulation as lung tissue, like brain tissue, granulocytes, and amniotic fluid, is rich in thromboplastin.

3. Acute Pancreatitis[64-67]

Recent reports have described the occurrence of respiratory complications, especially of respiratory distress syndrome, in the course of severe acute pancreatitis. At least some of these patients present a picture of pulmonary edema with normal pulmonary wedge pressures, excluding the possibility of circulatory overload. Speculations on the mechanism of pulmonary capillary injury in such patients include release of proteolytic enzymes from the pancreas or of phospholipase A which can inactivate alveolar surfactant (and can generate arachidonic acid, a precursor of prostaglandins); elevated levels of triglycerides; and systemic hypotension.

4. Trauma, Burns[68-71]

Extensive skin burns and other forms of trauma, unrelated to direct thoracic injury, may be followed by diffuse pulmonary lesions and respiratory distress. In these cases, too, humoral mediators may be released from injured tissue and induce pulmonary lesions, but these putative mediators remain to be identified.

H. Mediator Release by Other Mediators[31,72]

There are several reports of one vasoactive substance provoking the release of another, during passage through the pulmonary circulation. For example, serotonin infused in relatively large concentrations (0.05 to 1µg/mℓ) into the pulmonary artery of isolated lung from rats or dogs, stimulated the release from the lung of substances with the biological activity of prostaglandins and of the "slow-reacting substance" (i.e., contraction of guinea pig ileum in the presence of mepyramine and atropine) and other active substances. Infusions of tryptamine (0.5 to 2 µg/mℓ) had a similar releasing effect. This tyramine-induced release could be antagonized by methysergide, but was not dose related once a threshold had been reached. Tyramine and β-phenylethylamine, decarboxylation products of the amino acids 1-tyrosine and 1-phenylalanine, respectively, given in higher concentrations (10 to 100 µg/mℓ), also released PG-like substances and a slow-reacting substance from isolated cat and dog lungs. Acetylcholine (0.5 to 1 μg/mℓ) also has ben reported to induce the release of PG-like materials and a slow-reacting substance. Bradykinin releases prostaglandins and, in large doses (10 μg), RCS. Other examples of release of biologically active substances by other active agents are RCS and PGs by histamine, dihomo-γ linolenic and arachidonic acids, SRS-A, arachidonic acid, and by RCS.RF. Norepinephrine and angiotensin I and II have been shown to release PGs from the kidney. Whether such release may also occur in the lung is at present unknown. On the other hand, catecholamines may inhibit the release of PGs and their metabolites from the lung.

I. Chemical and Toxic Influences[49]

A larger number of chemicals and industrial toxins, including irritant gases and fumes (such as chlorine, ammonia, and nitrogen dioxide), oxidants (e.g., ozone), and oxygen itself, especially at high partial pressures, can induce acute lung injury in the form of tracheobronchitis, bronchitis, or edema.

Chemical and toxic factors may provoke the synthesis and release of mediators (e.g., prostaglandins and related lipids), may activate others (e.g., the kallikrein-kinin and complement systems), and may also interfere with the normal pulmonary inactivation of biologically active compounds. The latter action is exemplified by the depression of serotonin clearance and of prostaglandin metabolism by the lung following prolonged exposure to high partial pressures of oxygen. Moderate impairment of serotonin clearance occurred in rats exposed to 100% O_2 for at least 18 hr, and further impairment occurred with more prolonged exposure.[73] Similarly, metabolism of $PGF_{2\alpha}$ was markedly inhibited in lungs of guinea pigs that had breathed 100% O_2 for 48 hr.[74] These metabolic effects of hyperoxia appear to precede gross evidence of lung injury and may thus prove to be sensitive indicators of pulmonary oxygen toxicity.

J. Bronchogenic Tumors and Other Pulmonary Lesions[75,76]

Hypersecretion of hormones by pulmonary tumors may result in a variety of endocrine syndromes. These hormones are usually polypeptides or biogenic amines, but may include enzymes and prostaglandin-related compounds. The tumors are most often of the oat cell variety, but other cell types are more often associated with certain hormonal secretions. Table 8 gives a listing of the more common endocrine syndromes, together with the associated secretions and anatomic lesions.

IX. ADDENDUM

Since the preparation of this manuscript, important advances have been made in the field of mediators, including the chemical characterization of the leukotrienes and of "platelet activating factor," and the identification of additional peptides in lung tissue. For a summary of these advances, refer to *Ann. Rev. Physiol.*, 44, 1982; *Circ. Res.*, 1981; and *Ann. N. Y. Acad. Sci.* Symposium on Mechanism of Lung Injury, 1981.

Table 8

HORMONAL SECRETION BY PULMONARY TUMORS: PARANEOPLASTIC SYNDROMES[a]

Secretion	Syndrome	Lesion
ACTH	Hypokalemic alkalosis, edema, Cushing's syndrome	Oat cell carcinoma, adenoma
ADH (arginine vasopressin)	Hyponatremia (SIADH)	Oat cell carcinoma, adenoma; also, tuberculosis, pneumonia, aspergillosis
PTH or releated peptide	Hypercalcemia	Squamous cell carcinoma, adeno-carcinoma and large-cell undif-ferentiated carcinoma
Gonadotropins	Gynecomastia (adults), precocious puberty (children)	Large-cell anaplastic carcinoma
Calcitonin	No clinical findings	Adenocarcinoma, squamous and oat cell carcinoma
VIP or related peptide	Watery diarrhea or no symptoms	Squamous, oat or large-cell carci-noma
Growth hormone(?)	Hypertrophic osteoarthropathy	Squamous cell carcinoma
Serotonin, kinins (and PGs)	"Carcinoid"	Bronchial adenoma, oat cell carci-noma
Insulin-like peptide	Hypoglycemia	Mesenchymal cell tumors
Glucagon or related peptide	Diabetes	Fibrosarcoma
Prolactin	Galactorrhea (or no symptoms)	Anaplastic cell carcinoma
Combination of above	Multiple syndromes	Anaplastic cell carcinoma
Prostaglandins	Hypercalcemia	—
Enzymes (e.g., amylase, renin)	Hypertension	—

[a]   Abbreviations: ACTH, adrenocorticotropic hormone; SIADH, syndrome of inappropriate secretion of antidiuretic hormone; PTH, parathyroid hormone; PGs, prostaglandins; VIP, vasoactive intestinal poly-peptide.

REFERENCES

1. **Austen, K. F.,** Reaction mechanisms in the release of mediators of immediate hypersensitivity from human lung tissue, *Fed. Proc. Fed. Am. Soc. Exp. Biol.,* 33, 2256, 1974.
2. **Said, S. I.,** The lung as a metabolic organ, *N. Engl. J. Med.,* 279, 1330, 1968.
3. **Vane, J. R.,** The release and fate of vasoactive hormones in the circulation, *Br. J. Pharmacol.,* 35, 209, 1969.
4. **Said, S. I.,** The lung in relation to vasoactive hormones, *Fed. Proc. Fed. Am. Soc. Exp. Biol.,* 32, 1972, 1973.
5. **Gaddum, J. H.,** Technique of superfusion, *Br. J. Pharmacol. Chemother.,* 8, 321, 1953.
6. **Vane, J. R.,** The use of isolated organs for detecting active substances in the circulating blood, *Br. J. Pharmacol. Chemother.,* 23, 360, 1964.
7. **Vane, J. R.,** The release and assay of hormones in the circulation, in *The Scientific Basis of Medicine Annual Reviews,* Athlone Press, London, 1968, 366.
8. **Vane, J. R.,** Inhibition of prostaglandin synthesis as a mechanism of action for aspirin-like drugs, *Nature (London) New Biol.,* 231, 232, 1971.
9. **Robinson, H. J. and Vane, J. R.,** *Prostaglandin Synthetase Inhibitors — Their Effects on Physiolog-ical Functions and Pathological States,* Raven Press, New York, 1974.
10. **Samuelsson, B., Goldyne, M., Granström, E., Hamberg, M., Hammarström, S., and Malmsten, C.,** Prostaglandins and thromboxanes, *Annu. Rev. Biochem.,* 47, 997, 1978.
11. **Lewis, R. A. and Austen, K. F.,** Nonrespiratory functions of pulmonary cells: the mast cell, *Fed. Proc. Fed. Am. Soc. Exp. Biol.,* 36, 2676, 1977.

12. Lauweryns, J. M. and Cokelaere, M., Intrapulmonary neuro-epithelial bodies: hypoxia-sensitive neuro (chemo-) receptors, *Experientia,* 29, 1384, 1973.

13. Said, S. I., Humoral mediators in bronchial asthma: implications for therapy, in *New Directions in Asthma,* Stein, M., Ed., American College of Chest Physicians, Park Ridge, Ill., 1975, 261.

14. Erdös, E. G., The kinins — a status report, *Biochem. Pharmacol.,* 25, 1563, 1976.

15. Said, S. I., VIP: overview, in *Gut Hormones,* Bloom, S. R., Ed., Churchill Livingstone, New York, 1978, chap. 73.

16. Said, S. I. and Mutt, V., Relationship of spasmogenic and smooth muscle relaxant peptides from normal lung to other vasoactive compounds, *Nature (London),* 265, 84, 1977.

17. Cutz, E., Chan, W., Track, N. S., Goth, A., and Said, S. I., Release of vasoactive intestinal polypeptide in mast cells by histamine liberators, *Nature (London),* 275, 661, 1978.

18. Uddman, R., Alumets, J., Densert, O., Häkanson, R., and Sundler, F., Occurrence and distribution of VIP nerves in the nasal mucosa and tracheobronchial wall, *Acta Oto-Laryngol.,* 86, 443, 1978.

19. Sundler, F., Alumets, J., Brodin, E., Dahlberg, K., and Nilsson, G. Perivascular substance P-immunoreactive nerves in tracheobronchial tissue, in *Substance P,* von Euler, U. S. and Pernow, B., Eds., Raven Press, New York, 1977, 271.

20. Warton, J., Polak, J. M., and Bloom, S. R., Bombesin-like immunoreactivity in the lung, *Nature (London),* 273, 769, 1978.

21. Müller-Eberhard, H. J., Chemistry and function of the complement system, *Hosp. Pract.,* 12, 33, 1977.

22. Cohen S., Cell mediated immunity and the inflammatory system, *Hum. Pathol.,* 7, 249, 1976.

23. Hitchcock, M., Piscitelli, D. M., and Bouhuys, A., Histamine release from human lung by a component of cotton bracts, *Arch. Environ. Health,* 26, 177, 1973.

24. Mittman, C., Ed., *Pulmonary Emphysema and Proteolysis,* Academic Press, New York, 1972.

25. McCord, J. M. and Fridovich, I., Superoxide dismutase, *J. Biol. Chem.,* 244, 6049, 1969.

26. Said, S. I., Metabolic events in the lung, in *Pathophysiology: Altered Regulatory Mechanisms in Disease,* 2nd ed., Lippincott, Philadelphia, 1976, 189.

27. Heidelberger, C., Chemical carcinogenesis, *Annu. Rev. Biochem.,* 44, 79, 1975.

27a. Gryglewski, R. J., Korbut, R., and Ocetkiewicz, A., Generation of prostacyclin by lungs in vivo and its release into the arterial circulation, *Nature (London),* 273, 765, 1978.

28. Bach, M. K., Brashler, J. R., and Gorman, R. R., On the structure of slow-reacting substance of anaphylaxis: evidence of biosynthesis from arachidonic acid, *Prostaglandins,* 14, 21, 1977.

28a. Dawson, W., SRS-A and the leukotrienes, *Nature (London),* 285, 68, 1980.

29. Henson, P. M., Mechanisms of mediator release from inflammatory cells, in *Mediators of Inflammation,* Weissman, G., Ed., Plenum Press, New York, 1974, 9.

30. Piper, P. J. and Vane, J. R., Release of additional factors in anaphylaxis and its antagonism by anti-inflammatory drugs, *Nature (London),* 223, 29, 1969.

31. Piper, P. J., Release of biologically active materials from the lung: release induced by anaphylaxis, in *Metabolic Functions of the Lung,* Vol. 4, Bakhle, Y. S. and Vane, J. R., Eds., Marcel Dekker, New York, 1977, chap. 9.

32. Piper, P. J. and Vane, J. R., The release of prostaglandins from the lung and other tissues, *Ann. N. Y. Acad. Sci.,* 180, 363, 1971.

33. Piper, P. J. and Walker, J. L., The release of spasmogenic substances from human chopped lung tissue and its inhibition, *Br. J. Pharmacol.,* 47, 291, 1973.

34. Said, S. I., Kitamura, S., and Vreim, C., Prostaglandins: release from the lung during mechanical ventilation at large tidal volumes, *J. Clin. Invest.,* 51, 1972.

35. Said, S. I., Kitamura, S., Yoshida, T., Preskitt, J., and Holden, L. D., Humoral control of airways, *Ann. N.Y. Acad. Sci.,* 221, 103, 1974.

36. Kitamura, S., Preskitt, J., Yoshida, T., and Said, S. I., Prostaglandin release, respiratory alkalosis, and systemic hypotension during mechanical ventilation, *Fed. Proc. Fed. Am. Soc. Exp. Biol.,* 32, 341, 1973.

37. Palmer, M. A., Piper, P. J., and Vane, J. R., Release of rabbit aorta contracting substance (RCS) and prostaglandins induced by chemical or mechanical stimulation of guinea pig lungs, *Br. J. Pharmacol.,* 49, 226, 1973.

38. Comroe, Jr., J. H., Van Lingen, B., Stroud, R. C., and Roncoroni, A., Reflex and direct cardiopulmonary effects of 5-OH-tryptamine (serotonin). Their possible role in pulmonary embolism and coronary thrombosis, *Am. J. Physiol.,* 173, 379, 1953.

39. Gurewich, V., Cohen, M. D., and Thomas, D. P., Humoral factors in massive pulmonary embolism: an experimental study, *Am. Heart J.,* 76, 784, 1968.

40. Halmagyi, D. F. J., Starzecki, B., and Horner, G. J., Humoral transmission of cardiorespiratory changes in experimental lung embolism, *Circ. Res.,* 14, 546, 1964.

41. Weisbach, H., Waalkes, T. P., and Udenfriend, S., Presence of serotonin in lung and its implication in the anaphylactic reaction, *Science,* 125, 235, 1957.

42. Lindsey, H. E. and Wyllie, J. H., Release of prostaglandins from embolized lungs, *Br. J. Surg.,* 57, 738, 1970.
43. Rådegran, K., The effect of acetylsalicylic acid on the peripheral and pulmonary vascular responses to thrombin, *Acta Anaesthesiol. Scand.,* 16, 140, 1972.
44. Nakano, J. and McCloy, R. B., Jr., Effects of indomethacin on the pulmonary vascular and airway resistance responses to pulmonary microembolization, *Proc. Soc. Exp. Biol. Med.,* 143, 218, 1973.
45. Saldeen, T., The microembolism syndrome, *Forensic Sci.,* 1, 179, 1972.
46. Vaage, J., Bo, G., and Hognestad, J., Pulmonary responses to intravascular platelet aggregation in the cat, *Acta Physiol. Scand.,* 92, 546, 1974.
47. Vaage, J. and Piper, P. J., The release of prostaglandin-like substances during platelet aggregation and pulmonary microembolism, *Acta Physiol. Scand.,* 94, 8, 1975.
48. Said, S. I. and Yoshida, T., Release of prostaglandins and other humoral mediators during hypoxic breathing and pulmonary edema, *Chest,* 66, 12S, 1974.
49. Said, S. I., Environmental injury of the lung: role of humoral mediators, *Fed. Proc. Fed. Am. Soc. Exp. Biol.,* 37, 2504, 1978.
49a. Matsuzaki, Y., Oyamada, M., Hara, N., Tai, H.-H., and Said, S. I., Increased thromboxane generation by the lung during alloxan-induced pulmonary edema, *Clin. Res.,* 28, 530a, 1980.
50. Said, S. I., Yoshida, T., Kitamura, S., and Vreim, C., Pulmonary alveolar hypoxia: release of prostaglandins and other humoral mediators, *Science,* 185, 1181, 1974.
51. Said, S. I. and Hara, N., Prostaglandins and the pulmonary vasoconstrictor response to alveolar hypoxia, *Science,* 189, 899, 1975.
52. Said, S. I., Release of biological active materials from the lung: release induced by physical and chemical stimuli, in *Metabolic Functions of the Lung,* Vol. 4, Bakhle, Y. S. and Vane, J. R., Eds., Marcel Dekker, New York, 1977, chap. 10.
53. Hopewell, P. C. and Murray, J. F., The adult respiratory distress syndrome, *Annu. Rev. Med.,* 27, 343, 1976.
54. Erdös, E. G., Hinshaw, L. B., and Gill, C. C., Effect of indomethacin in endotoxin shock in the dog, *Proc. Soc. Exp. Biol. Med.,* 125, 916, 1967.
55. Greenway, C. V. and Murthy, V. S., Mesenteric vasoconstriction after endotoxin administration in cats pretreated with aspirin, *Br. J. Pharmacol.,* 43, 259, 1971.
56. Herman, A. G. and Vane, J. R., Release of renal prostaglandins during endotoxin-induced hypotension, *Eur. J. Pharmacol.,* 39, 79, 1976.
57. Hjort, P. F. and Rapaport, S. I., The Shwartzman reaction: pathogenetic mechanisms and clinical manifestations, *Annu. Rev. Med.,* 16, 135, 1965.
58. McKay, D. G., Experimental aspects of the Shwartzman phenomenon, in *Coagulation Disorders in Obstetrics,* Proc. Dijkzigt Conf., Excerpta Medica Foundation, Amsterdam, 1966.
59. Thomas, L. and Good, R. A., Studies on the generalized Shwartzman reaction. I. General observations concerning the phenomenon, *J. Exp. Med.,* 96, 605, 1952.
60. Horn, R. G. and Collins, R. D., Studies on the pathogenesis of the generalized Shwartzman reaction. The role of granulocytes, *Lab. Invest.,* 18, 101, 1968.
61. Niemetz, J. and Fani, K., Role of leukocytes in blood coagulation and the generalized Shwartzman Reaction, *Nature (London) New Biol.,* 232, 247, 1971.
62. Goodnight, S. H., Jr., Disseminated intravascular coagulation: proteases and pathology, in *Proteases and Biological Control,* Reich, E., Rifkin, D. B., and Shaw, E., Eds., Cold Spring Harbor Laboratory, Cold Spring Harbor, N.Y., 1975, 191.
63. Colman, R. W., Robboy, S. J., and Minna, J. D., Disseminated intravascular coagulation (DIC): an approach, *Am. J. Med.,* 52, 679, 1972.
64. Intenario, B., Staurd, I. D., and Hyde, R. W., Acute respiratory distress syndrome in pancreatitis, *Ann. Intern. Med.,* 77, 923, 1972.
65. Kellum, J. M., DeMeester, T. R., Elkins, R. C., and Zuidema, G. D., Respiratory insufficiency secondary to acute pancreatitis, *Ann. Surg.,* 175, 657, 1972.
66. Warshaw, A. L., Lesser, P. B., Rie, M., and Cullen, D. J., The pathogenesis of pulmonary edema in acute pancreatitis, *Ann. Surg.,* 182, 505, 1975.
67. Rovner, A. J. and Westcott, J. L., Pulmonary edema and respiratory insufficiency in acute pancreatitis, *Radiology,* 118, 513, 1976.
68. Moore, F. D., Lyons, J. H., and Pierce, E. C., Jr., *Post-traumatic Pulmonary Insufficiency,* W. B. Saunders, Philadelphia, 1969.
69. Nash, G., Foley, F. D., and Langlinais, P., Pulmonary interstitial edema and hyaline membranes in adult burn patients. Electron microscopic observations, *Hum. Pathol.,* 5, 149, 1974.
70. Teplitz, C., The ultrastructural basis for pulmonary pathophysiology following trauma, *J. Trauma,* 8, 700, 1968.
71. Pietra, G. G., The lung in shock, *Hum. Pathol.,* 5, 121, 1974.

72. Bakhle, Y. S. and Vane, J. R., Pharmacokinetic function of the pulmonary circulation, *Physiol. Rev.*, 54, 1007, 1974.

73. Block, E. R. and Fisher, A. B., Depression of serotonin clearance by rat lungs during oxygen exposure, *J. Appl. Physiol.*, 42, 33, 1977.

74. Parkes, D. G. and Eling, T. E., The influence of environmental agents on prostaglandin biosynthesis and metabolism in the lung, *Biochem. J.*, 146, 549, 1975.

75. Hall, T. C.,Ed., Paraneoplastic syndromes, *Ann. N.Y. Acad. Sci.*, 230, 1, 1974.

76. Odell, W., Wolfsen, A., Yoshimoto, Y., Weitzman, R., Fisher, D., and Hirose, F., Ectopic peptide synthesis: a universal concomitant of neoplasia, *Trans. Assoc. Am. Physicians*, 90, 204, 1977.

Chapter 4

METABOLIC ACTIVATION OF PULMONARY TOXINS

Michael R. Boyd

TABLE OF CONTENTS

I. INTRODUCTION

A. Metabolic Activation and Chemical Toxicity

The in vivo biotransformation of relatively inert chemicals to highly reactive metabolites underlies the toxicities of many types of chemicals, including industrial products, naturally occurring toxicants, and drugs. Highly reactive, toxic metabolites may interact with cells in numerous potentially detrimental ways, such as by binding covalently with essential cellular constituents and/or by stimulating the peroxidative decomposition of cellular lipids.[1-17]

Because of its major role in xenobiotic metabolism and its relative ease for study, the liver has received much attention as a target organ for cytotoxins and carcinogens requiring metabolic activation. However, extrahepatic tissues frequently are equally or more prominent than the liver as target organs for toxic chemicals. Therefore, increasing attention is being directed toward these tissues as sites for the metabolic activation of potentially toxic foreign compounds.

B. The Lung as a Potential Target Organ for Toxicities by Chemicals Requiring Metabolic Activation

The lung is a prominent target organ for numerous chemical-induced pathological changes.[18] Moreover, the lungs, like the liver, contain active enzyme systems capable of metabolizing drugs and other chemicals.[19-26] The lungs also are situated in a primary site for exposure to xenobiotics or their blood-borne metabolites. They are exposed to such substances both externally by the inspired air and internally by the circulation. The lungs also contain active uptake and concentrating systems for some endogenous substances as well as for certain exogenously administered chemicals.[22-26] For these reasons, it is not surprising that the metabolic activation of chemical toxins has important potential roles in the pathogenesis of xenobiotic-induced pulmonary injury.

C. Mechanisms of Chemical-Induced Lung Injury Involving Metabolic Activation

Three potential mechanisms of lung toxicity in which metabolic activation plays a crucial role have been described (see Figure 1).[13] Mechanism I depicts a reaction in which an "inert" parent compound is metabolized to a highly reactive ultimate toxin *in situ* in the lung. In Mechanism II, the ultimate toxin also is a highly reactive metabolite of the parent compound, but it is formed primarily in the liver and is transported to the lung by the circulation. In Mechanism III, the parent compound undergoes a cyclic reduction/oxidation leading to the "activation" of molecular oxygen and the consumption of cellular-reducing equivalents (e.g., NADPH). Thus, in the latter mechanism, the parent compound participates only indirectly in the toxic reaction. Presumably, the activated oxygen species (such as $^-O_2$ and derivatives thereof) could act as the ultimate toxin(s). In addition, or alternatively, the deficits in cellular energy metabolism, and/or diminished defense mechanisms resulting from depletion of essential cofactors, could lead to pulmonary damage. The relatively high oxygen tensions in pulmonary tissue conceivably could contribute to the preferential damage of the lungs by agents acting through Mechanism III.

It should be emphasized that Mechanisms I, II, and III are highly simplified representations of early metabolic events involved in undoubtedly complex sequences leading to lung damage by chemical toxins. Other critical determinants of cell and tissue susceptibility to metabolically activated toxins include the availability of metabolic detoxication pathways and other cellular defense mechanisms, as well as the capacities for target cells and tissues to repair themselves after chemical-induced insults. The further elucidation of all of these critical determinants of susceptibility should be a major goal for future studies.

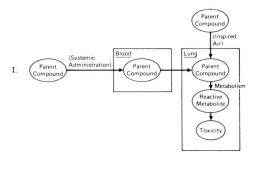

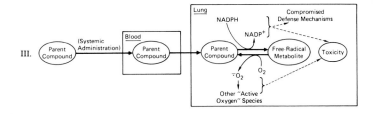

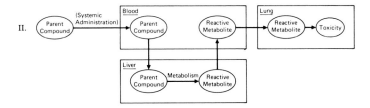

FIGURE 1.   Schematic representations of mechanisms of chemical-induced lung injury involving metabolic activation.

The experimental data from which Mechanisms I, II, and III are derived were obtained largely from studies on model pulmonary toxins which generally are chemically homogeneous, stable, simple in structure, and which cause pulmonary toxicity highly reproducibly in laboratory animals. An extensive review of these metabolically activated lung toxins, as well as a discussion of the experimental approaches and methodologies involved in the study of pulmonary toxicities occurring by the various mechanisms, already has been presented.[13] Therefore, the present review will emphasize only one each of the best available examples of toxicities occurring by the mechanisms shown in Figure 1. Studies with 4-ipomeanol, monocrotaline, and paraquat are shown to illustrate Mechanisms I, II, and III, respectively.

II. EXAMPLE OF PULMONARY TOXICITY BY MECHANISM I; STUDIES WITH 4-IPOMEANOL

A. Background; Nature of Toxicity
4-Ipomeanol [1- (3-furyl) -4-hydroxypentanone]

is a naturally occurring, toxic furan derivative. The compound was isolated and identified originally from moldy sweet potatoes. 4-Ipomeanol appears to be responsible for the potentially lethal pulmonary injury which has occurred in cattle consuming moldy sweet potatoes. The compound also has been detected in human food products, although the public health significance of this observation is not known.

A characteristic lesion produced by 4-ipomeanol after ingestion or injection in several laboratory animal species (e.g., rat, mouse, and hamster) is necrosis of the nonciliated pulmonary bronchiolar (Clara) cells.[36] The initial damage to this cell population appears to be highly selective. In the early stages, no other toxic manifestations are apparent. Even the adjacent ciliated bronchiolar cells remain intact. Relatively late-occurring manifestations of lung toxicity after comparatively large doses of 4-ipomeanol sometimes may include pulmonary edema, pleural effusions, vascular congestion and hemorrhage, and scattered necrosis of other lung cell types. It is possible that some or all of the latter changes occur as the result of the initial damage to Clara cells, but this possibility needs further investigation.

4-Ipomeanol has proved to be an immensely valuable tool in experimental lung toxicology. In particular, studies with this model pulmonary toxin have provided the first definitive evidence to validate a mechanism of pulmonary toxicity primarily involving the *in situ* generation of an active metabolite.[10,13-17,36-44] Moreover, these studies also have shown the importance of a specific lung cell population, the Clara cells, in mediating the activation of 4-ipomeanol and have led directly to the view that the Clara cells are an important site of cytochrome P-450 monooxygenase activity in the lung.[36] This finding has major implications for pulmonary toxicology and carcinogenesis.[13,16,17,36]

B. Distribution and Excretion

The distribution and excretion of toxic doses of radiolabeled 4-ipomeanol were studied after i.p. administration in rats.[39] After 96 hr, approximately half the administered ^{14}C-labeled material appeared in the urine, and radioactivity in the feces amounted to 15 to 20% of the administered dose. Excretion of radioactive material into the expired air totaled less than 5% of the administered dose. The concentrations of radioactive compound(s) in most tissues reached maximal levels within the first hour. However, the highest level of radioactivity in the GI tract (including contents) occurred 2 to 8 hr after administration of the radiolabeled 4-ipomeanol, possibly reflecting the accumulation of metabolites in the feces. Carcass and gut contained the greatest total percentage of radioactivity. Liver contained a maximum of about 10% of the total administered radioactivity, whereas the amounts in lungs, kidneys, and blood reached maxima of about 1 to 4%. All other tissues contained less than 1% of the administered dose. A maximum of 1 to 2% of the administered 4-ipomeanol was recovered from peritoneal fluid after 0.5 hr, and only traces of radioactivity were found at later times, indicating that the compound was absorbed rapidly from the site of injection.

C. Covalent Binding to Tissues In Vivo

Much of the residual radioactivity in rats 24 hr after administration of radiolabeled 4-ipomeanol was tightly bound to lung macromolecules.[38,39] Extensive organic solvent extraction of homogenates of the lungs failed to remove the residual activity. Repeated solubilization and reprecipitation of the labeled homogenates did not release the bound material. Sephadex® chromatography of samples of the solubilized residues indicated that the radioactivity eluted primarily with the protein fractions. Thin-layer chromatography of the solubilized protein fractions revealed that no radioactivity moved from the origin of silica gel plates, even when such plates were eluted with polar solvents such as methanol and acetone. By all these criteria, therefore, the residual radioactivity appeared to be bound covalently to the protein fractions.

The time courses of colvalent binding, pulmonary edemagenesis, and lethality were studied in rats after administration of ^{14}C-4-ipomeanol.[38] When toxic doses were given i.p., the maximal levels of covalently bound compound were attained by 80 min. After i.v. administration, the amount of covalently bound material reached a peak within 40 min. It therefore appeared not only that 4-ipomeanol was absorbed rapidly from the peritoneal cavity, but also that the covalent binding of the compound occurred rapidly after absorption. Lung fluid accumulation (wet weight to dry weight ratios) peaked 16 to 24 hr after toxin administration. Interestingly, this also was the time at which the lethally dosed animals began to die, suggesting that lung damage was the primary cause of death.

The dose-dependence of covalent binding, pulmonary edemagenesis, and lethality of 4-ipomeanol were examined in rats.[38] Although the amount of product bound covalently to the lung increased relatively constantly over the range of doses tested, a pronounced threshold effect was observed in the rate of change of the pulmonary wet weight to dry weight ratios. Doses of 4-ipomeanol in the range of 2 to 10 mg/kg produced only a slight increase in lung fluid, whereas doses above 10 to 15 mg/kg produced striking increases. Deaths occurred only in the animals receiving the higher range of doses, again suggesting that the lung lesions were the primary cause of death.

D. Metabolic Activation by Microsome Preparations In Vitro

In vitro studies[40] led to the conclusion that cytochrome P-450-dependent monooxygenase enzymes in rat lung and liver could mediate the formation of 4-ipomeanol metabolite(s) capable of alkylating tissue proteins. When ^{14}C-4-ipomeanol was incubated in the presence of NADPH with various subcellular fractions of rat lung and liver, radioactive material became covalently bound predominantly in the microsomal fractions. The microsomal covalent binding was inhibited by carbon monoxide or cytochrome c, but was not inhibited by the addition of cyanide. No binding occurred in the absence of NADPH or oxygen or when heat-denatured microsomes were used or when the incubations were performed at 1 to 2°C. These experiments indicated that, without prior metabolism, 4-ipomeanol was not sufficiently reactive to alkylate tissue components. The covalent binding of material from ^{14}C-4-ipomeanol thus represented the formation of a chemically reactive metabolite.

Several monoxygenase enzyme inhibitors decreased the covalent binding of 4-ipomeanol in rat lung and liver microsomes in vitro.[40] Pyrazole, piperonyl butoxide, or β-diethylaminoethyldiphenylpropyl acetate (SKF 525-A) inhibited the covalent binding; piperonyl butoxide was the most potent of these three agents. The covalent binding of 4-ipomeanol was decreased markedly in lung and liver microsomes from rats pretreated with cobaltous chloride. An antibody prepared against purified rat liver NADPH-cytochrome c reductase inhibited both the NADPH-cytochrome c reductase activity and the covalent binding of 4-ipomeanol in incubation mixtures containing rat lung or liver microsomes.[41] Thus, all the various inhibitor studies supported the view that cytochrome P-450-dependent microsomal enzymes mediated the metabolic activation of 4-ipomeanol in vitro.

The pretreatment of rats with phenobarbital did not increase rat pulmonary cytochrome P-450, nor the in vitro lung microsomal alkylation by 4-ipomeanol. In contrast, 3-methylcholanthrene pretreatment increased lung cytochrome P-450, but produced either no significant change or, in some experiments, a slight decrease in the amount of 4-ipomeanol bound covalently in vitro to lung microsomes.[40] Both pretreatments produced the expected increases in hepatic cytochromes P-450 and likewise increased the in vitro hepatic microsomal covalent binding of 4-ipomeanol.

In vitro kinetic studies[40] indicated the K_m for the covalent binding pathway was more than tenfold lower in rat lung microsomes (2.9×10^{-5} M) than in rat hepatic microsomes, suggesting a possible basis for the lung-specific alkylation and toxicity of 4-ipomeanol in vivo. Maximal rates of hepatic and pulmonary microsomal alkylation were of about equal magnitude (V_{max}, 0.45 and 0.51 nmol bound per milligram protein per minute, respectively) when expressed per milligram of microsomal protein. These findings seemed remarkable, considering the much lower cytochrome P-450 content of rat lung microsomes, compared to rat liver microsomes. Moreover, other experiments[13] have shown that, under conditions where maximal rates were obtained, the ratios of the amounts of 4-ipomeanol bound covalently compared to the total amounts of 4-ipomeanol metabolized were about the same for hepatic and pulmonary microsomes. Thus, the high rate of lung microsomal alkylation by 4-ipomeanol did not seem to be due to a deficiency in a lung microsomal detoxication pathway.

Immunochemical studies have suggested that cytochrome b_5 also may play an important role in the metabolic activation of 4-ipomeanol in the lung.[41] An anticytochrome b_5 antibody strikingly inhibited both the NADH-mediated reduction of cytochrome c and the NADPH-mediated metabolic activation of 4-ipomeanol by lung microsomes. In contrast, the inhibition of NADH-mediated cytochrome c reduction in liver microsomes was accompanied by only very small decreases in the rate of 4-ipomeanol activation. Preincubation of the anticytochrome b_5 antibody with purified cytochrome b_5 abolished its inhibitory effect on the NADH-mediated reduction of cytochrome c and on the activation of 4-ipomeanol in lung microsome preparations. In another experiment, it was shown that the anticytochrome b_5 antibody strongly inhibited both the disappearance and the covalent binding of 4-ipomeanol, whether the cofactor present was NADPH or NADH or a mixture of the two. With NADH alone as the cofactor, nearly 30% of the maximal activity (expressed either as covalent binding or as total metabolism of 4-ipomeanol) was obtained. The stimulatory effects of NADPH and NADH were not synergistic; indeed, they were not even additive. Based on the results of these studies, a mechanism for the in vitro metabolic activation of 4-ipomeanol was proposed which involved a two-electron transfer, in which one or both electrons could be derived from NADPH by cytochrome c reductase, but in which transfer of the second electron by cytochrome b_5 was rate limiting in lung microsomes. Whether such a mechanism is operative in vivo, and therefore whether cytochrome b_5 is important in the in vivo target organ metabolism and toxicity of 4-ipomeanol, cannot yet be assessed.

E. Evidence for Role of Metabolic Activation in Covalent Binding and Toxicity In Vivo; Studies with Inhibitors of Metabolism

Pretreatments with pyrazole or cobaltous chloride, which previously had been shown to inhibit the microsomal activation of 4-ipomeanol in vitro,[40] markedly decreased both the in vivo covalent binding and the toxicity of 4-ipomeanol in rats.[38] Pretreatment with another inhibitor of 4-ipomeanol metabolism, piperonyl butoxide,[40] caused a striking increase in both the blood and the pulmonary levels of unmetabolized 4-ipomeanol,[36] but produced a marked decrease in the amount of toxin bound covalently in the lung and the liver.[36,38] The selective pulmonary alkylation by 4-ipomeanol did not appear to be due to selective uptake and accumulation of the parent compound, since pulmonary concentrations of unmetabolized 4-ipomeanol were similar to the blood concentrations both in the controls and in the animals pretreated with piperonyl butoxide.[36] Although both the pulmonary and the hepatic binding were decreased by these inhibitor pretreatments, lung binding still predominated; lung remained the target organ when larger doses of toxin were given to the pretreated animals. SKF 525-A inhibited the in vitro metabolism and covalent binding of 4-ipomeanol,[40] but had no significant effect on the covalent binding or toxicity of 4-ipomeanol in rats in vivo.[38] It is possible that SKF 525-A either inhibited detoxifying metabolic pathways in vivo as well as toxifying ones or that its concentration in vivo was too low to inhibit the toxifying pathway.

Thus, these experiments demonstrated an excellent correlation between the degree of toxicity and the amount of covalent binding of toxin to the lung. Furthermore, the demonstrated in vitro inhibitory effects of these agents on 4-ipomeanol activation could satisfactorily account for the in vivo findings. 4-Ipomeanol toxicity therefore clearly seemed due to the formation of a chemically reactive metabolite(s) in vivo which could alkylate tissue.

F. In Vivo Evidence for Role of *In Situ* Metabolic Activation in Covalent Binding and Toxicity of 4-Ipomeanol; Studies with Inducers of Metabolism

The highly preferential alkylation of lung such as occurred with 4-ipomeanol in rats would be difficult to explain by a mechanism in which the alkylating metabolite binding to the extrahepatic tissue was formed primarily in the liver and reached the lungs by the circulation. Studies with animals pretreated with the inducer, 3-methylcholanthrene, indicated that the extrahepatic tissue alkylation and toxicity by 4-ipomeanol involved the *in situ* generation of highly reactive 4-ipomeanol metabolites primarily within the target tissue itself.[17,38]

In methylcholanthrene-induced rats, the relative proportion of 4-ipomeanol bound covalently in the liver was markedly increased, whereas it was decreased in the lung, over a wide range of administered doses of 4-ipomeanol. Consistent with these alterations in binding patterns, toxic doses of 4-ipomeanol frequently caused severe centrilobular hepatic necrosis in methylcholanthrene-pretreated rats (no liver damage occurs in control rats). The pulmonary toxicity of 4-ipomeanol was relatively less pronounced in the pretreated rats compared to controls.

The finding that methylcholanthrene could increase greatly the formation and covalent binding of reactive 4-ipomeanol metabolites in the liver, without increasing the amount of 4-ipomeanol binding in extrahepatic tissues, argues strongly against the possibility that a major proportion of alkylating metabolites formed in the liver could escape that organ and bind covalently to extrahepatic tissues. In fact, the inducer pretreatment invariably caused a decrease in the levels of 4-ipomeanol bound covalently in the lungs; it is probable that this decrease was due to an increased rate of hepatic clearance and shortened biological half-life of the 4-ipomeanol in the induced animals.[17,38]

Phenobarbital pretreatment did not alter the target organ for covalent binding and toxicity of 4-ipomeanol in rats in vivo, although it did significantly increase the LD_{50} value.[17,38] Covalent binding was decreased to similar extents both in the lungs and the livers of the pretreated animals compared to controls. It appeared that phenobarbital treatment enhanced detoxifying pathways in vivo more than toxifying ones.[17]

G. Possible Role of Glutathione in Pulmonary Toxicity by 4-Ipomeanol

Reduced glutathione (GSH) has been shown to participate in the detoxication of highly reactive, hepatotoxic metabolites generated in the liver.[45-47] Because 4-ipomeanol appeared to cause lung damage only after metabolic activation *in situ*, the compound has been used in studies exploring the possible protective role of GSH in pulmonary toxicity initiated by a reactive metabolite.[42-44]

In vitro studies[40,43] showed that GSH reacted with the electrophilic, alkylating metabolite(s) of 4-ipomeanol to form water-soluble conjugates. These reactions thereby prevented the covalent binding of 4-ipomeanol to tissue macromolecules in vitro, and they did so without altering the rate of formation of the alkylating metabolites. A method recently has been developed for the qualitative and quantitative analysis of 4-ipomeanol/GSH conjugates;[43] at least two different conjugates were formed in incubation mixtures containing rat lung or liver microsomes, NADPH, 4-ipomeanol, and GSH. This method will facilitate further investigations of the possible role that GSH and GSH-transferases may have as potential detoxication pathways for 4-ipomeanol and also should permit the isolation of sufficient quantities of the conjugates for detailed structural studies.

Other studies indicate GSH may modulate the covalent binding and toxicity of 4-ipomeanol in vivo.[42] In rats, toxic doses of 4-ipomeanol preferentially depleted lung GSH, and this effect was prevented by pretreatment of the animals with piperonyl butoxide. Administration of sulfhydryl reagents such as cysteine or cysteamine decreased both the tissue covalent binding and the toxicity of 4-ipomeanol.

Treatment of rats with diethyl maleate, which depleted lung GSH,[42,44] markedly enhanced the pulmonary covalent binding and toxicity of 4-ipomeanol. To clarify the mechanism of this effect, the distribution and metabolism of 4-ipomeanol were studied in control and diethyl maleate-treated rats.[44] Diethyl maleate had no significant effect on the tissue distribution or blood levels of unmetabolized 4-ipomeanol (relative levels present were in order: blood > lung > liver). In control rats, the relative levels of both the covalently bound and the noncovalently bound 4-ipomeanol metabolites were in the order: lung > liver >>> blood; diethyl maleate pretreatment markedly enhanced the pulmonary levels of both of these types of metabolites. Radioactivity appearing in the urine of both the control and the diethyl maleate-treated groups consisted primarily of 4-ipomeanol metabolites. The total urinary metabolite pool was significantly less in the pretreated group. These results are consistent with the view that diethyl maleate enhances the pulmonary covalent binding and toxicity of 4-ipomeanol by depleting lung GSH and not by altering the tissue distribution of the parent compound.

H. Nature of Chemically Reactive Furan Metabolites

The furan moiety of 4-ipomeanol clearly is essential for its covalent binding and toxicity. Analogues of 4-ipomeanol in which the furan ring was replaced by phenyl or methyl substituents did not undergo NADPH-mediated covalent binding in incubations with rat lung or liver microsomes in vitro.[40] Neither of the analogues became bound covalently to rat lungs or livers in vivo, and they were nontoxic at doses greater than 800 mg/kg.[38]

Data from other laboratories also support the conclusion that furan derivatives are potentially toxic by virtue of their metabolic activation in vivo. Studies by Swenson and colleagues[48] indicated that rat and human hepatic microsomes mediated the formation of an epoxide of the dihydrofuran moiety of aflatoxin B1. The epoxide is thought to be responsible for the carcinogenicity of this potent hepatocarcinogen. Studies by Mitchell and co-workers[49,50] suggested that metabolic activation of the furan ring of the diuretic agent furosemide was responsible for renal and hepatic necrosis it produced in laboratory animals. Further investigations by McMurtry and Mitchell[51] showed a relationship between the metabolism and the renal and hepatic toxicity of several other furan derivatives and related compounds. Wirth and colleagues[52] found that a furosemide analogue containing a tetrahydrofuran moiety, instead of the unsaturated furan ring, did not become bound covalently when incubated with liver microsomes in the presence of NADPH. This suggested that, unlike the intact furan ring, the tetrahydrofuran group could not be metabolized to a reactive epoxide. The covalent binding of furosemide was enhanced in the presence of an epoxide hydrase inhibitor, 1,1,1-trichloropropene oxide, suggesting further that the irreversible binding of the drug was mediated by an arene oxide intermediate.

It likewise has been suggested that an epoxide may be formed during the metabolic activation of 4-ipomeanol in vitro and in vivo.[38-40] However, definitive evidence supporting this possibility is not available. Two inhibitors of epoxide hydrase (1,1,1-trichloropropene oxide and cyclohexene oxide) failed to alter the covalent binding of 4-ipomeanol in incubation mixtures containing rat lung or liver microsomes.[40] This suggested either that an epoxide was not involved in the covalent binding or that deactivation of a furan epoxide of 4-ipomeanol by microsomal epoxide hydrase was not a significant pathway. Further studies are needed to clarify the precise chemical identity of the ultimate toxic metabolite(s) of 4-ipomeanol.

I. Cellular Specificity for Metabolism of 4-Ipomeanol in the Lung In Vivo

The pulmonary cellular specificity for the metabolic activation of 4-ipomeanol in vivo was studied by autoradiography.[36] The covalently bound metabolite was most heavily concentrated in epithelial cells of the small airways. Identical results were obtained using both tritium and ^{14}C-labeled 4-ipomeanol, indicating that the binding did indeed represent covalently bound metabolite, as previous biochemical studies had indicated, and was not due to nonspecific tritium exchange or carbon incorporation.

In several animal species tested (rat, mouse, and hamster), 4-ipomeanol was covalently bound preferentially to the nonciliated bronchiolar (Clara) cells of the terminal airways. As discussed earlier, 4-ipomeanol caused necrosis of Clara cells. It thus appeared that the Clara cell was a specific cellular target of 4-ipomeanol.

In order to determine whether metabolism of 4-ipomeanol was required to produce the tissue-bound radioactivity seen in the autoradiograms, animals were pretreated with piperonyl butoxide prior to administration of the radiolabeled toxin. Histologic examination of the lungs from these animals revealed a striking decrease in covalently bound radioactivity in the bronchiolar cells and the total absence of bronchiolar necrosis, even though both the blood and the pulmonary concentrations of the unmetabolized compound were elevated markedly by the inhibitor. This experiment illustrated further that a highly reactive metabolite of 4-ipomeanol which became bound covalently within the target cells and which could be localized by autoradiography was responsible for the Clara cell necrosis.

In studies of the dose-dependency of bronchiolar binding and necrosis by 4-ipomeanol, it was apparent that the sensitivity to the compound decreased as airway size increased. With minimally toxic doses, covalently bound radioactivity was concentrated primarily in the small airways, and the subsequent development of bronchiolar necrosis was restricted to those areas. As doses were increased, proportionately larger airways also were labeled and eventually showed epithelial cell necrosis. It was suggested that the apparently greater sensitivity of the smaller airways might be related to the fact that the relative proportion of Clara cells to the less sensitive ciliated bronchiolar cells increased as airway size decreased. Alternatively, the nonciliated cells of the terminal airways actually may have been more active in the metabolism of 4-ipomeanol than were the cells of the larger airways. Another possibility is that cells in the larger airways (and possibly other pulmonary cells) might also have been capable of activating 4-ipomeanol, but could more effectively detoxify the reactive 4-ipomeanol metabolite and thereby prevent its covalent binding.

Previous studies showing that the toxic 4-ipomeanol metabolite formed in vivo during cytochrome P-450-dependent oxidative metabolism was formed *in situ* in the lung, in conjunction with the finding that the toxic metabolite was covalently bound preferentially in pulmonary Clara cells, led to the conclusion that the Clara cells are a locus of cytochrome P-450-dependent mixed-function oxidase activity in lung.[36]

J. Studies of the Metabolic Activation of 4-Ipomeanol In Vitro in Systems Containing Intact Pulmonary Cells

4-Ipomeanol was metabolized and bound covalently in incubation mixtures containing mouse lung slices and in isolated whole mouse lungs suspended in, and perfused

intratracheally with, oxygenated Krebs solution.[53] Covalent binding was time dependent and was concentration dependent up to 0.25 to 0.50 mM 4-ipomeanol, at which
concentrations the maximal rates of binding were achieved. Heat-denatured tissues did
not mediate the covalent binding of 4-ipomeanol. In vitro covalent binding was markedly decreased in lung preparations from animals pretreated in vivo with piperonyl
butoxide. In lung tissue preparations from animals pretreated in vivo with diethyl maleate, the in vitro covalent binding of 4-ipomeanol was enhanced markedly. Autoradi-
ographic studies indicated that 4-ipomeanol covalently bound in these in vitro systems
was located predominantly in the nonciliated bronchiolar cells.[16] Thus, all of these in
vitro results are fully consistent with previous in vivo studies which indicated the involvement of *in situ* metabolic activation in the preferential damage to pulmonary
Clara cells by 4-ipomeanol.

III. EXAMPLE OF PULMONARY TOXICITY BY MECHANISM II; STUDIES WITH MONOCROTALINE

A. Background; Nature of Toxicity

Monocrotaline

is a member of the pyrrolizidine family of compounds. Pyrrolizidines are natural products occurring worldwide in many different kinds of plants. Several of these compounds are highly toxic, and their ingestion, especially by grazing animals, has caused
numerous outbreaks of poisonings. These compounds also are potentially toxic to
man. A detailed account of the occurrence and many features of the toxicology of this
class of compounds has been provided by McLean.[54]

A prominent target organ for damage by pyrrolizidines is the liver. However, some
pyrrolizidines also cause major toxicity in extrahepatic tissues. In particular, monocrotaline causes severe lung injury, in addition to hepatic damage, when ingested by or
when injected into animals. A major initial site of damage within the lung is the pulmonary vascular endothelium. Other pathological changes, including pulmonary hypertension and right heart failure, may follow the initial destruction of the vascular
endothelial cells.

B. Role of Metabolism in Toxicity

Studies by Mattocks[55] first suggested a metabolic basis for pyrrolizidine toxicity,
and subsequent investigations by others also have contributed substantially to the development of this concept. Reviews by Mattocks[55,56] describe many of the relevant
experimental studies and hypothetical concepts which support a theory of pyrrolizidine
toxicity involving the in vivo generation of highly reactive pyrrolic derivatives as the
ultimate toxins. In the present review, some general aspects of the "pyrrole theory"
of pyrrolizidine toxicity are outlined briefly, with an emphasis on the potential implications this theory has specifically for a mechanism of lung injury by monocrotaline.

Chemically, the pyrrolizidine alkaloids are relatively nonreactive. However, toxic
pyrrolizidine alkaloids are metabolized both in vitro and in vivo to pyrrole derivatives

which avidly bind to macromolecular tissue constituents. The pyrrole derivatives are potent alkylating agents, and their reactivity is enhanced greatly by the presence of ester groups at or adjacent to ring positions 1 and 7. As envisaged by Mattocks,[55] the ester groups are the most reactive sites due to conjugation with the ring nitrogen atom. The ester group(s) therefore could be lost readily, leaving a positively charged dihydro-pyrrolizine moiety which could react with nucleophilic groups such as amines or thiols to form relatively stable alkylation products. The highly reactive pyrrole-esters hydro-lyze very rapidly (seconds) in water to give hydroxy derivatives which are much less reactive, (and much less toxic) but which still are capable of undergoing alkylation reactions, albeit at much slower rates. Although the esterified pyrrole derivatives can be prepared chemically and isolated in pure form from the parent alkaloids, their extreme reactivity in physiological media makes their isolation from biological systems difficult or impossible. However, in some instances their hydrolysis products have been detected in biological systems in vitro (e.g., dehydroheliotridine from heliotridine-based pyrrolizidines in rat liver microsomes)[57] and in vivo (dehydroretronecine in tissues and excreta of monocrotaline-treated rats),[58] suggesting that the highly reactive esterfied pyrrolic metabolites indeed could have been formed initially in these systems.

Mattocks and White[59] examined the in vitro characteristics of pyrrolic metabolite production in rat liver microsome preparations. The reaction had characteristics typical of a cytochrome P-450-dependent microsomal mixed-function oxidation: pyrrole formation required oxygen and NADPH, was inhibited by carbon monoxide and SKF 525-A, and was increased in microsomes from phenobarbital-pretreated rats. Although dehydrogenation is not a common reaction catalyzed by microsomal enzymes, Mattocks and White[59] speculated that an initial hydroxylation at the 3 or the 8 position of the pyrrolizidine ring could lead to unstable oxygenated product(s) which could degrade spontaneously to form the pyrrole structure.

Largely by elimination of other possibilities, the likelihood that the esterified pyrrolic metabolites are responsible for pyrrolizidine toxicities seems great. Other known or possible metabolites, such as hydrolysis products, 1,2-epoxides or N-oxides, are much less toxic than the parent alkaloids. On the other hand, the corresponding de-hydro-alkaloids (pyrroles) are extremely toxic and produce severe tissue damage when injected i.v. into the afferent circulations to target organs (such as the liver through the mesenteric vein or the lung through the systemic venous circulation). Because of their instability in aqueous media, the pyrroles used in toxicologic studies have been prepared by chemical dehydrogenation and have been administered as solutions in non-aqueous solvents such as N,N-dimethylformamide. The pyrroles are ineffective when given orally, since they are decomposed rapidly by the aqueous acid in the stomach. If administered i.p. they cause local effects, such as inflammation and peritonitis; in this instance, the pyrrolic materials apparently become bound primarily at the injection site and therefore do not survive long enough to reach vital organs.

C. Pulmonary Toxicity of Parent Alkaloid

As reviewed by McLean[54] and also more recently by others,[60-64] some of the pyrrol-izidines cause severe pulmonary injury, in addition to liver damage, after oral, s.c., or i.p. administration. With a large series of different pyrrolizidines and related compounds, Culvenor and co-workers[65] found that lung lesions were produced only in animals that developed chronic liver lesions. Moreover, the minimum dose levels required to cause lung lesions were never below those for liver toxicity (in some cases they were as much as fourfold higher). Culvenor and colleagues[65] suggested that these results were to be expected if the same toxic metabolites causing both the liver and lung lesions were produced in the liver. As summarized by McLean,[54] the pathological changes which may occur in the lungs of pyrrolizidine-poisoned animals include

1.   Dilated lymphatics, intraalveolar and interstitial edema, alveolar hemorrhage (all of which are suggestive of early increases in vascular permeability)
2.   Proliferation of cells of the alveolar wall
3.   Pulmonary hypertension (and presumed manifestations of increased pulmonary vascular pressure, including thickened muscular coats of arteries, pulmonary arteritis, right cardiac ventricular hypertrophy, and terminal right heart failure)

In attempting to elucidate mechanisms of lung injury, it is especially important to differentiate between the earliest pathological changes, or the initiating events, from changes which occur secondarily. Experiments on pyrrolizidine lung toxicity[54,61-64] which showed striking and early occurring damage to the walls of arteries, capillaries, and veins indicated that these vascular walls were primary targets for the pyrrolizidines. This would not be surprising if indeed the lung injury by pyrrolizidines were due to highly reactive alkylating agents (i.e., pyrrolic metabolites) reaching the lungs by way of the bloodstream after formation in the liver.

D. Pulmonary Toxicity of Pyrrolic Metabolites

Consistent with and strongly supportive of a mechanism of pyrrolizidine-induced lung injury involving vascular damage by pyrrolic metabolites are studies[66-71] which showed that, when injected i.v. into the afferent circulation to the lungs, the chemically prepared dehydropyrrolizidines caused lung injury with features very similar to those caused by the parent pyrrolizidines (when the latter compounds are given orally, i.p., or s.c.). Butler and colleagues[66] found that the i.v. injection of monocrotaline pyrrole or retrorsine pyrrole caused early (within 1 to 3 days) signs of increased pulmonary vascular permeability (dilatation of lymphatics, edema, effusions, and hemorrhage). After 3 to 4 weeks, cellular proliferation was prominent in the alveoli.

Butler[67] examined the ultrastructural features of dehydromonocrotaline-induced lung damage. The earliest changes apparently involved the alveolar capillary endothelium, where initially there were marked nuclear and cytoplasmic alterations which later progressed to hyperplasia and sometimes complete occlusion of the capillaries. The capillary alterations were prominent at times (1 to 2 weeks after injection) when the alveolar epithelium clearly was normal or minimally altered, indicating that the alveolar cell proliferation which was seen after 3 weeks possibly was a secondary reaction.

Carbon-labeling studies (i.v. injection of colloidal carbon shortly after administration of monocrotaline pyrrole) showed carbon deposition adjacent both to capillaries and to venules[68,69] (there is some disagreement as to which is the primary site),[68-70] indicating these were probable sites of damage and increased permeability caused by the pyrrolic derivative.

Studies by Chesney and co-workers[71] of monocrotaline pyrrole toxicity in rats also indicated that the vascular endothelium of the lungs was a primary target for damage by the i.v.-administered pyrrole derivative. Moreover, pulmonary hypertension and right cardiac ventricular hypertrophy were shown to occur secondarily to the pyrrole-induced vascular damage, as it did with the parent alkaloids. The development of pulmonary hypertension may lead to a variety of other secondary pathological effects (e.g., vasculitis) which may contribute significantly to the spectrum of changes seen in the lungs several weeks after poisoning with the pyrrolizidines or their pyrrolic derivatives.

E. Role of Metabolism in Pulmonary Toxicity

The findings that the i.v. administration of low doses of dehydropyrrolizidines caused lung damage closely mimicking that produced by much larger doses of the parent alkaloids led to the view that similar pyrrolic derivatives, produced in vivo by hepatic metabolism of the pyrrolizidines, were the ultimate toxins responsible for pyrrolizidine-induced pulmonary vascular damage.[55,66]

The possibility that the pyrrolizidine metabolites damaging the pulmonary vascular system were produced exclusively (or at least predominantly) in the liver was supported further by in vitro studies which indicated that lung preparations had little if any capacity to convert pyrrolizidine alkaloids to pyrrolic metabolites. Mattocks and White[59] found that Ehrlich-positive (pyrrolic) products were not produced when either retrorsine or monocrotaline were incubated with rat lung microsomes in the presence of NADPH. Similar studies with rat liver microsomes yielded large amounts of Ehrlich-reactive material. These experiments were validated further by the demonstration that the lung microsomes were metabolically active toward a different substrate (e.g., N-demethylation of dimethylaniline).

Allen and colleagues[72] found that pretreatment of rats with phenobarbital prior to the administration of monocrotaline considerably enhanced the amounts of pyrrolic metabolites in the livers and lungs in vivo and likewise potentiated the acute pulmonary toxicity. As shown by Chesney and co-workers,[73] the in vitro production of pyrrolic derivatives from monocrotaline was enhanced greatly in liver microsomes from phenobarbital-pretreated rats.

On the other hand, chloramphenicol pretreatment just prior to administration of monocrotaline markedly decreased the tissue pyrrole concentrations and the acute pulmonary toxicity. In vitro experiments[73] demonstrated that chloramphenicol was a good inhibitor of pyrrole formation from monocrotaline in rat hepatic microsomes. Therefore, collectively the metabolic studies described by Mattocks and White,[59] Allen et al.,[72] and Chesney et al.[73] provide good evidence that pyrrolic metabolites were responsible for monocrotaline-induced lung toxicity in vivo and likewise support the view that the toxic metabolites were produced primarily in the liver.

Recent studies by Huxtable and co-workers[74] also agree with the view that the pyrrolizidine metabolites damaging the pulmonary vascular endothelium reach the lungs by the circulation after formation in the liver. The uptake of serotonin (a pulmonary endothelial cell function) was markedly and specifically depressed in isolated perfused lungs from rats treated in vivo with monocrotaline. In contrast, the direct perfusion of monocrotaline through isolated perfused lung preparations from untreated rats caused no apparent alterations in endothelial cell functions. Moreover, the in vivo administration (or direct perfusion into the isolated lungs from control animals) of dehydroretronecine, a de-esterified pyrrolic derivative of monocrotaline, caused an increased rate of release of serotonin metabolites from the corresponding isolated lung preparations. On the other hand, there was a decreased rate of release of serotonin metabolites from lungs of monocrotaline-treated rats. These results were consistent with the view that dehydroretronecine (which has been identified in tissues and excreta of animals administered monocrotaline) was not the metabolite primarily responsible for the pulmonary endothelial damage caused in vivo by monocrotaline.

IV. EXAMPLE OF PULMONARY TOXICITY MECHANISM III; STUDIES WITH PARAQUAT

A. Background; Nature of Toxicity

Paraquat is a quaternary bipyridyl compound, most commonly manufactured as the dichloride salt (1,1′-dimethyl-4,4′-dipyridilium dichloride).

$$H_3C-\overset{+}{N}\diagup\hspace{-6pt}\diagdown\hspace{-2pt}=\hspace{-2pt}\diagup\hspace{-2pt}\overset{+}{N}-CH_3$$

$$2Cl^-$$

It is a widely used broad-spectrum herbicide. The compound has caused profound and usually lethal pulmonary toxicity in man after suicide attempts and also in man and domestic animals after accidental ingestion.[75-79] Moreover, because of its capacity for reproducibly causing lung injury in laboratory animals after feeding or injection, paraquat is one of the most extensively studied pulmonary toxins. Despite this intensive investigation, however, many mysteries still remain as to the ultimate mechanism(s) by which paraquat causes lung damage. Nonetheless, considerable information has been accumulated which suggests that the enzymatically catalyzed cyclic reduction/oxidation of paraquat underlies its pulmonary toxicity. Unlike the pulmonary toxins discussed in the preceding sections of this review, a reactive (free-radical) metabolite of paraquat does not appear to damage the lungs directly. Instead, according to current views, the transient production of this free radical may lead to lung toxicity through "oxygen activation" (i.e., generation of reactive and potentially toxic oxygen derivatives) and/or through the depletion of essential cofactors(e.g., NADPH) which are required for cellular energy metabolism and for cellular protective (antioxidant) mechanisms.

B. Pathological Changes in Lungs

Lungs of animals 12 to 36 hr after receiving toxic doses (10 to 60 mg of paraquat per kilogram i.v. or i.p. in the rat, the most commonly studied species) frequently appear enlarged, edematous, and plum colored. The lungs generally are much heavier than normal, and light microscopic examinations usually reveal extensive edema and hemorrhage. Animals surviving this acute, "destructive" phase may progress through a "proliferative" phase in which intraalveolar fibrosis is the result.[78] Many of the features of the destructive and the proliferative phases described in laboratory and domestic animals also have been documented in man after paraquat poisoning.

Several ultrastructural studies of paraquat toxicity have been presented.[75-78] There seems to be general agreement that during the destructive phase both the Type I and the Type II pneumocytes were damaged severely (including necrosis), although Type I cells appeared to be affected earlier than the Type II cells. In contrast, there was no ultrastructural evidence of primary changes in pulmonary capillary endothelial cells. This is of interest considering the edema and apparent hemorrhaging which frequently can be observed macroscopically (see pages 67 to 69, Reference 76). During the proliferative phase, ultrastructural studies have demonstrated the invasions of profibroblasts into alveoli, their transformations into fibroblasts, and finally the development of intraalveolar fibrosis.

C. Tissue Distribution: Selective Accumulation in Lung

A number of investigators[80-87] have demonstrated a transient, preferential accumulation of paraquat in vivo in the lungs of several different animal species after i.v. or oral dosing. In contrast, diquat, a related bipyridyl compound which was not preferentially toxic to the lungs, did not accumulate to a significant extent in pulmonary tissue.[80,81,86,87] On the other hand, studies by Ilett and co-workers[83] suggested that the selective pulmonary accumulation of paraquat was not sufficient in itself for lung toxicity, since the lungs of rabbits, a species relatively resistant to paraquat, accumulated the compound to levels comparable to those in rats (although the levels did appear to decline somewhat more rapidly from rabbit lungs than from rat lungs).

Studies by Rose and co-workers[88-90] demonstrated the presence of an energy-dependent accumulation process for paraquat in vitro in slices of rat lung and, to a much smaller extent, rat brain. In medium containing a concentration of 10^{-6} M paraquat, lung slices accumulated the compound to concentrations nearly ten times that of the medium, and brain slices accumulated concentrations double that of the medium.

Slices from other organs showed little, if any, ability to accumulate paraquat in vitro. None of the tissues examined significantly accumulated diquat. The energy-dependent in vitro accumulation of paraquat occurred to a comparable degree in lung slices from dog, monkey, rabbit, and man and therefore did not appear to be species specific. Paraquat did not accumulate in brain in vivo, possibly due to poor penetration of the compound through the blood-brain barrier.

Rose and co-workers[86.88.89] determined that the rate of accumulation of paraquat by rat lung in vivo was about one seventh of that predicted by in vitro studies. Because this difference might have been due to inhibitors of paraquat accumulation present in the circulation, Lock and co-workers[91] studied the effects of rat plasma, several endogenous amines, amino acids, and drugs on paraquat accumulation by rat lung slices. Rat plasma inhibited paraquat accumulation in a concentration-dependent, but time-independent, manner. An ultrafiltrate of plasma also inhibited paraquat uptake, indicating that the inhibitory factor(s) was a low molecular weight compound(s). A number of endogenous amines, including norepinephrine, 5-hydroxytryptamine, and histamine, as well as several drugs, including imipramine, propranolol, burimamide, and betazole, all inhibited paraquat uptake by lung slices in vitro. Lock and colleagues[91] emphasized that although paraquat accumulation could be inhibited by various compounds, it did not necessarily follow that agents which inhibited were themselves accumulated or that they necessarily interacted directly with the lung at the site of the paraquat accumulation process. This contention was supported by the observation that diquat was not accumulated by lung slices in vitro, although it was an effective inhibitor of paraquat uptake. It was speculated that the structural similarity between paraquat and diquat might result in competition for a recognition site on the cell membrane.

Studies by Smith and co-workers[92] on the relationship between lung uptake processes for paraquat and 5-hydroxytryptamine (5HT) were indirectly suggestive of some cellular specificity for paraquat accumulation and toxicity in lung. The uptake both of 5HT and of paraquat by lung slices was energy dependent, but the accumulation processes apparently were different for the two compounds. For example, cyanide strongly inhibited paraquat uptake, but only moderately inhibited 5HT uptake. Likewise, a sodium-deficient medium inhibited 5HT uptake, whereas it strongly enhanced paraquat uptake. Lung slices from animals pretreated with paraquat accumulated 5HT in vitro as efficiently as did lung slices from control rats. However, the in vitro uptake of paraquat itself was decreased markedly in lung slices from paraquat-pretreated rats. Since the pretreatment doses of paraquat damaged Type I and Type II pneumocytes,[93] Smith and colleagues[92] speculated that the progressive destruction of these two cell types was responsible for the inhibition of paraquat accumulation. Moreover, since paraquat given in vivo did not alter the uptake of 5HT by lung slices in vitro, it was unlikely that the alveolar epithelial cells were a major site of accumulation of 5HT. Because other investigations have implicated the capillary endothelial cells as the major site of uptake of 5HT in the lung, it likewise seems probable that these cells are not a major site of energy-dependent paraquat uptake in lung.

In summary, the relatively selective concentration of paraquat in lungs apparently is an important factor in the pulmonary toxicity of the compound. However, it also seems clear that other critical factors are required to produce the lung lesions. Other studies suggest that the cellular metabolism of paraquat may be one critical factor.

D. Metabolic Transformation of Paraquat

Quantitatively significant amounts of stable paraquat metabolites have not been detected in tissues or excreta from animals dosed with paraquat.[94] However, gut flora apparently can degrade a significant proportion of orally administered paraquat.[94]

Ilett and co-workers[83] reported that paraquat was not bound covalently to lungs of rats in vivo. This contrasted paraquat with other pulmonary toxins such as 4-ipomeanol, 3-methylfuran and other furans, α-naphthylthiourea, and bromobenzene.[13] On the other hand, Hollinger and Giri[95] reported that the incubation of rat lung slices with radiolabeled paraquat led to the binding of radioactivity to acid-precipitable protein. However, there was no evidence that the binding (exceedingly low levels) required metabolic activity, nor that this binding occurred in vivo, nor that it might be involved in the toxicity of paraquat. Rose and Smith[86] found that paraquat did not bind irreversibly to macromolecules when incubated with lung homogenates. Moreover, when paraquat was incubated with lung slices, it was not bound to any small molecular weight materials. Thus, Rose and Smith[86] concluded that the accumulation and retention of paraquat by lung was not related to any binding phenomenon. It appears highly unlikely that the pulmonary toxicity of paraquat involves the irreversible binding of the parent compound or its metabolite(s) to target tissue.

Bus and colleagues[96] found that phenobarbital pretreatment partially protected animals from paraquat toxicity. However, this effect apparently was present only when phenobarbital concentrations in the tissues were relatively high, suggesting that the protection was not due to induction of drug-metabolizing enzymes.

Ilett and co-workers[83] found no evidence of N-demethylation of paraquat by 9000 × g supernatant fractions from livers or lungs either from rats or from rabbits. These tissues had measurable N-demethylase activity when codeine or ethylmorphine were used as substrates.

Gage[97] found that a stable, blue-colored, free-radical metabolite was produced when paraquat was incubated under anaerobic conditions with fresh rat liver homogenate. The formation of the radical was prevented by heating or by dialyzing the homogenate. The production of paraquat free-radicals also was demonstrated with preparations of mitochondrial fragments and microsomes from liver. NADH was a required cofactor for the mitochondrial preparation, whereas NADPH was required for the reduction of paraquat to a free radical in the microsomes. The addition of paraquat or diquat to incubations of microsomes under aerobic conditions caused a pronounced and simultaneous stimulation both of the oxygen uptake and of the oxidation of NADPH, although under these conditions there was no net reduction of paraquat or diquat. Diquat was more effective in producing these effects than was paraquat. Carbon monoxide did not inhibit the reactions. It was concluded that, under anaerobic conditions in the presence of microsomes, the NADPH reduced the dipyridilium compounds to free-radical products. Under aerobic conditions, the high rates of oxidation of NADPH were due to the cyclic reduction and reoxidation of the dipyridilium compound. It was suggested that since the initial rate of stimulated oxygen uptake was about one half of the initial rate of disappearance of NADPH, one molecule of oxygen must have oxidized two molecules of NADPH.

Ilett and co-workers[83] confirmed the stimulatory effect of paraquat on NADPH oxidation in rat liver microsomes and found a similar effect in rabbit liver microsomes. Moreover, paraquat stimulated the oxidation of NADPH in aerobic incubations with either rat or rabbit lung microsomes. The stimulation of NADPH oxidation was not blocked by carbon monoxide. It therefore was suggested that paraquat acted as an uncoupler in the microsomal electron transport chain by receiving electrons from cytochrome *c* reductase. This contention was supported by the observation that paraquat inhibited the in vitro microsomal metabolism of bromobenzene, even though it apparently did not bind with cytochrome P-450.

The experiments by Ilett and co-workers[83] suggested that a cyclic reduction/oxidation of paraquat, as Gage[97] described for liver microsomes, also occurred in lung microsomes under aerobic conditions. This view was supported by the subsequent finding by Bus and co-workers[98] that, under anaerobic conditions, paraquat was reduced to a free-radical metabolite by NADPH in the presence of lung microsomes.

Bassett and Fisher[99] found that during the perfusion of isolated rat lungs with medium containing 1.5 mM paraquat, the activity of the pentose cycle was increased greatly (evidenced by 182% increase in $^{14}CO_2$ from 1-^{14}C-glucose) while glucose utilization, CO_2 production from mitochondrial metabolism, and lactate production all showed much smaller (<40%) increases. Pyruvate production and the lactate-to-pyruvate ratio were not altered significantly. These results suggested that the interaction of paraquat with the lung resulted in an increased turnover of cytoplasmic NADPH and an increase in the metabolic activity of the mitochondria, but did not result in a significant change in the cytoplasmic redox state. The findings were compatible with the intracellular enzymatic reduction of paraquat by an NADPH-requiring reductase.

Baldwin and colleagues[100] examined the rates of radical formation from paraquat, diquat, and morfamquat in homogenates of rat lung, kidney, and liver. These studies were undertaken to explore the hypothesis that differing rates of radical formation might account for the organ selectivities of the various dipyridilium compounds. However, in each organ homogenate the order of rates found was morfamquat > diquat > paraquat. For each herbicide, the order of rates was liver > lung > kidney. Carbon monoxide inhibited the rate of appearance of the diquat radical in all three organ homogenates. In contrast, the rates of radical formation from paraquat and morfamquat were not altered, suggesting that these two compounds were reduced by a different electron-transferring agent than that reducing diquat. These results were inconsistent with the hypothesis that selectively enhanced rates of radical production in the target tissues were responsible for the respective target organ toxicities.

Ilett and co-workers[83] found evidence of paraquat-dependent H_2O_2 formation (measured indirectly by the conversion of methanol to formaldehyde) in liver and lung microsomes from rats and rabbits. This seemed to be an apparent discrepancy with the suggestion by Gage[97] that H_2O_2 was not produced in similar preparations. However, other studies suggest that H_2O_2 may be a product formed secondarily from an initially formed, reactive oxygen species generated by the reaction of oxygen with the paraquat radical.[101]

Using the technique of pulse radiolysis to generate the paraquat radical, Farrington and co-workers[101] demonstrated that a short-lived species of oxygen, the superoxide anion radical ($^-O_2$), was formed from the reduction of oxygen by the paraquat radical. This observation led to the suggestion that superoxide might be responsible for the herbicidal activity of paraquat. Not surprisingly, the possibility that superoxide, or some species derived therefrom, likewise might be involved in the mammalian toxicity of paraquat also has become an issue of considerable interest. Davies and Davies[102] found that superoxide was produced by the reaction of oxygen with the paraquat radical which was generated during aerobic incubations of paraquat with liver microsomes (the oxidation of adrenaline to adrenochrome was used to monitor $^-O_2$ production). Similarly, Montgomery[103] showed that paraquat stimulated the production of superoxide in rat lung microsomes. The dismutation of $^-O_2$ by the ubiquitous enzyme, superoxide dismutase, can produce H_2O_2 which can react further to produce the hydroxyl radical ($\cdot OH$) and other oxygenated products. The observation that superoxide dismutase did not alter the net oxygen uptake stimulated by the addition of paraquat to aerobically incubated lung microsomes led Mason and Holtzman[104] to suggest that hydrogen peroxide also could be produced by the direct reduction of superoxide by the paraquat radical.

Thus, in summary, all of the evidence described indicated that several potentially toxic moieties could be derived from oxygen during the enzymatic reduction and reoxidation of paraquat.

E. Role of Oxygen in Toxicity

The acute pathological changes in the lungs after paraquat poisoning resemble in some ways the lesions produced by prolonged inhalation of pure oxygen. Interestingly, oxygen appears to be an important modulator of paraquat toxicity.

Fisher and co-workers[105] found that the toxicity of paraquat was enhanced markedly in rats exposed to oxygen-enriched atmospheres. Moreover, there were similarities in the lung lesions in rats either after receiving paraquat alone or after exposure to pure oxygen or after receiving the combination of the two pulmonary toxins. These findings led to the suggestion that paraquat injured the lung by potentiating the toxic effects of oxygen. Bus and Gibson[106] and Witschi et al.[87] likewise found that the toxicity of paraquat was enhanced in mice and rats, respectively, in oxygen-enriched atmospheres.

The validity of a mechanism of paraquat toxicity involving oxygen seemed strengthened further by the finding that the toxicity of the compound was diminished in animals exposed to atmospheres relatively deficient in oxygen. Rhodes et al.[107] found greater lethality and more severe histologic damage in the lungs of paraquat-poisoned mice kept in room air as compared to those kept in a 10% oxygen atmosphere. If animals surviving in the hypoxic atmosphere were exposed briefly to air, they quickly died. On the other hand, Smith and Rose[108] found that rats placed in 10% oxygen after lethal doses of paraquat died faster than comparable controls left in room air. Moreover, the pulmonary concentrations of paraquat in the animals placed in 10% oxygen were much higher than those in the control animals kept in room air. It was speculated that this might have been due to increased cardiac output (and therefore greater exposure of the lungs to paraquat) induced by the relative hypoxia. Thus, the effects of 10% oxygen atmospheres in experiments with rats were opposite to those reported for mice,[107] and these results led Smith and Rose[108] to suggest that the treatment of paraquat poisoning by lowering the inspired oxygen concentrations might be contraindicated.

Although several mechanisms of oxygen toxicity have been proposed (e.g., Reference 109), Crapo and Tierney[110] suggested that the superoxide radical ($\dot{-}O_2$) actually might be the species responsible for the lung lesions produced in animals exposed to high oxygen concentrations. The possibility that superoxide also might be involved in paraquat toxicity seemed to be supported by the report by Autor[111] that the i.v. administration of the enzyme, superoxide dismutase (SOD), provided partial protection against paraquat toxicity. The conversion of superoxide to H_2O_2 is catalyzed by SOD. The activity of SOD in the lung is relatively low as compared to other tissues, and it has been suggested that this may be a significant factor in the pulmonary specificity of paraquat.[103]

Goldstein et al.[112] reported that the toxicity of paraquat was potentiated in mice by the prior administration of diethyldithiocarbamate (DDC), an inhibitor of superoxide dismutase. However, the interpretation of these results was made equivocal by the additional finding that DDC inhibited glutathione peroxidase, another important component of the antioxidant defenses of the lungs.

Since the herbicidal activity of paraquat in plants had been ascribed to the accumulation of H_2O_2 during the cyclic reduction/oxidation of paraquat,[113] Ilett and co-workers[83] also considered the possible role of H_2O_2 in paraquat-induced damage to animal cells. Paraquat stimulated the formation of H_2O_2 in liver and lung microsomes from rats and rabbits in vitro, but the rate of H_2O_2 formation was actually highest in the tissues of the rabbit, a species very resistant to paraquat. Moreover, catalase activities were similar in rat and rabbit lungs. Therefore, it was not likely that a difference in the activity of this H_2O_2 detoxication enzyme could have led to a higher steady state concentration of H_2O_2 in rat lung in vivo.

In summary, a relative deficiency of SOD, in addition to the relatively high oxygen tension in lung and the preferential accumulation of paraquat in lung cells capable of metabolizing it to its free radical form, all seem to be consistent both with the involvement of superoxide in paraquat toxicity and with the target organ selectivity of the compound. However, the actual mode of toxic action of superoxide is less certain, and other potential mechanisms, not requiring the participation of superoxide, have not yet been eliminated.

F. Possible Role of Lipid Peroxidation in Toxicity

Investigations by Pederson and Aust[114] suggested that singlet oxygen derived from the spontaneous dismutation of superoxide could cause the peroxidative decomposition of lipids in vitro. This led Bus et al.[96,98,115-117] to propose that paraquat caused lung lesions by stimulating pulmonary lipid peroxidation. Similar mechanisms also have been proposed to be involved in paraquat-induced damage in plants.[118,119] Although singlet oxygen, derived from superoxide produced during the redox cycling of paraquat, originally was suggested to be the "activated" species responsible for initiating lung damage,[116] recently the potential role of singlet oxygen as an initiator of peroxidative lipid decomposition has been questioned.[120,121]

Several in vivo studies seem to be consistent with a peroxidative mechanism of paraquat toxicity. In accord with the view that antioxidants should modulate peroxidative lung damage by paraquat, Bus et al.[115] found that vitamin E-deficient mice were sensitized to paraquat, as measured by the single-dose 7-day i.p. LD_{50}. Likewise, mice fed a selenium-deficient diet were sensitized to paraquat.[115] Since selenium is required for glutathione peroxidase activity[122] and glutathione peroxidase is thought to be a modulator of lipid peroxidation,[123] this experiment was supportive of a peroxidative mechanism of paraquat toxicity. Further support also seemed to be afforded by the finding that pretreatment of mice with diethylmaleate, which depleted tissues of reduced glutathione (GSH), significantly enhanced paraquat toxicity,[115] as also did tri-o-cresyl phosphate, an inhibitor of GSH-peroxidase.[117] It was speculated that the enhancement of paraquat toxicity by diethylmaleate was caused by the loss of reducing equivalents necessary for GSH-peroxidase activity or possibly by the loss of the intrinsic antioxidant activity of GSH.[115,116] Consistent with the findings of Bus et al.,[116] who studied the effect of selenium deficiency on paraquat toxicity in mice, Omaye et al.[124] likewise found that the toxicity of paraquat was greater in selenium-deficient rats, as evidenced by decreased survival times, increased lung weights, increased activities of several lung enzymes (superoxide dismutase, catalase, GSH-reductase), and an increase in thiobarbituric acid (TBA)-reactive products. The report by Omaye et al.[124] appears to be the only one in which an increase in TBA-reactive materials was found in vivo in lungs after paraquat, although in selenium-deficient animals only.

Paraquat caused significant decreases in the concentration of the water-soluble antioxidant, GSH, in the liver, but not in the lung.[96] It was suggested that this decrease could have resulted from increased utilization of GSH by GSH-peroxidase in detoxifying lipid hydroperoxides or possibly from the direct utilization of GSH as an antioxidant in terminating free-radical reactions.

In contrast to its effects on pulmonary and hepatic levels of GSH, paraquat decreased the level of lipid-soluble antioxidants (primarily vitamin E) in the lung, but not in the liver. The paraquat-induced depression in pulmonary lipid-soluble antioxidants was very prolonged; recovery to control levels required nearly 200 hr.[96] Bus and co-workers[96] suggested that the differential organ effects of paraquat on GSH and lipid-soluble antioxidants might have reflected differences in the cellular site(s) of paraquat toxicity or in the available pools of antioxidant in the liver and lung tissue.

Bus et al.[96] investigated oxygen-induced tolerance to paraquat. A 3-week exposure of rats to 100 ppm of paraquat in the drinking water resulted in significant increases in pulmonary glucose-6-phosphate dehydrogenase and GSH-reductase activities. However, the pretreatment with paraquat had no effect on lung GSH-peroxidase activity. Pretreatment of rats for 7 days with 85% oxygen, which induced tolerance to subsequent exposure to 100% oxygen, caused elevations in pulmonary activities of G-6-P dehydrogenase, superoxide dismutase, and GSH-peroxidase. The average survival time after a toxic dose of paraquat was increased in oxygen-tolerant rats as compared to control rats. These experiments seemed consistent with the lipid peroxidation hypothesis for paraquat toxicity, since the enzyme activities known to be induced by O_2 pretreatment conceivably could have been involved as defenses against peroxidative lipid damage.

Studies of paraquat-induced lipid peroxidation in vitro have yielded contradictory results. Bus et al.[98] showed that paraquat markedly stimulated the in vitro peroxidation of lipids (as evidenced by malondialdehyde production) when added to preparations of highly purified NADPH-cytochrome *c* reductase and lipid, in the presence of NADPH and oxygen. Similarly, Talcott et al.[125] found that lipid peroxidation rates, as assessed in vitro either by the malondialdehyde assay or by the measurement of conjugated dienes, were stimulated markedly by the addition of paraquat to incubation mixtures containing mouse lung microsomes. However, in similar preparations, diquat (much less lung-toxic than paraquat) was a more potent stimulator of lipid peroxidation than was paraquat. Moreover, other reports[83,126,127] indicated that paraquat did not stimulate (in fact, it could inhibit) the in vitro peroxidation of lipids in liver or lung microsomes from rats (a species highly susceptible to paraquat lung toxicity).

Direct in vivo evidence of damaged lipids in paraquat-poisoned animals has not yet been forthcoming. It is possible that the sensitivities of methods used thus far do not permit the measurement of quantitatively small, but possibly toxicologically significant, rates of lipid peroxidation. More sensitive methods must be applied before the lipid peroxidation hypothesis of paraquat-induced lung damage can be tested further. Moreover, if paraquat-induced lipid peroxidation eventually can be demonstrated conclusively in the lungs, then the relationship between the altered lipids and the pathological changes in the target tissue will have to be established. It is conceivable that lipid destruction could lead directly to the tissue lesions, but the possibility that altered lipids could be a manifestation occurring secondarily to another mode of primary tissue damage also will have to be considered. While a lipid peroxidative mechanism for paraquat-induced lung damage certainly is attractive, and much indirect evidence appears to support it, critical and definitive evidence for the mechanism still seems to be lacking.

G. Possible Role of NADPH Depletion in Toxicity

It is possible that the depletion of intracellular NADPH, which might occur in vivo during the redox cycling of paraquat, could lead to the disruption of vital cell processes, including defenses against free-radical assault.[87,90,108,128] From their in vitro and in vivo studies of the stimulation of the pentose phosphate pathway by paraquat and diquat, Rose and co-workers[128] concluded there was no simple relationship between the stimulation of this pathway (and, by implication, free-radical generation) and lung damage. Both paraquat and diquat entered lung cells and stimulated the pentose phosphate pathway, indicating that both compounds underwent catalytic reduction and reoxidation (which presumably resulted in the oxidation of NADPH and the activation of oxygen). However, since there seemed to be little or no damage to the lung following the i.v. administration of diquat to rats, even though there was evidence for free-radical generation, it seemed likely that the generation of radicals was not sufficient in itself to cause cell damage. However, the possibility could not be excluded that a greater rate of radical generation in the specific cell type(s) which accumulated paraquat (possibly alveolar cell types I and II) could lead to damage to those cells. More-over, the accumulation of paraquat by pulmonary target cells could have led to exceptionally high intracellular concentrations of paraquat which could have produced such fast rates of NADPH oxidation that cell death would have resulted from an inability of the cells to maintain normal levels of NADPH and ATP. It was suggested[128] that this hypothesis, which did not require damage to the cell by superoxide, hydrogen peroxide, or singlet oxygen, might explain the difficulties that have been encountered in demonstrating lipid peroxidation in the lung following paraquat.

Because fatty acid synthesis requires NADPH, Smith and Rose[108] studied the effects of paraquat and diquat on the in vitro and in vivo incorporation of ^{14}C-acetate into pulmonary fatty acids. In lung slices in vitro and after i.v. administration in vivo paraquat markedly inhibited pulmonary fatty acid synthesis, whereas diquat did not. Because putrescine, an inhibitor of the active uptake of paraquat into lung tissue, prevented the inhibitory effect of paraquat on fatty acid synthesis in lung slices, it seemed likely that the accumulation of paraquat in the lung resulted in the inhibition of fatty acid synthesis. Moreover, if indeed paraquat was accumulated in Types I and II pneumocytes, then the measurement of changes in fatty acid synthesis caused by paraquat might have reflected changes in metabolic activities in these particular cell types.

To elucidate further the possible role of excessive NADPH oxidation in bipyridylium-induced lung damage, Witschi and co-workers[87] studied the in vivo oxidation of NADPH in rats administered similar i.v. doses of paraquat and diquat. An initial experiment confirmed that, with the doses tested and with the particular animals used, there was a selective accumulation and retention of paraquat, but not diquat, in the lungs. Interestingly, both compounds caused rapid and persistent decreases in the NADPH/NADP$^+$ ratios in the lungs. Only paraquat, however, caused a decrease (albeit small) in the total amounts of NADPH and NADP$^+$. After administration of either paraquat or diquat, there were no significant changes in the capacity of the lungs to synthesize adenine nucleotides *de novo*.

Because diquat had been presumed not be significantly toxic to the lungs, but yet it decreased the NADPH/NADP$^+$ ratios as did paraquat, Witschi and co-workers[87] reevaluated the possibility that diquat could damage the lungs. Electronmicroscopic examinations of lungs of diquat-poisoned rats showed damage to Type I pneumocytes similar to that caused by paraquat. However, the injury was less severe, and Type II cells which were damaged extensively by paraquat did not apparently suffer primary damage by diquat.

Witschi and co-workers[87] compared the effect of oxygen on NADPH oxidation and on the enhancement of bypyridylium toxicity. The exposure of rats to an atmosphere of 100% oxygen increased the lethality of both paraquat and diquat. However, oxygen did not enhance substantially the bipyridylium-induced changes in the pulmonary NADPH/NADP$^+$ ratios when relatively high doses (40 mg/kg) of the compounds were given, although it seemed to amplify slightly the effects of relatively small (5 mg/kg) doses.

Thus, Witschi and colleagues[87] concluded that there was not a straightforward relationship between the oxidation of NADPH in vivo and the pathogenesis of bipyridylium-induced lung damage. However, the possible importance of the Type II alveolar epithelial cell as a target for a paraquat toxicity seemed apparent. Both paraquat and diquat caused Type I alveolar cell damage, but only paraquat damaged Type II pneumocytes. Since only paraquat is transported actively into lung cells, it is possible that Type II pneumocytes are the predominat cell type into which accumulation occurs. In vitro studies by other investigators[129,130] showed that only paraquat, and not diquat, had toxic effects on isolated Type II alveolar cell preparations, but both paraquat and diquat adversely affected preparations containing alveolar macrophages.

V. SUMMARY AND PERSPECTIVE

As an example of Mechanism I (see Figure 1), the studies with 4-ipomeanol showed that the relatively "inert" parent compound reaching the lungs through the circulation was converted *in situ* in the lung to a highly reactive, ultimate toxic metabolite. This biotransformation occurred predominantly within the pulmonary Clara cells and led to the selective destruction of this family of bronchiolar cells. The investigations with 4-ipomeanol led to the conclusion that the pulmonary Clara cells are an important site of cytochrome P-450-dependent monooxygenase activity in lung. This discovery led to the view that the Clara cells are likely targets for many different kinds of toxic and/ or carcinogenic chemicals which reach the lungs through the bloodstream or through the inspired air. Support for this view is afforded by investigations, reviewed previously,[13] which confirm the susceptibility of Clara cells to such diverse agents as furans and related heterocyclic compounds, halocarbons such as carbon tetrachloride, aromatic hydrocarbons and their halogenated derivatives, and certain carcinogenic nitrosamines.

Mechanism II was illustrated by studies with the pyrrolizidine alkaloids, particularly monocrotaline. The available evidence strongly suggests that a pyrrolic alkylating agent which probably is the ultimate toxic metabolite of monocrotaline, is formed primarily in the liver. The toxic metabolite, although having considerable chemical reactivity, nonetheless is sufficiently stable to survive at least transiently in the circulation. The pulmonary vascular endothelium therefore is exposed to the circulating pyrrolic metabolite, resulting in severe vascular injury. Indeed, when chemically prepared monocrotaline pyrrole was injected i.v. into the afferent circulation to the lungs, lung lesions were produced which were very similar to those caused when monocrotaline itself was injected i.p. or administered orally.

Mechanism III was illustrated by the investigations with paraquat. The available evidence suggests that the redox cycling of paraquat in certain lung cells leads to the consumption of cellular NADPH and the "activation" of molecular oxygen. The specific toxicologic consequences of these effects still are not certain. There is considerable circumstantial evidence to suggest that the intracellular generation of superoxide and its derivatives (such as singlet oxygen, H_2O_2, and .OH) may lead to cell damage by stimulating the peroxidative decomposition of cellular lipids. Alternatively, or in addition, the consumption of cofactors such as NADPH conceivably could contribute to lung cell damage by the disruption of essential cellular metabolic pathways.

Mechanisms I, II, and III described herein, which have been derived largely from experimental studies in laboratory animals, may provide useful models for future investigations of chemical agents causing pulmonary disease in man. It should be emphasized that these models are based on information currently available, and as further knowledge is gained, they may be subject to modifications. In addition, other altogether new models of chemical-induced lung injury by compounds requiring metabolic activation may become apparent. Nevertheless, even the available models offer potentially useful bases for predictions of what kinds of chemicals are likely to undergo metabolic transformations leading to specific types of pulmonary damage.

The problem of chemically induced lung disease is an increasingly important one, especially as industrialization progresses and more and more manmade potential toxicants are released into the environment. Moreover, there now are precedents to suggest that there may be less obvious, but nevertheless potentially important, natural environmental sources of agents harmful to the lung.[13-15] It also is becoming appreciated increasingly that many drugs are capable of causing serious lung injury as a side effect in patients.[131-137] As a drug class, the cancer chemotherapeutic agents are especially prominent as a cause of iatrogenic lung disease.[137]

The further refinement of mechanistic models such as those shown in Figure 1, as well as the investigation of alternative models, should be an area of future emphasis for experimental pulmonary toxicologists. Not only are further studies needed of toxication and detoxication pathways relevant to each mechanism, but also the subsequent biologic events leading to or modifying irreversible cell damage should receive increased attention. Such investigations would benefit greatly from more multidisciplinary interest in this research area. The development and application of new technologies and research approaches surely would contribute to accelerated progress.

REFERENCES

1. Miller, E. C. and Miller, J. A. Mechanisms of chemical carcinogenesis: nature of proximate carcinogens and interactions with macromolecules, *Pharmacol. Rev.*, 18, 805, 1966.
2. Miller, J. A., Carcinogenesis by chemicals: an overview — G.H.A. Clowes Memorial Lecture, *Cancer Res.*, 30, 559, 1970.
3. Miller, E. C., Some current perspectives on chemical carcinogenesis in humans and experimental animals: presidential address, *Cancer Res.*, 38, 1479, 1978.
4. Magee, P. N., Activation and inactivation of chemical carcinogens and mutagens in the mammal, *Essays Biochem.*, 10, 105, 1974.
5. Rechnajel, R. O. and Glende, E. A., Carbon tetrachloride hepatotoxicity: an example of lethal cleavage, *CRC Crit. Rev. Toxicol.*, 2, 263, 1973.
6. Gillette, J. R., Mitchell, J. R., and Brodie, B. B., Biochemical mechanisms of drug toxicity, *Annu. Rev. Pharmacol.*, 14, 271, 1974.
7. Gillette, J. R., A perspective on the role of chemically reactive metabolites of foreign compounds in toxicity. I. Correlation of changes in covalent binding of reactive metabolites with changes in the incidence and severity of toxicity, *Biochem. Pharmacol.*, 23, 2785, 1974.
8. Gillette, J. R., A perspective on the role of chemically reactive metabolites of foreign compounds in toxicity. II. Alterations in the kinetics of covalent binding, *Biochem. Pharmacol.*, 23, 2927, 1974.
9. Nelson, S. D., Boyd, M. R., and Mitchell, J. R., Role of metabolic activation in chemical-induced tissue injury, in *Drug Metabolism Concepts*, Jerina, D. M., Ed., American Chemical Society, Washington, D.C., 1977, chap. 8.
10. Boyd, M. R., Role of metabolic activation in the pathogenesis of chemically induced pulmonary disease: mechanism of action of the lung-toxic furan, 4-ipomeanol, *Eviron. Health Perspect.*, 16, 127, 1976.
11. Weisburger, J. H. and Weisburger, E. K., Biochemical formation and pharmacological, toxicological and pathological properties of hydroxylamines and hydroxamic acids, *Pharmacol. Rev.*, 25, 1, 1973.
12. Judah, J. D., McLean, A. E., and McLean, E. K., Biochemical mechanism of liver injury, *Am. J. Med.*, 49, 609, 1970.
13. Boyd, M. R., Biochemical mechanisms in chemical-induced lung injury: roles of metabolic activation, *CRC Crit. Rev. Toxicol.*, 7, 103, 1980.
14. Boyd, M. R., Biochemical mechanisms in pulmonary toxicity of furan derivatives, in *Reviews in Biochemical Toxicology*, Hodgson, E., Bend, J., and Philipot, R., Eds., Elsevier/North-Holland, New York, 1980, 71.
15. Boyd, M. R., Dutcher, J. S., Buckpitt, A. R., Jones, R. B., and Statham, C. N., Role of metabolic activation in extrahepatic target organ alkylation and cytotoxicity by 4-ipomeanol, a furan derivative from moldy sweet potatoes: possible implications for carcinogenesis, in *Naturally Occurring Carcinogens — Mutagens and Modulators of Carcinogenesis*, Miller, E. C., et al., Eds., University Park Press, Baltimore, in press.
16. Boyd, M. R., Buckpitt, A. R., Jones, R. B., Statham, C. N., and Longo, N. S., Metabolic activation of toxins in extrahepatic target organs and target cells, in *The Scientific Basis of Toxicity Assessment*, Witschi, H., Ed., Elsevier/North Holland, New York, in press.
17. Boyd, M. R., Effects of inducers and inhibitors on drug-metabolizing enzymes and drug toxicity in extrahepatic tissues, in *Drug-Metabolizing Enzymes and Environmental Chemicals: Toxic Interactions*, Ciba Foundation Symposium No. 76, Excerpta Medica, Amsterdam, in press.

18. Witschi, H. and Côté, M. G., Primary pulmonary responses to toxic agents, *CRC Crit. Rev. Toxicol.,* 5, 23, 1977.
19. Hook, G. E. R. and Bend, J. R., Pulmonary metabolism of xenobiotics, *Life Sci.,* 18, 279, 1976.
20. Gram, T. E., Comparative aspects of mixed function oxidation by lung and liver of rabbits, *Drug Metab. Rev.,* 2, 1, 1973.
21. Remmer, H., Pulmonary drug-metabolizing enzymes, in *Lung Metabolism,* Junod, A. F. and de-Haller, R., Eds., Academic Press, New York, 1975, 133.
22. Junod, A. F., Uptake, release, and metabolism of drugs in the lungs, *Pharmacol. Ther. B,* 2, 511, 1976.
23. Junod, A. F., Mechanisms of drug accumulation in the lung, in *Lung Metabolism,* Junod, A. F. and deHaller, R., Eds., Academic Press, New York, 1975, 219.
24. Philpot, R. M., Anderson, M. W., and Eling, T. M., Uptake, accumulation, and metabolism of chemicals by the lung, in *Metabolic Functions of the Lung,* Bakhle, Y. S. and Vane, J. R., Eds., Marcel Dekker, New York, 1977, chap. 5.
25. Brown, E. A. B., The localization, metabolism, and effects of drugs and toxicants in lung, *Drug Metab. Rev.,* 3, 33, 1974.
26. Alabaster, V. A., Inactivation of endogenous amines in the lungs, in *Metabolic Functions of the Lung,* Bakhle, Y. S. and Vane, J. R., Eds., Marcel Dekker, New York, 1977, chap. 1.
27. Wilson, B. J., Yang, D. T. C., and Boyd, M. R., Toxicity of mould-damaged sweet potatoes (*Ipomoea batatas*), *Nature (London),* 227, 521, 1970.
28. Wilson, B. J., Boyd, M. R., Harris, T. M., and Yang, D. T. C., Lung oedema factor from moldy sweet potatoes (*Ipomoea batatas*), *Nature (London),* 231, 52, 1971.
29. Boyd, M. R., Harris, T. M., and Wilson, B. J., Confirmation by chemical synthesis of the structure of 4-ipomeanol, a lung-toxic metabolite of the sweet potato (*Ipomoea batata*), *Nature (London) New Biol.,* 236, 158, 1972.
30. Boyd, M. R. and Wilson, B. J., Isolation and characterization of 4-ipomeanol, a lung-toxic furanoterpenoid produced by sweet potatoes, *J. Agric. Food Chem.,* 20, 428, 1972.
31. Wilson, B. J. and Boyd, M. R., Sweet potato toxins stimulated by *Fusarium solani* and *Ceratocystis fimbriata,* in *Mycotoxins,* Purchase, I. F. H., Ed., Elsevier, New York, 1974, chap. 15.
32. Boyd, M. R., Burka, L. T., Harris, T. M., and Wilson, B. J., Lung-toxic furanoterpenoids produced by sweet potatoes (*Ipomoea batatas*) following microbial infection, *Biochim. Biophys. Acta,* 337, 184, 1974.
33. Peckham, J. C., Mitchell, F., Jones, O. H., and Doupnik, B., Atypical interstitial pneumonia in cattle fed moldy sweet potatoes, *J. Am. Vet. Med. Assoc.,* 160, 169, 1972.
34. Doster, A. R., Mitchell, F. E., Farrell, R. L., and Wilson, B. J., Effects of 4-ipomeanol, a product from mold-damaged sweet potatoes, on the bovine lung, *Vet. Pathol.,* 15, 367, 1978.
35. Boyd, M. R. and Wilson, B. J., Preparative and analytical gas chromatography of ipomeamarone, a toxic metabolite of sweet potatoes (*Ipomoea batatas*), *J. Agric. Food Chem.,* 19, 547, 1971.
36. Boyd, M. R., Evidence for the Clara cell as a site of cytochrome P450-dependent mixed-function oxidase activity in lung, *Nature (London),* 269, 713, 1977.
37. Dutcher, J. S. and Boyd, M. R., Species and strain differences in target organ alkylation and toxicity by 4-ipomeanol; predictive value of covalent binding in studies of target organ toxicities by reactive metabolites, *Biochem. Pharmacol.,* 28, 3367, 1980.
38. Boyd, M. R. and Burka, L. T., *In vivo* studies on the relationship between target organ alkylation and the pulmonary toxicity of a chemically reactive metabolite of 4-ipomeanol, *J. Pharmacol. Exp. Ther.,* 207, 687, 1978.
39. Boyd, M. R., Burka, L. T., and Wilson, B. J., Distribution, excretion, and binding of radioactivity in the rat after intraperitoneal administration of the lung-toxic furan, 4-ipomeanol-^{14}C, *Toxicol. Appl. Pharmacol.,* 32, 147, 1975.
40. Boyd, M. R., Burka, L. T., Wilson, B. J., and Sasame, H. A., *In vitro* studies on the metabolic activation of the pulmonary toxin, 4-ipomeanol, by rat lung and liver microsomes, *J. Pharmacol. Exp. Ther.,* 207, 677, 1978.
41. Sasame, H. A., Gillette, J. R., and Boyd, M. R., Effects of anti-NADPH-cytochrome *c* reductase and anti-cytochrome b₅ antibodies on the hepatic and pulmonary microsomal metabolism and covalent binding of the pulmonary toxin, 4-ipomeanol, *Biochem. Biophys. Res. Commun.,* 84, 389, 1978.
42. Boyd, M., Statham, C., Stiko, A., Mitchell, J., and Jones, R., Possible protective role of glutathione in pulmonary toxicity by 4-ipomeanol, *Toxicol. Appl. Pharmacol.,* 48, A66, 1979.
43. Buckpitt, A. R. and Boyd, M. R., Determination of electrophilic metabolites produced during microsomal metabolism of 4-ipomeanol by high-pressure anion exchange chromatography of the glutathione adducts, *Fed. Proc. Fed. Am. Soc. Exp. Biol.,* 38, 692, 1979.
44. Statham, C. N. and Boyd, M. R., Distribution and metabolism of the pulmonary toxin 4-ipomeanol in control and diethylmaleate-treated rats, *Pharmacologist,* 21, 195, 1979.

45. Mitchell, J. R., Jollow, D. J., Potter, W. Z., Gillette, J. R., and Brodie, B. B., Acetaminophen-induced hepatic necrosis. IV. Protective role of glutathione, *J. Pharmacol. Exp. Ther.,* 187, 211, 1973.

46. Jollow, D. J., Mitchell, J. R., Zampaglione, N., and Gillette, J. R., Bromobenzene-induced liver necrosis. Protective role of glutathione and evidence for 3,4-bromobenzene oxide as the hepatotoxic intermediate, *Pharmacology,* 11, 151, 1974.

47. Mitchell, J. R. and Boyd, M. R., Dose thresholds, host susceptibility, and pharmacokinetic considerations in the evaluation of toxicity from chemically reactive metabolites, in *Proc. 1st Int. Congr. Toxicology,* Plaa, G. I. and Duncan, W. A. M., Eds., Academic Press, New York, 1978, 169.

48. Swenson, D. H., Miller, E. C., and Miller, J. A., Aflatoxin B1-2,3-oxide: evidence for its formation in rat liver *in vivo* and by human liver microsomes *in vitro, Biochem. Biophys. Res. Commun.,* 60, 1036, 1974.

49. Mitchell, J. R., Potter, W. Z., Hinson, J. A., and Jollow, D. J., Hepatic necrosis caused by furosemide, *Nature (London),* 251, 508, 1974.

50. Mitchell, J. R., Nelson, S. D., Potter, W. Z., Sasame, H. A., and Jollow, D. J., Metabolic activation of furosemide to a chemically reactive, hepatotoxic metabolite, *J. Pharmacol. Exp. Ther.,* 199, 41, 1976.

51. McMurtry, R. J. and Mitchell, J. R., Renal and hepatic necrosis after metabolic activation of 2-substituted furans and thiophenes, including furosemide and cephaloridine, *Toxicol. Appl. Pharmacol.,* 42, 285, 1977.

52. Wirth, P. J., Bettis, C. J., and Nelson, W. L., Microsomal metabolism of furosemide. Evidence for the nature of the reactive intermediate involved in covalent binding, *Mol. Pharmacol.,* 12, 759, 1976.

53. Longo, N. and Boyd, M., *In vitro* metabolic activation of the pulmonary toxin 4-ipomeanol by lung slices and isolated whole lungs, *Toxicol. Appl. Pharmacol.,* 48, A130, 1979.

54. McLean, E. K., The toxic actions of pyrrolizidine (Senecio) alkaloids, *Pharmacol. Rev.,* 22, 429, 1970.

55. Mattocks, A. R., Toxicity and metabolism of Senecio alkaloids, in *Phytochemical Ecology,* Harborne, J. B., Ed., Academic Press, New York, 1972, chap. 11.

56. Mattocks, A. R., Mechanisms of pyrrolizidine alkaloid toxicity, in *Proc. 5th Int. Congr. Pharmacology,* Vol. 2, S. Karger, Basel, 1973, 114.

57. Jago, M. V., Edgar, J. A., Smith, L. W., and Culvenor, C. J., Metabolic conversion of heliotridine-based pyrrolizidine alkaloids to dehydroheliotridine, *Mol. Pharmacol.,* 6, 402, 1970.

58. Hsu, I. C., Allen, J. R., and Chesney, C. F., Identification and toxicological effects of dehydroretronecine, a metabolite of monocrotaline, *Proc. Soc. Exp. Biol. Med.,* 144, 834, 1973.

59. Mattocks, A. R. and White, I. N. H., The conversion of pyrrolizidine alkaloids to N-oxides and to dihydropyrrolizine derivatives by rat liver microsomes, *in vitro, Chem. Biol. Interact.,* 3, 383, 1971.

60. Allen, J. R. and Carstens, L. A., Pulmonary vascular occlusions initiated by endothelial lysis in monocrotaline-intoxicated rats, *Exp. Mol. Pathol.,* 13, 159, 1970.

61. Kay, J. M., Heath, D., Smith, P., Bras, G., and Summerell, J., Fulvine and the pulmonary circulation, *Thorax,* 26, 249, 1971.

62. Chesney, C. F. and Allen, J. R., Monocrotaline-induced pulmonary vascular lesions in non-human primates, *Cardiovasc. Res.,* 7, 508, 1973.

63. Wagenvoort, C. A., Wagenvoort, N., and Dijk, H. J., Effect of fulvine on pulmonary arteries and veins of the rat, *Thorax,* 29, 522, 1974.

64. Kay, J. M., Smith, P., Heath, D., and Will, J. A., Effects of phenobarbitone, cinnarizine, and zoxazolamine on the development of right ventricular hypertrophy and hypertensive pulmonary vascular disease in rats treated with monocrotaline, *Cardiovasc. Res.,* 10, 200, 1976.

65. Culvenor, C. J., Edgar, J. A., Jago, M. V., Outteridge, A., Peterson, J. E., and Smith, L. W., Hepato- and pneumotoxicity of pyrrolizidine alkaloids in relation to molecular structure, *Chem. Biol. Interact.,* 12, 299, 1976.

66. Butler, W. H., Mattocks, A. R., and Barnes, J. M., Lesions in the liver and lungs of rats given pyrrole derivatives of pyrrolizidine alkaloids, *J. Pathol.,* 100, 169, 1970.

67. Butler, W. H., An ultrastructural study of the pulmonary lesion induced by pyrrole derivatives of the pyrrolizidine alkaloids, *J. Pathol.,* 102, 15, 1970.

68. Pleština, R. and Stoner, H. B., Pulmonary oedema in rats given monocrotaline pyrrole, *J. Pathol.,* 106, 245, 1972.

69. Hurley, J. V. and Jago, M. V., Pulmonary oedema in rats given dehydromonocrotaline: a topographic and electron microscope study, *J. Pathol.,* 117, 23, 1975.

70. Pleština, R., Stoner, H. B., Jones, G., Butler, W. H., and Mattocks, A. R., Vascular changes in the lungs of rats after intravenous injection of pyrrole carbamates, *J. Pathol.,* 121, 9, 1977.

71. Chesney, C. F., Allen, J. R., and Hsu, I. C., Right ventricular hypertrophy in monocrotaline-treated rats, *Exp. Mol. Pathol.,* 20, 257, 1974.

72. Allen, J. R., Chesney, C. F., and Frazee, W. J., Modifications of pyrrolizidine alkaloid intoxication resulting from altered hepatic microsomal enzymes, *Toxicol. Appl. Pharmacol.*, 23, 470, 1972.
73. Chesney, C. F., Hsu, I. C., and Allen, J. R., Modifications of the *in vitro* metabolism of the hepatotoxic pyrrolizidine alkaloid monocrotaline, *Res. Commun. Chem. Pathol. Pharmacol.*, 8, 567, 1974.
74. Huxtable, R., Ciaramitero, D., and Einstein, D., The effect of a pyrrolizidine alkaloid, monocrotaline, and a pyrrole, dehydroretronecine, on the biochemical functions of the pulmonary endothelium, *Mol. Pharmacol.*, 14, 1189, 1978.
75. Smith, P. and Heath, D., Paraquat, *CRC Crit. Rev. Toxicol.*, 4, 411, 1976.
76. Autor, A. P., Ed., *Biochemical Mechanisms of Paraquat Toxicity*, Academic Press, New York, 1977.
77. Pasi, A., *The Toxicology of Paraquat, Diquat, and Morfamquat*, Hans Huber, Bern, 1978.
78. Heath, D. and Smith, P., The pathology of the lung in paraquat poisoning, in *Biochemical Mechanisms of Paraquat Toxicity*, Autor, A. P., Ed., Academic Press, New York, 1977, 39.
79. Conning, D. M., Fletcher, K., and Swan, A. A. B., Paraquat and related bipyridyls, *Br. Med. Bull.*, 25, 245, 1969.
80. Sharp, C. W., Ottolenghi, A., and Posner, H. S., Correlation of paraquat toxicity with tissue concentrations and weight loss in the rat, *Toxicol. Appl. Pharmacol.*, 22, 241, 1972.
81. Litchfield, M. H., Daniel, J. W., and Longshaw, S., The tissue distribution of the bipyridylium herbicides diquat and paraquat in rats and mice, *Toxicology*, 1, 155, 1973.
82. Murray, R. E. and Gibson, J. E., Paraquat disposition in rats, guinea pigs and monkeys, *Toxicol. Appl. Pharmacol.*, 27, 283, 1974.
83. Ilett, K. F., Stripp, B., Menard, R. H., Reid, W. D., and Gillette, J. R., Studies on the mechanism of the lung toxicity of paraquat: comparison of tissue distribution and some biochemical parameters in rats and rabbits, *Toxicol. Appl. Pharmacol.*, 28, 216, 1974.
84. Bus, J. S., Preache, M. M., Cagen, S. Z., Poseur, H. S., Eliason, B. C., Sharp, C. W., and Gibson, J. E., Fetal toxicity and distribution of paraquat and diquat in mice and rats, *Toxicol. Appl. Pharmacol.*, 33, 450, 1975.
85. Molnar, I. G. and Hayes, W. J., Distribution and metabolism of paraquat in the rat, *Toxicol. Appl. Pharmacol.*, 19, 405, 1971.
86. Rose, M. S. and Smith, L. L., Tissue uptake of paraquat and diquat, Gen. Pharmacol., 8, 173, 1977.
87. Witschi, H., Kacew, S., Hirai, K., and Côte, M., *In vivo* oxidation of reduced nicotinamide-adenine dinucleotide phosphate by paraquat and diquat in rat lung, *Chem. Biol. Interact.*, 19, 143, 1977.
88. Rose, M. S., Smith, L. L., and Wyatt, I., Evidence for the energy dependent accumulation of paraquat into the lung, *Nature (London)*, 252, 314, 1974.
89. Rose, M. S., Lock, E. A., Smith, L. L., and Wyatt, I., Paraquat accumulation. Tissue and species specificity, *Biochem. Pharmacol.*, 25, 419, 1976.
90. Rose, M. S. and Smith, L. L., The relevance of paraquat accumulation by tissues, in *Biochemical Mechanisms of Paraquat Toxicity*, Autor, A. P., Ed., Academic Press, New York, 1977, 71.
91. Lock, E. A., Smith, L. L., and Rose, M. S., Inhibition of paraquat accumulation in rat lung slices by a component of rat plasma and a variety of drugs and endogenous amines, *Biochem. Pharmacol.*, 25, 1769, 1976.
92. Smith, L. L., Lock, E. A., and Rose, M. S., The relationship between 5-hydroxytryptamine and paraquat accumulation into rat lung, *Biochem. Pharmacol.*, 25, 2485, 1976.
93. Sykes, B. I., Purchase, I. F. H., and Smith, L. L., Pulmonary ultrastructure after oral and intravenous dosage of paraquat to rats, *J. Pathol.*, 121, 233, 1977.
94. Daniel, J. W. and Gage, J. C., Absorption and excretion of diquat and paraquat in rats, *Br. J. Ind. Med.*, 23, 133, 1966.
95. Hollinger, M. A. and Giri, S. N., Binding of radioactivity from [^{14}C] paraquat to rat lung protein, *in vitro*, *Res. Commun. Chem. Pathol. Pharmacol.*, 19, 329, 1978.
96. Bus, J. S., Cagen, S. Z., Olgaard, M., and Gibson, J. E., A mechanism of paraquat toxicity in mice and rats, *Toxicol. Appl. Pharmacol.*, 35, 501, 1976.
97. Gage, J. C., The action of paraquat and diquat on the respiration of liver cell fractions, *Biochem. J.*, 109, 757, 1968.
98. Bus, J. S., Aust, S. D., and Gibson, J. E., Superoxide- and singlet oxygen-catalyzed lipid peroxidation as a possible mechanism for paraquat (methyl viologen) toxicity, *Biochem. Biophys. Res. Commun.*, 58, 749, 1974.
99. Bassett, D. J. P. and Fisher, A. B., Alterations of glucose metabolism during perfusion of rat lung with paraquat, *Am. J. Physiol.*, 234, E653, 1978.
100. Baldwin, R. C., Pasi, A., MacGregor, J. T., and Hine, C. H., The rates of radical formation from the dipyridylium herbicides paraquat, diquat, and morfamquat in homogenates of rat lung, kidney, and liver: an inhibitory effect of carbon monoxide, *Toxicol. Appl. Pharmacol.*, 32, 298, 1975.

101. Farrington, J. A., Ebert, M., Land, E. J., and Fletcher, K., Bipyridylium quaternary salts and related compounds. V. Pulse radiolysis studies of the reaction of paraquat radical with oxygen. Implications for the mode of action of bipyridyl herbicides, *Biochim. Biophys. Acta,* 314, 372, 1973.

102. Davies, D. S. and Davies, D. L., Effect of *d*-propranolol and superoxide dismutase on paraquat reduction and adrenochrome formation by rat liver microsomes, *Fed. Proc. Fed. Am. Soc. Exp. Biol.,* 33, 228, 1974.

103. Montgomery, M. M., Interactions of paraquat with the pulmonary microsomal fatty acid desaturase system, *Toxicol. Appl. Pharmacol.,* 36, 543, 1976.

104. Mason, R. P. and Holtzman, J. L., The role of catalytic superoxide formation in the O_2 inhibition of nitroreductase, *Biochem. Biophys. Res. Commun.,* 67, 1267, 1975.

105. Fisher, H. K., Clements, J. A., and Wright, R. R., Enhancement of oxygen toxicity by the herbicide paraquat, *Am. Rev. Respir. Dis.,* 107, 246, 1973.

106. Bus, J. S. and Gibson, J. E., Postnatal toxicity of chronically administered paraquat in mice and interactions with oxygen and bromobenzene, *Toxicol. Appl. Pharmacol.,* 33, 461, 1975.

107. Rhodes, M. L., Zavala, D. C., and Brown, D., Hypoxic protection in paraquat poisoning, *Lab. Invest.,* 35, 496, 1976.

108. Smith, L. L. and Rose, M. S., Biochemical changes in lungs exposed to paraquat, in *Biochemical Mechanisms of Paraquat Toxicity,* Autor, A. P., Ed., Academic Press, New York, 1977, 187.

109. Clark, J. M. and Lambertson, C. J., Pulmonary oxygen toxicity: a review, *Pharmacol. Rev.,* 23, 37, 1971.

110. Crapo, J. D. and Tierney, D. F., Superoxide dismutase and pulmonary oxygen toxicity, *Am. J. Physiol.,* 226, 1401, 1974.

111. Autor, A. P., Reduction of paraquat toxicity by superoxide dismutase, *Life Sci.,* 14, 1309, 1974.

112. Goldstein, B. D., Rozen, M. G., Quintavalla, J. C., and Amoruso, M. A., Decrease in mouse lung and liver glutathione peroxidase activity and potentiation of the lethal effects of ozone and paraquat by the superoxide dismutase inhibitor, diethyldithiocarbamate, *Biochem. Pharmacol.,* 28, 27, 1979.

113. Calderbank, A., The bipyridylium herbicides, *Adv. Pest Control Res.,* 8, 127, 1968.

114. Pederson, T. C. and Aust, S. D., The role of superoxide and singlet oxygen in lipid peroxidation promoted by xanthine oxidase, *Biochem. Biophys. Res. Commun.,* 52, 1071, 1973.

115. Bus, J. S., Aust, S. D., and Gibson, J. E., Lipid peroxidation: a possible mechanism for paraquat toxicity, *Res. Commun. Chem. Pathol. Pharmacol.,* 11, 31, 1975.

116. Bus, J. S., Aust, S. D., and Gibson, J. E., Paraquat toxicity: proposed mechanism of action involving lipid peroxidation, *Environ. Health Perspect.,* 16, 139, 1976.

117. Bus, J. S., Aust, S. D., and Gibson, J. E., Lipid peroxidation as a proposed mechanism for paraquat toxicity, in *Biochemical Mechanisms of Paraquat Toxicity,* Autor, A. P., Ed., Academic Press, New York, 1977, 157.

118. Dodge, A. D. and Harris, N., The mode of action of paraquat and diquat, *Biochem. J.,* 118, 43, 1970.

119. Dodge, A. D., The mode of action of the bipyridylium herbicides, paraquat and diquat, *Endeavour,* 30, 130, 1971.

120. King, M. M., Lai, E. K., and McCay, P. B., Singlet oxygen production associated with enzyme-catalyzed lipid peroxidation in liver microsomes, *J. Biol. Chem.,* 250, 6496, 1975.

121. Svingen, B. A., O'Neal, F. O., and Aust, S. D., The role of superoxide and singlet oxygen in lipid peroxidation, *Photochem. Photobiol.,* 28, 803, 1978.

122. Rotruck, J. T., Pope, A. L., Ganther, H. E., Swanson, A. B., Hafeman, D. G., and Hoekstra, W. G., Selenium: biochemical role as a component of glutathione peroxidase, *Science,* 179, 588, 1973.

123. Christopherson, B. O., Reduction of linolenic acid hydroperoxide by a glutathione peroxidase, *Biochim. Biophys. Acta,* 176, 463, 1969.

124. Omaye, S. T., Reddy, K. A., and Cross, C. E., Enhanced lung toxicity of paraquat in selenium-deficient rats, *Toxicol. Appl. Pharmacol.,* 43, 237, 1978.

125. Talcott, R. E., Shu, H., and Wei, E. T., Dissociation of microsomal oxygen reduction and lipid peroxidation with the electron acceptors, paraquat and menadione, *Biochem. Pharmacol.,* 28, 665, 1979.

126. Shu, H., Talcott, R. E., Rice, S. A., and Wei, E. T., Lipid peroxidation and paraquat toxicity, *Biochem. Pharmacol.,* 28, 327, 1979.

127. Steffen, C. and Netter, K. J., On the mechanism of paraquat action on microsomal oxygen reduction and its relation to lipid peroxidation, *Toxicol. Appl. Pharmacol.,* 47, 593, 1979.

128. Rose, M. S., Smith, L. L., and Wyatt, I., The relevance of pentose phosphate pathway stimulation in rat lung to the mechanism of paraquat toxicity, *Biochem. Pharmacol.,* 25, 1763, 1976.

129. Schmitt, S. L., Van Orden, L. S., and Autor, A. P., Effect of paraquat on alveolar macrophages and type II pneumocytes isolated from rat lungs, *Fed. Proc. Fed. Am. Soc. Exp. Biol.,* 36, 413, 1977.

130. Witschi, H., Kacew, S., Hirai, K., and Côté, M., *In vivo* oxidation of reduced nicotinamide-adenine dinucleotide phosphate by paraquat and diquat in rat lung, *Chem. Biol. Interact.,* 19, 143, 1977.

131. Brettner, A., Heitman, E. R., and Woodin, W. G., Pulmonary complications of drug therapy, *Radiology*, 96, 31, 1970.
132. Rosenow, E. C., The spectrum of drug-induced pulmonary disease, *Ann. Intern. Med.*, 77, 977, 1972.
133. Whitcomb, M. E., Drug-induced lung disease, Chest, 63, 418, 1973.
134. Cole, P., Drug-induced lung disease, *Drugs*, 13, 422, 1977.
135. Lippman, M., Pulmonary reactions to drugs, *Med. Clin. North Am.*, 61, 1353, 1977.
136. Shanies, H. M., Noncardiogenic pulmonary edema, *Med. Clin. North Am.*, 61, 1319, 1977.
137. Sostman, H. D., Matthay, R. A., and Putnam, C. E., Cytotoxic drug-induced lung disease, *Am. J. Med.*, 62, 608, 1977.

Mechanisms Involved in Late Responses

Chapter 5

LUNG CONNECTIVE TISSUE

Stephen I. Rennard, Victor J. Ferrans, Kathryn H. Bradley, and Ronald G. Crystal

TABLE OF CONTENTS

I. INTRODUCTION

The connective tissue of lung is comprised of several classes of macromolecules that together represent approximately 25% of the dry weight of the entire organ.[1] By virtue of their unique properties, relative abundance, and distribution, these macromolecules exert a profound effect on lung structure and function.

The major lung connective tissue components are collagen, elastic fibers, and proteoglycans. Collagen is the most abundant, comprising 6 to 20% of lung dry weight and 60 to 70% of the connective tissue mass (see Table 1). There are at least five different types of collagen in lung, each with specific composition, form, and location. The term "elastic fiber" is used to describe at least two intimately associated connective tissue components, elastin and microfibrils, that together make up approximately 3 to 5% of lung dry weight. Proteoglycans are complex, heterogeneous macromolecules composed of long carbohydrate chains of variable length usually associated with one or more proteins. Together with other glycoproteins, proteoglycans form the "ground substance" and comprise approximately 5% of the entire lung connective tissue mass.

In order to appreciate the role played by connective tissue in maintaining the integrity and function of the lung, it is necessary to understand the uniqueness of these macromolecules. We will begin this review, therefore, by briefly summarizing current knowledge concerning the structure, form, and location of each component with respect to the lung. With this as a backgound, we will detail what is known about how the lung produces and destroys each connective tissue component and briefly outline what is known about lung connective tissue in disease. For the reader interested in more details about connective tissue in general, several recent reviews are available.[1-6]

II. STRUCTURE, FORM, AND LOCATION OF LUNG CONNECTIVE TISSUE COMPONENTS

A. Collagen

Collagen is the best-characterized component of pulmonary connective tissue. Although there are several types of collagen in lung (see below), the major types have several common properties. Each collagen molecule is a rod-like unit composed of three polypeptides coiled about each other in a triple helix. These triple-helical structures tend to aggregate to form fibrils and sometimes larger fibers. The structure of these fibrils is stabilized by covalent cross-links within and between the component collagen molecules.[2]

In general, all collagen polypeptide chains contain certain characteristic amino acids. For more than 90% of the length of each polypeptide chain, every third amino acid is glycine. Of the remaining amino acids, approximately 20% are proline, about half of which are modified to hydroxyproline after the polypeptide chain has been assembled. In addition, 3 to 5% of the amino acids are lysine. Some of the hydroxylysine residues also have sugar side chains in the form of galactosyl-hydroxylysine or glucosyl-galactosyl-hydroxylysine. Like the hydroxylation of proline, modifications to lysine residues in the collagen chain occur after the polypeptide has been assembled.[2]

The position of the glycine, proline, and hydroxyproline within the collagen chain is important to the overall structure of the molecule. In general, these occur in form of Gly-Pro-X, where X can be any amino acid, but is commonly hydroxyproline.[2] Although the specific interactions are still not completely understood, it is generally accepted that each of these amino acids plays an important role in forming and stabilizing the triple helix. In contrast, the position of the lysine residues within each collagen chain does not seem to be critical to the structure of the triple-helical molecule.

Table 1
CLASSES OF CONNECTIVE TISSUE MACROMOLECULES
PRESENT IN LUNG

Class	Number of known types	General chemical nature		Amount in lung (% dry weight)
		Protein	Carbohydrate	
Collagen	5	95%	<5	6—25%
Elastic fiber	1[a]	100	?	3—5
Proteoglycans	>3[b]	10—30[c]	70—90[c]	<1
Other glycoproteins	?	70—80[c]	20—30[c]	<1

[a]   Recent evidence suggests the existence of more than one elastic fiber type.

[b]   Intact proteoglycans have not been studied in detail in lung; proteoglycans are composed of variable aggregates of protein and complex lung carbohydrates termed glycosaminoglycans; there are seven subtypes of glycosaminoglycans known, all of which are present in lung.

[c]   There is a variable amount of protein and carbohydrate in these macromolecules, most of which have not been characterized in detail.

However, the presence of lysine and hydroxylysine is important, since these residues form the covalent cross-links that link collagen molecules together.

The fact that a large proportion of proline residues are hydroxylated has been used by investigators desiring to quantitate the amounts of collagen present in various tissues.[7] With minor exceptions, this amino acid is unique for collagen and thus is used as a biochemical marker for collagen. In lung, hydroxyproline is also found in elastin,[3,4] the C1q component of complement,[8] two proteins present in epithelial surface fluid,[9,10] and possibly in acetylcholinesterase.[11] It is estimated, however, that these sources of hydroxyproline constitute less than 5% of all lung hydroxyproline, and, in practice, the error introduced by considering hydroxyproline unique for collagen is negligible.[12] By weight, collagen contains approximately 120 μg hydroxyproline per milligram of collagen, and thus a quantitative measurement of the amount of hydroxyproline in the lung can be converted to a close estimate of the collagen content of the organ.[7]

Pulmonary collagen content has been estimated in a number of species and ranges from 6.4% of dry weight in mouse[13] to about 20% in human lung.[14] For most species, however, adult lung collagen content is in the 10 to 20% range.[15-22] It is likely that the large variations noted are truly species differences, since various investigators tend to agree on the collagen content in a given species. However, there is some controversy over the relative abundance of collagen in different lung structures within a given species.[23,24]

Most of the collagen in lung is insoluble. Some intact collagen can be obtained from lung with a variety of extracting solutions, such as neutral salt, 0.5 M acetic acid, or guanidine.[2,19] Limited pepsin digestion[19,25,26] is also a useful technique to obtain nearly intact collagen molecules. For the normal adult, however, at most, 20 to 30% of the total collagen can be recovered by these methods; larger amounts can be extracted from fetal lung. By cleaving lung with cyanogen bromide (a chemical that disrupts peptide bonds at methionine residues), most of the collagen can be extracted. This collagen, however, is no longer intact, although the cyanogen bromide derived fragments are characteristic of the collagen.

Several studies have attempted to evaluate the "quality" of lung collagen by estimating the relative extractability of the total lung collagen mass by various techniques.[18,19,28-33] However, the reasons for the relative insolubility of lung collagen are poorly understood and likely involve complex intermolecular interactions in addition to covalent cross-links.[18,31,34-37] Thus, the significance of the amount of lung collagen solubilized by one technique or another is unclear and should not be interpreted too closely until these intermolecular interactions are better understood.

Five different types of collagen have been characterized to date, and all types have been identified in lung.[19,25,26,38,39] These collagen types vary in amino acid sequence of the component polypeptide chains and in the types of polypeptide chains making up the triple helix. In addition to differences in amino acid sequence, collagen types differ in the relative degree of prolyl hydroxylation, lysyl hydroxylation, glycosylation of the hydroxy-lysine residues, presence of disulfide cross-links, and lysine-derived covalent cross-links. As a result, the ability and propensity of the various collagen types to aggregate into fibrils differs, giving each type a different macromolecular structure.

Type I collagen is the most abundant collagen type present in pulmonary tissues.[27,40] This collagen type is composed of two $\alpha_1(I)$ chains and one α_2 chain.[2] It has been identified in lung by direct extraction with salt,[19] acetic acid,[19] and pepsin,[19,26] and fragments of Type I collagen have been extracted from lung with cyanogen bromide.[27] Type I collagen is widely distributed in lung, including the alveolar interstitium, pleura, and external to the basement membrane of arteries, veins, and airways.[26,39] Chemical studies suggest that the primary amino acid sequence of Type I collagen isolated from lung is identical to Type I collagen isolated from other organs. However, some investigators have suggested that lung Type I collagen may have some unique modifications to its primary amino acid sequence such as an increased hydroxylation of its lysine residues.[14,19,27] The exact structure and location of Type I carbohydrate side chains and Type I covalent cross-links have not been described. It is known, however, that lung Type I collagen forms thick fibers as it does in other organs.[41] Although there is little direct proof, most investigators feel that Type I collagen is the major collagen type seen by light microscopy and that it stains blue with Masson-trichrome and yellow with Movat-pentachrome.[42] By electron microscopy, lung Type I collagen appears as 20- to 200-nm-wide fibers with a 67-nm repeating periodicity along their longitudinal axes. Although light microscopy shows little Type I collagen in the alveolar interstitium (see Figure 1), it is quite apparent on electron microscopy[41] (see Figure 2). In addition, Type I fibers are arranged in a branching helical array that surrounds the vasculature and airways[43,44] (see Figures 3 and 4). In the pleura, it is present as a series of sheets that branch into the interlobular septa. Type I collagen likely forms a continuum throughout the lung, such that the collagen arrays of interlobular septa, blood vessels, and airways are connected through the alveolar interstitium.[43,45]

Type II collagen is the collagen present in cartilage, both in the lung and elsewhere[38] (see Figure 5). Lung Type II collagen is composed of three identical $\alpha_1(II)$ chains and appears to be identical to other cartilage collagens, including a relative abundance of hydroxylysine residues and absence of cysteine residues.[2] Little more is known about this macromolecule in the lung. It appears to form thin, nonbanded fibrils that are embedded within the proteoglycan matrix of the cartilage[46] (see Figures 6A and B).

Type III collagen is made up of three identical $\alpha_1(III)$ polypeptide chains.[2] In general, Type III is found in locations similar to Type I. Although the primary sequence of lung Type III is similar to that of other tissues, some workers have reported that lung Type III has a higher hydroxylysine content than does Type III from the skin of the same species.[47] Like Type III from other sources, lung Type III differs from both Type I and II in that the mature molecule contains disulfide cross-links formed through cysteine residues.[47] The staining and macromolecular structural characteristics of Type III collagen are not well understood, but it is thought that it corresponds to the "reticulin"[48] demonstrable by light microscopy.

Types IV and V collagen have only been described within the last few years, and little is known about their structure, form, and location in lung.[25,26,39] Both are unique

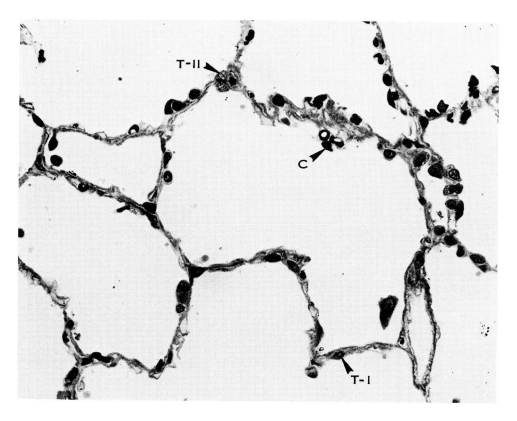

FIGURE 1. Histologic section of normal rabbit lung, inflated to physiological pressure, showing the alveolar architecture. Alveoli are lined by Type I (T-I) and Type II (T-II) epithelial cells, and the alveolar walls contain capillaries (C), interstitial cells, and extracellular components of connective tissue, including collagen, elastic fibers, and proteoglycans. Alkaline toluidine blue stain. (Magnification × 400.)

collagens in that their component polypeptide chains are distinct from that found in collagens I, II, and III. The chains of Type IV collagen are about 140,000 daltons, and those of Type V are estimated at 95,000 daltons. Type IV collagen is likely composed of at least two different polypeptides [currently termed α(C) and α(D)], as is Type V [termed α(A) and α(B)].[49-51] However, there is controversy as to whether the triple helix of Type IV is made up of a mixture of α(C) and α(D) or whether more than one type of Type IV exists [e.g., all α(C) and all α(D)].[49,50,52] Likewise, while α(A) and α(B) chains are found in a 1:2 ratio, respectively, it is unclear as to whether they are present in one macromolecule or two.[25,51] Both collagen IV and V differ from collagens I, II, and III in that they possess a significant number of hydroxyproline residues that are hydroxylated in the 3 position of the proline.[51,52] Collagens IV and V also have a high degree of hydroxylysine residues, many of which are glycosylated.[51,52] Studies of these collagen types in lung are just beginning, but all available evidence indicates they will be similar to their counterparts elsewhere in the body.[25,26,39] Immunofluorescence studies with antibodies prepared against Type IV have shown that it is present only in epithelial and endothelial basement membranes and not in interstitial structures.[26,39] The same may be true for Type V, but this is less clear and Type V may be also present in the interstitium.[26] The fibril structure and orientation of these collagen types have not been studied in detail, and nothing is known about their staining characteristics in pulmonary tissue (see Figure 7).

There has been a great deal of interest in quantitating the relative amount of each collagen type in lung, but there are a number of technical problems that hamper such

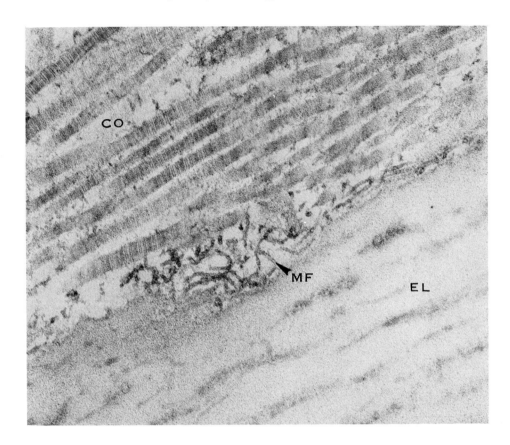

FIGURE 2.   Collagen fibrils (CO) with typical periodic banding are adjacent to a large elastic fiber. The elastin component (EL) is very lightly stained; the microfibrils (MF) are few in number and are peripherally located. (Magnification × 60,000.)

studies. Quantitation of collagen types by most methods requires extraction, yet available extraction methods yield only 15 to 30% of all lung collagen present. In addition, since the types are unevenly distributed among various pulmonary anatomic structures, sampling techniques (e.g., contamination of parenchyma with airways and blood vessels) lead to other errors. However, the best estimates suggest that Type I collagen is the most abundant, representing approximately 60% of the total. Next is Type III (about 30%), followed by Types II, IV, and V (each less than 5%).[26,27,53]

In addition to collagen Types I to V, several other types of "unique" collagen have been proposed.[9,10,54] However, the existence of such additional collagens has not been proven, and they have not been characterized in lung.

B. Elastic Fibers

Elastic fibers have long been recognized as prominent components of lung connective tissue. They are known to be composed of at least two components, elastin and microfibrils.[3,4]

Elastin is composed of large and extremely insoluble polymers. Each polymer is made up of a cross-linked array of identical protein subunits called tropoelastin. Each tropoelastin polypeptide has a mol wt of 72,000 daltons and contains large proportions of nonpolar amino acids, including leucine, proline, and valine.[3,4] Like collagen, tropoelastin has hydroxyproline residues, but these are rarer in tropoelastin, representing only 1% of all amino acids.[3,4] In addition, tropoelastin contains no hydroxylysine,

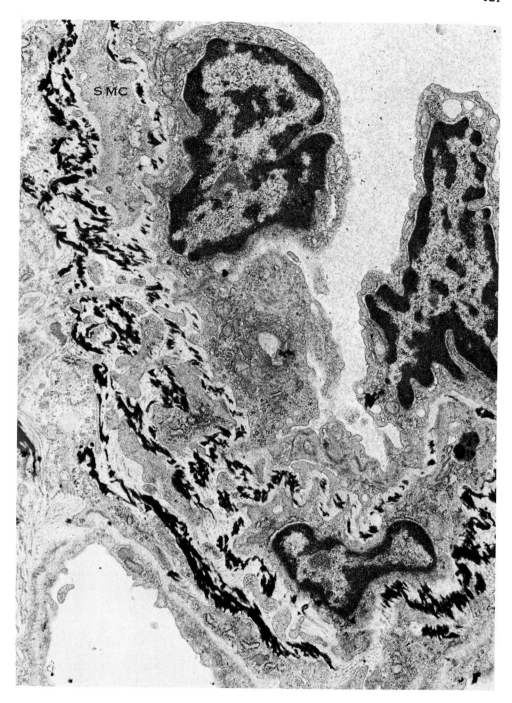

FIGURE 3. Electron micrograph of part of small pulmonary vessel from normal rabbit. Elastic fibers (stained black) are found just beneath the endothelium and surrounding the smooth muscle cells (SMC) in the media. Section stained according to the method of Kajikawa et al.[62] (Magnification × 15,000.)

methionine, cysteine, histidine, or tryptophan.[3,4] Unlike other connective tissue components, elastin contains no carbohydrate. In elastin, the tropoelastin subunits are linked together by covalent bonds through lysine residues.[3,4] Two of these cross-linking structures, termed desmosine and isodesmosine, are unique to elastin; a third, termed lysinonorleucine, is also present in collagen.[2]

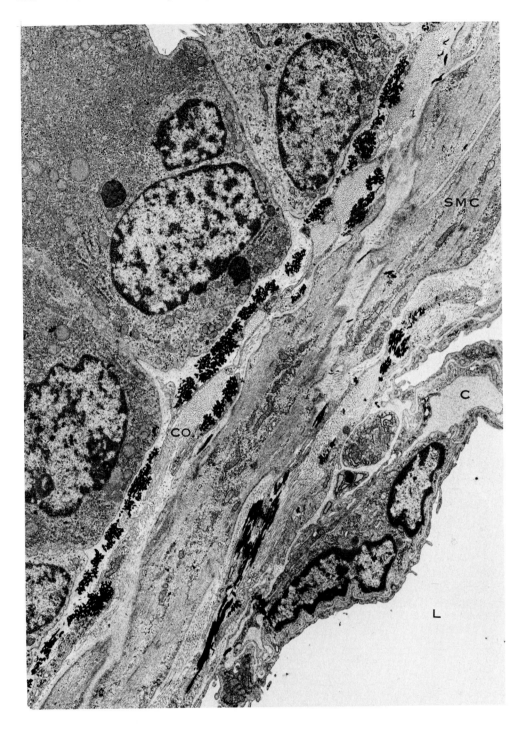

FIGURE 4.   Electron micrograph of wall of bronchiole in normal rabbit lung. The epithelial cell layer is composed of Clara cells and ciliated cells. Subjacent to these cells is a layer of elastic tissue (stained black) and collagenous fibrils (CO) and a layer of smooth muscle cells (SMC). A capillary (C) and the lumen (L) of an alveolus are shown at lower right. Section stained according to the method of Kajikawa et al.[62] (Magnification × 9000.)

Although there is not much information available concerning lung elastin structure, current evidence suggests the tropoelastin monomer is similar throughout the lung.

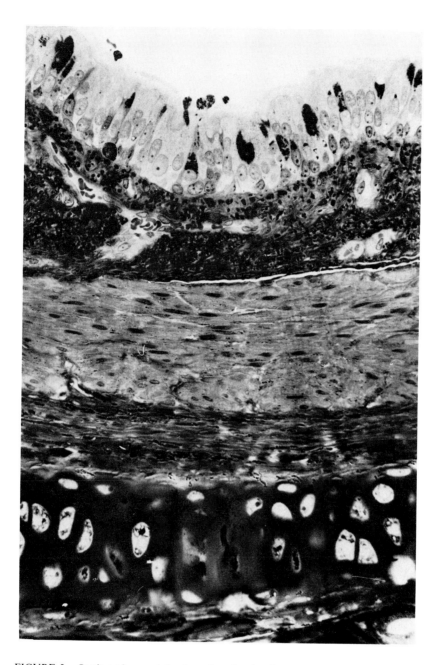

FIGURE 5. Section of normal dog bronchus showing from top to bottom the epithelial cell layer, the submucosal layer, the muscularis, a layer of fibrous connective tissue, and the cartilage layer. Alkaline toluidine blue stain. (Magnification × 400.)

The possibility of lung elastin polymorphism should remain open, however, as at least two types of elastin have now been described in other organs.[55] In addition, it has been suggested that the types of cross-links of elastin from parenchyma and pleura differ in relative amount.[56]

The microfibrillar component of elastic fibers has not been well characterized chemically. Although it has been assigned a mol wt of approximately 250,000 daltons,[57] it

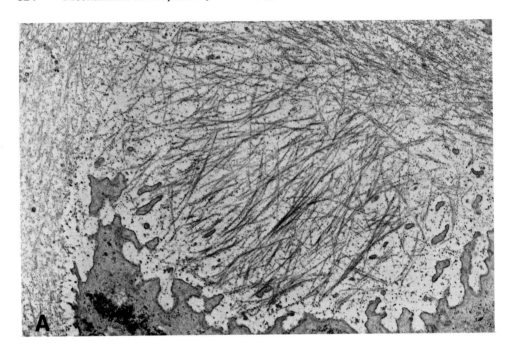

A

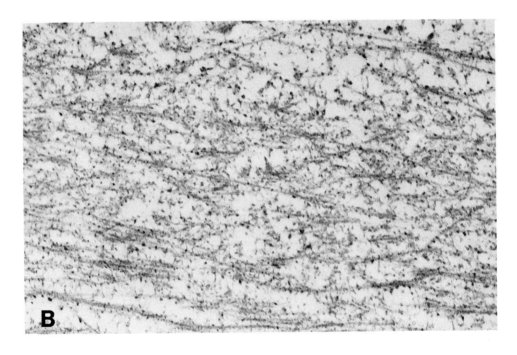

B

FIGURE 6.   Low (A) and high (B) magnification views of tracheal cartilage from Syrian golden hamster, showing chondrocytes surrounded by abundant Type II collagen (unbanded fibrils) and electron-dense proteoglycan granules. (Magnification × 13,500 and × 35,600, respectively.)

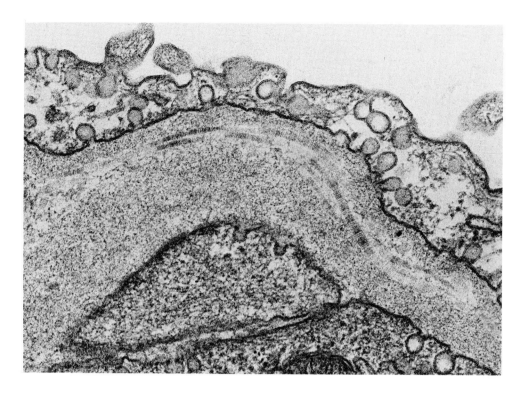

FIGURE 7. The cytoplasm of a Type I alveolar epithelial cell (top) rests upon a basal lamina composed of finely filamentous material. Interstitial cell (middle) and capillary endothelial cell (bottom) also are surrounded by basal lamina composed of similar material. The basal laminae of the epithelial and endothelial basement membranes contain collagen Types IV and V as well as other connective tissue proteins. A few banded collagen fibrils (likely Type I collagen) are adjacent to the epithelial basal lamina. (Magnification × 52,000.)

may be composed of various subunits. Unlike elastin, the microfibrillar component has a large proportion of polar, acidic amino acids and significant amounts of carbohydrate side chains.[58] It has no hydroxyproline or hydroxylysine, but does contain methionine, cysteine, and tryptophan. The cysteine residues are probably important to the overall microfibrillar structure because of their ability to form disulfide crosslinks within and between these molecules.[57]

At the light microscopy level, elastic fibers can be stained with a number of dyes, including the Weigert, Verhoeff, and Gomori methods. In the alveolar interstitium, they appear as a branching fiber network. At the ultrastructural level, elastic fibers appear cylindrical or as fenestrated sheets. On electron microscopic study of routinely fixed and stained tissues (fixation with glutaraldehyde, postfixation with osmium tetroxide, and staining of sections with uranyl acetate and lead citrate), the elastin component appears either unstained or very pale gray, while the microfibrils are more darkly stained (see Figures 2 and 8). The elastin component can be stained selectively in ultrathin sections of routinely processed tissues. Several methods give satisfactory results, including the silver tetraphenylporphin sulfonate,[59] modified Verhoeff iron hematoxylin[60] and orcein[61] methods, and the tannic acid, uranyl acetate, and p-nitrophenol technique of Kajikawa et al.[62] In our experience, the latter technique gives the best results: it is simple, highly reproducible, it imparts a high electron density to the elastin, and it permits clear visualization of other tissue components (see Figures 3 and 4). Elastin appears as an amorphous material that forms the cores of the elastic fibers (see Figure 8). The microfibrillar component appears as cylinders or cables 10 to 12

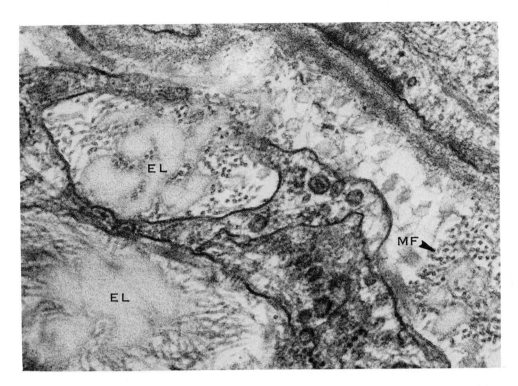

FIGURE 8.   View of three elastic fibers subjacent to epithelial cell layer in dog bronchus. Fiber at lower right contains abundant microfibrils (MF) and only small amounts of elastin (EL). Fibers at upper and lower left contain much more elastin and fewer microfibrils; thus, they are presumed to be more mature. (Magnification × 75,000.)

nm in diameter. The microfibrils appear to have central hollow cores and may show an axial periodicity (see Figure 8). Early in lung development, the microfibrils are scattered throughout the entirety of each elastic fiber and are proportionally in much greater abundance than is the elastin component. With maturity, the microfibrillar component decreases in relative amount and becomes localized to the periphery of the fiber; elastin forms the central core and becomes the dominant component. In the mature lung, elastic fibers are found in close association with collagen fibers and proteoglycans (see Figure 2).

Quantitation of elastic fibers in tissue presents technical difficulties. Most methods used for elastin quantitation rely on a variation of the Lansing procedure,[63] which involves extracting the tissue with solvents followed by heating to 100°C in a 0.1 M NaOH solution and defining the residue as "elastin". However, even though mature elastin is extremely insoluble, some may be lost during the extraction, particularly uncross-linked material.[6,56,64] Other methods estimate elastin content by quantitating the elastin-specific cross-links desmosine and isodesmosine[15,65] or exploit the relative resistance of elastin to various proteolytic agents. At this time, no method has been developed for quantitating the microfibrillar component of the elastic fiber.

Reports of parenchymal elastin content vary with species and with the methodology used; in the same specimen, as much as a twofold difference is obtained with different analytic techniques.[56] In general, however, elastin content for the lung parenchyma is thought to be 3 to 6% of dry weight.[16,20,22,56,66] When expressed as a fraction of connective tissue mass, lung elastin varies from 10 to 30%.[20,56,66] In addition to the lung parenchyma, elastic fibers are also found in blood vessels (see Figure 3), airways (see Figure 4), and pleura (see Figure 9). Some investigators have suggested that the pleural

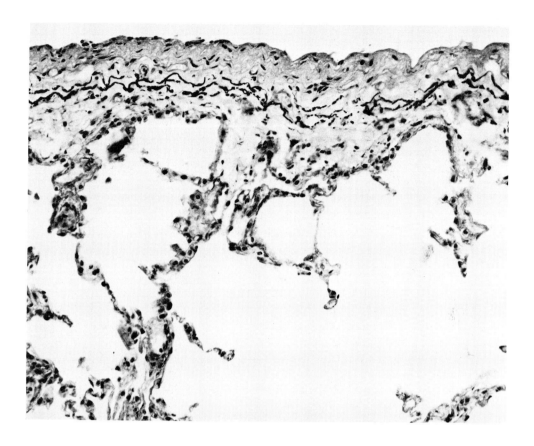

FIGURE 9. Pleura of human lung showing elastic tissue (black) and collagenous fibers arranged parallel to the surface. Movat pentachrome stain. (Magnification × 100.)

elastin content is higher than that of parenchyma, but this remains controversial.[23,24,56,67] With development, lung elastin content increases.[68,69] Although quantitative measurements of lung microfibrillar component have not been made, Keeley et al. noted that the elastic fiber fraction of human lung contains relatively less microfibrillar-type amino acids with increasing age.[69] While indirect, such data are consistent with the morphologic observation that as the lung matures, there is proportionally more elastin in the elastic fibers.[68]

C. Proteoglycans

Proteoglycans are macromolecules that make up the bulk of "ground substance". These macromolecules are comprised of a protein core to which a number of carbohydrate side chains are covalently attached.[5,6] In general, approximately 10 to 30% of the mass is protein and 70 to 90% carbohydrate.[5,6]

The carbohydrate side chains are repeating disaccharide subunits known as glycosaminoglycans, each of which contains an amino sugar and an acidic sugar. There are seven known types of glycosaminoglycans, each defined by the type of sugars comprising the disaccharide subunit.[5,6] The amino sugar can be N-acetylglucosamine, N-acetylgalactosamine, or a sulfated derivative of these. For most glycosaminoglycans, the acidic sugar is a uronic acid, either glucuronic acid or iduronic acid. The one exception is keratan sulfate, a glycosaminoglycan found only in cartilage; in this case, the acidic sugar is replaced by galactose. The approximate number of disaccharides in each glycosaminoglycan varies. Hyaluronic acid is the longest with 500 to 2500. Chondroitin

4-sulfate, chondroitin 6-sulfate, and dermatan sulfate have 60 to 80 disaccharides each. The smallest glycosaminoglycans are keratan sulfate (10 to 20 disaccharides), heparan heparan sulfate (10 to 20), and heparin (10 to 20).[1,5,6]

Much less is known about the protein component of the proteoglycans. In general, each glycosaminoglycan is thought to be associated with at least one core protein with approximately 30 to 100 glycosaminoglycans per protein.[5,6] The exceptions are hyaluronic acid (thought to exist without a protein core) and the cartilage-type proteoglycan. The latter is composed of keratan sulfate, a large core protein, at least two link proteins, and hyaluronic acid, giving a combined mol wt of $>10^6$ daltons.

There are no specific stains for the proteoglycans. Glycosaminoglycans stain positively at the light level with periodic acid-Schiff, alcian blue, and toluidine blue and at the ultrastructural level with ruthenium red. However, these stains are not specific for the glycosaminoglycans, as they also stain other acidic or carbohydrate materials.[70,71] With conventional ultrastructural techniques, proteoglycans appear as fine, electron-dense granules (see Figure 6A and B).

All seven types of glycosaminoglycans are present in lung; together they make up approximately 0.2 to 0.4% of total lung dry weight. Current evidence suggests that keratan sulfate is confined to the cartilage in the tracheobronchial tree while the other six are found in the lung parenchyma. In adult rabbit lung parenchyma, heparan sulfate plus heparin make up approximately one third as does dermatan sulfate. Approximately 20% is chrondroitin 6-sulfate, with the remainder comprised of chondroitin 4-sulfate plus hyaluronic acid.[72] These proportions are known to vary with maturity.

The number of lung proteoglycans is unknown. Recent studies of lung parenchyma suggest that at least two proteoglycan species are present with a third found in pleura.[73-76] In addition, one study suggests that cartilage-like proteoglycan can be found in noncartilage containing lung tissue.[77] The significance of this is unknown and this material needs to be studied in more detail. In addition, at least one proteoglycan is found in lung basement membrane.[78]

D. Other Connective Tissue Components

In recent studies, several additional connective tissue components have been described in lung.

Fibronectin, a major cell surface protein, is present in basement membranes and the alveolar interstitium.[79-82] This glycoprotein has monomer subunits of 240,000 daltons and exists as disulfide-linked fibers on the surface of cells and in the extracellular space.[70-81] The form of these fibers is not well understood, but fibronectin may be at least one component of reticulin.[83] Fibronectin has a number of properties including the ability to mediate cell-cell adhesion and cell-matrix interactions. In regard to the latter, fibronectin interacts with collagen, fibrin, and some glycosaminoglycans.[79-81]

Laminin is a newly described connective tissue glycoprotein found in basement membranes, including those of the lung.[84-86] This macromolecule is comprised of 400,000- and 220,000-dalton subunits that polymerize with disulfide bonds into aggregates of greater than 10^6 daltons. It has a high content of acidic amino acids and small amount of sugars. The amount of laminin in the lung is unknown.

Anchoring fibrils are 4000- to 6000-Å-long, 200- to 600-Å-wide connective tissue structures found in normal bronchial tree, but not in alveolar structures or blood vessels.[87] The biochemical composition of these structures is unknown, but they have transverse banding which is symmetric about the center and is clearly different from the banding of collagen fibers (see Figure 10). One characteristic of anchoring fibrils is that one or both ends insert into the basement membrane forming arcs. The function of these structures is unknown.

The distinction between "true" connective tissue components and molecules merely

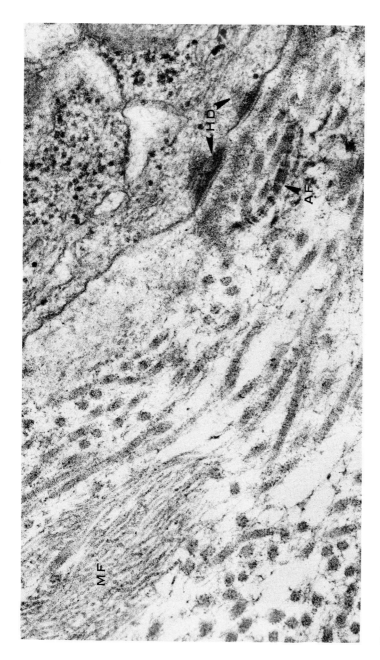

FIGURE 10. Epithelial cell and subepithelial region in small bronchiole from patient with idiopathic pulmonary fibrosis. A bundle of microfibrils is shown at upper left; at lower right, two hemidesmosomes (HD) are in close proximity to an anchoring fibril (AF) which shows typical banding and forms an arc, the two ends of which terminate in the basal lamina. (Magnification × 75,000.)

"in transit" in the extracellular space is an arbitrary one, depending largely on time. Undoubtedly, the number of lung extracellular "connective tissue" macromolecules will increase with further studies, and arbitrary distinctions of what is truly connective tissue will be less relevant when the biology and physiology of the extracellular space is better understood.

III. PRODUCTION OF LUNG CONNECTIVE TISSUE COMPONENTS

A. General Considerations

The biosynthesis of extracellular connective tissue components is complex. The process involves transcription of DNA into RNA, translation of RNA into protein, modification of amino acids in the resulting polypeptides, addition of carbohydrate side chains, assembly of subunits, partial cleavage by proteases, secretion from the cell, assembly into structural units, and stabilization by cross-links. These steps involve the coordinated action of many enzymes and cellular activities and are modulated by a complex system of metabolic control. Although the complete pathway is not known for all the connective tissue components, a considerable amount of information has been accumulated. Most of these studies have involved nonpulmonary tissue, but it is generally assumed that these processes are similar in all tissues. These studies have been reviewed elsewhere; the current discussion will be directed toward those studies relevant to connective tissue production in lung.

B. Collagen

Several in vivo and in vitro techniques have been developed to evaluate lung collagen production. In vivo, these include administration of tracer i.v.,[88] i.p.,[28,89,90] or intratracheally,[32] and in vitro, they include studies of lung slices[12,91-94] and minces,[21,38] cultured cells,[95] and cell-free components.[96]

In most species, the lung parenchyma of the adult utilizes 2 to 5% of its total protein-synthesizing machinery to produce collagen. Once maturity is reached, lung collagen production seems to be independent of age.[12,88] In contrast, there are marked shifts in collagen production during lung development, particularly in the last trimester and early neonatal period, when the relative collagen synthesis may be increased several-fold.[12] This shift toward increased collagen production seems to occur whenever the lung "grows". For example, when 3-month-old rabbits undergo unilateral pneumonectomy, the remaining lung increases collagen production at least twofold such that, after several weeks, collagen content has almost doubled.[97]

The control of lung collagen production is complex and likely involves modulating factors both within and external to the lung. Sex steroids,[98,99] glucocorticoids,[99] thyroxine,[100] α-adrenergic depletion,[101] and hypophysectomy[99,101] have all been examined for their effect on lung collagen production, but the results are inconsistent and no clear picture has emerged. It has been recently suggested that collagen production is normally suppressed by components of the β-adrenergic system.[102,103] In this context, collagen production in lung could be modulated by the relative concentration of β-agonists in the vicinity of collagen-producing cells. This process seems to work through the cyclic AMP system; when β-agonists are present, intracellular cyclic AMP increases while collagen production decreases and vice versa.[102-104] Other controls on lung collagen production probably include modulation by prostaglandins[104] and by inflammatory and immune effector cells.[105]

Different lung structures produce different collagen types, consistent with observations concerning the heterogeneity of collagen types in various locations. For example, lung parenchyma synthesizes collagen Types I,[12] III,[38] and IV,[106] while airways containing cartilage synthesize Type II.[38] In addition, evaluation of cultured lung cells has shown that each cell type produces a characteristic set of collagen types. Fibroblasts derived from the parenchyma produce collagen Types I and III,[95] and Type I epithelial cells may do so as well[107] (see Table 2). Although lung endothelial cells, smooth muscle cells, and chondrocytes have not been directly studied, these cell types have been evaluated in other organs. Aortic[108] and umbilical cord[109] endothelial cells produce Type IV collagen (and possibly Types I and III),[110] aortic and umbilical cord smooth muscle cells produce Types I, III, and V collagens,[111,112] and articular chondrocytes produce Type II collagen;[113] it is likely that lung endothelial cells, smooth muscle cells, and chondrocytes follow these patterns. Preliminary studies suggest alveolar Type II epithelial cells produce little, if any, collagen, but this has not been evaluated in detail.[114]

The function of lung collagen within the matrix is critically dependent upon its form. Following in vivo labeling, newly synthesized lung collagen is progressively more difficult to extract;[32] presumably this reflects progressive cross-linking and maturation of newly formed collagen fibers. It has been suggested that the extracellular assembly of collagen fibers is modulated by the relative abundance of different collagen types and by the presence of specific proteoglycans, but this has not been studied in detail.

C. Elastic Fibers

All studies concerned with evaluating lung elastic fiber production have concentrated on the elastin component; there is nothing known about the synthesis of the microfibrillar component in lung tissue. Like collagen, lung elastin production can be demonstrated in vivo[33,89] and in vitro.[115] However, even though minces of lung parenchyma incorporate radioactive tracers into elastin, the cells responsible for elastin synthesis in the parenchyma have not been identified.

It has been reported that lung endothelial cells produce elastin,[116] but this has not been confirmed. Smooth muscle cells derived from arteries produce elastin,[117] but smooth muscle cells are rarely found in the alveolar structures. As far as is known, lung fibroblasts and epithelial cells do not normally produce this macromolecule.

Although morphologic studies suggest lung elastin production progressively increases with fetal maturation,[68,118] there have been no biochemical studies that have quantified such changes. However, it has been shown that once maturity is reached elastin synthesis continues, but at a relatively slow rate. The turnover of lung elastin is very slow; for the rat, Pierce et al. estimated it to be approximately 1 year.[89]

D. Proteoglycans

Nothing is known about the synthesis of the protein components of lung proteoglycans, but the production of the glycosaminoglycan components has been evaluated both in vivo and in vitro.

The lung parenchyma actively synthesizes glycosaminoglycans; following the in vivo administration of labeled precursors, labeled lung glycosaminoglycans can be readily detected.[119,120] The cell sources of parenchymal glycosaminoglycans likely include mesenchymal, endothelial, and epithelial cells. Mixed populations of cultured parenchymal lung cells produce all forms of glycosaminoglycans except keratan sulfate.[121] Lung fibroblasts actively synthesize heparan sulfate, chondroitin sulfates, and dermatan sulfate,[122,123] and at least one line of lung endothelial cells produces all types of glycosaminoglycans found within the alveolar structures. Lung epithelial cells have not been evaluated for production of these macromolecules, but epithelial cells from other organs are active in this regard.[124] In addition, smooth muscle cells have been reported to produce glycosaminoglycans,[125] so these cells may contribute to lung glycosaminoglycans wherever they are found.

There are marked changes in the production of parenchymal glycosaminoglycans with lung development. In the rabbit, total glycosaminoglycan synthesis peaks about

Table 2

CONNECTIVE TISSUE COMPONENTS OF NORMAL LUNG

Class	Types	Structure	Form	Histology	Location in lung	Relative abundance[a]	Cells of origin in lung
Collagen	I	Trimer $[\alpha_1(I)]_2\alpha_2$ triple helical rod with small nonhelical ends	Polymerized, lysine-derived cross-linked, >45% insoluble	Cross-banded fibers in parallel arrays	Alveolar interstitium, blood vessels, airways, pleura	50%	Fibroblasts, smooth muscle cells, ? endothelial cells, ? epithelial cells
	II	Trimer $[\alpha_1(II)]_3$ triple helical rod with small nonhelical ends	Polymerized, lysine-derived cross-linked, insoluble	Thin dispersed fibrile	Cartilage	<3%	Chondrocytes
	III	Trimer $[\alpha_1(III)]_3$ triple helical rod with small nonhelical ends	Polymerized, cysteine and lysine-derived cross-linked, insoluble	Thin fibrils, τ reticulum	Alveolar interstitium, blood vessels, airways, pleura	20%	Fibroblast, smooth muscle cells, ? endothelial cell, ? epithelial cell
	IV	$[\alpha(C)][\alpha(D)]$[b]	Insoluble, likely cross-linked	?	Alveolar, endothlial and airway basement membranes	<5%	? Epithelial cell, ? endothelial cell
	V	$[\alpha(A)][\alpha(B)]$[c]	Insoluble, likely cross-linked	?	Alveolar, endothelial and airway basement membranes, ? alveolar interstitium	<5%	Smooth muscle cell, ? others
Elastic fiber Elastin	1[d]	Polymer of 72,000-dalton tropoelastin subunits	Insoluble, lysine-desmosine cross-links	Amorphous	Alveolar interstitium, pleura, airways, vessel walls	25%	Smooth muscle cell, endothelial cell
Microfibrillar component	1	Polymer of 250,000 dalton subunits; structure not established	?	10—12 nm cables in periphery of amorphous elastin	Alveolar interstitium, pleura, airways, vessel walls	?	Smooth muscle cell, ? endothelial cell
Proteoglycans	Cartilage	Protein core with keratan sulfate and chondroitin sulfate side chains	Aggregated around a hyaluronic acid core and bound by specific link proteins	Ground substance	Cartilage	<1%	Chondrocytes

	Subunit	Properties	Distribution	Percentage[a]	Cell of origin
Other, probably >3	Unknown; 7 types of glycosaminoglycan side chains are described	?	Ground substance throughout	<1%	?
Other glycoproteins					
Fibronectin	240,000-dalton monomer	Polymerized in fibers, disulfide cross-links, binds to collagen, heparin, hyaluronic acid	Branching fibers, Basement membrane, alveolar interstitium	<1%	Fibroblast, smooth muscle cell, endothelial cell, ? others
Laminin	220,000-dalton and 400,000 dalton subunits	Polymerized into disulfide linked aggregates	Basement membrane	?	?

a Expressed as percentage of connective tissue dry weight.

b Chain composition and structure of Type IV collagen is unclear at this time. Models with heterogeneous and homogeneous chain composition have been proposed. Likely consist of multiple triple helical regions separated by nonhelical domains within each chain.

c Chain composition unclear; current evidence favors $[\alpha(A)][\alpha(B)]_2$ structure.

d A second type of elastin has been reported from bovine ear cartilage; to date only a single type has been described in lung.

6 weeks after birth.[72] This increase involves all parenchymal glycosaminoglycan types, but the changes in the production of hyaluronic acid and the chondroitin sulfates are the most significant. It is important to note, however, that the content of lung glycosaminoglycans does not necessarily parallel these changes in production, further emphasizing that many factors likely control the type, quantity, and form of lung connective tissue components.[126]

E. Other Connective Tissue Components

There is very little information available concerning the production of lung connective tissue components other than collagen, elastic fibers, and proteoglycans.

Lung fibroblasts produce fibronectin in large quantities; besides collagen, it is the major secretory product of these cells.[127] Endothelial cells,[128] epithelial cells,[129] smooth muscle cells,[130] and chondrocytes[131] from other organs produce similar macromolecules and probably also do so in lung. The fate of newly synthesized lung fibronectin is not known. Some likely remains locally, but it may also contribute to a plasma form of fibronectin called cold-insoluble globulin.

No formation is available concerning the production of lung laminin or anchoring fibrils.

IV. DESTRUCTION OF LUNG CONNECTIVE TISSUE COMPONENTS

A. General Considerations

In most species, the total amount of each lung connective tissue component remains constant once adulthood is reached. This requires that synthesis must be balanced by degradation. Like the control of connective tissue production, the mechanisms for connective tissue destruction are complex and involve a number of processes that are only partly understood.

B. Collagen

The normal, triple helical collagen molecule is remarkably resistant to proteolysis. However, specific enzymes, called collagenases, are capable of functioning under certain conditions in the extracellular milieu and of cleaving the collagen triple helix.[132] These enzymes attack the collagen molecules at a specific site approximately three quarters of the distance from the N-terminal end of the molecule. Once the collagen molecule has been cleaved, the resulting pieces denature, the triple helical structure is lost, and the remaining polypeptides can be degraded by nonspecific neutral proteases. The collagenase-sensitive site of collagen is distinctive in several respects:

1. It is adjacent to a "hole" left by staggered adjacent collagen molecules in the collagen fiber.[132]
2. It has no proline or hydroxyproline residues for a short distance on either side of the collagenase-sensitive site of the collagen polypeptide chain.[133]
3. This region of the molecule also is the site where fibronectin interacts with collagen.[133]

Thus, the collagenase-sensitive site is likely "accessible" to collagenase under some circumstances, but situations are possible where the enzyme cannot get at its substrate, thus preventing collagen destruction.

Several different collagenases have been described,[132] many of which are present in lung. Alveolar macrophages from several species produce a collagenase which attacks collagen Types I, II, and III,[143] and lung fibroblasts do so as well.[135] The neutrophil, a cell present in lung in a variety of lung diseases, contains a collagenase which is more specific; it readily attacks Type I, but not Type III collagen.[136] In addition, a separate collagenase for Type IV collagen has been reported in certain rat tumors;[137] this collagenase has not been evaluated in reference to lung cells. No information is available concerning the susceptibility of lung Type V collagen to these various collagenases.

Many collagenases are secreted in an inactive form. This is true for alveolar macrophages,[134] lung fibroblasts,[135] and at least some of the neutrophil enzyme.[138] The likely mechanism for activation of these enzymes is by cleavage by other neutral proteases; such a system has been described for rabbit alveolar macrophage collagenase.[139] It is not clear whether these inactive forms are precurors (i.e., "proenzymes") or complexes between active enzymes and inhibitors. However, in either case, it is apparent that there are numerous controls modulating lung collagen degradation by collagenase.

The antiprotease regulation of collagenase activity in lung is not clear. α_2-macroglobulin is a major serum antiprotease with anticollagenase activity, but it is a very large macromolecule (mol wt 725,000 daltons)[140] and thus is probably too large to diffuse into lung. It has been suggested that mononuclear phagocytes and fibroblasts produce α_2-macroglobulin,[141] but α_2-macroglobulin is not normally detected in human bronchoalveolar lavage fluid, suggesting that if it is present it must be in very low amounts. α_1-antitrypsin, another major serum antiprotease, has a mol wt of 48,000 daltons and readily diffuses through lung tissue. Although it has been reported that α_1-antitrypsin can inhibit collagenase,[142] most studies suggest this antiprotease has little effect on most mammalian collagenases.[132] Another circulating antiprotease, a β_1-globulin,[143] will inhibit collagenase and theoretically could diffuse through lung (mol wt 40,000 daltons), but it is present in such small quantities that it is likely unimportant in lung protease-antiprotease homeostasis.

Besides collagenase, the lung has other mechanisms to degrade collagen. Neutral proteases such as elastase can degrade the ends of the collagen molecule (the so-called "teleopeptide" segments) and thus release it from the fiber. It is also possible that lung cells phagocytize collagen and degrade it within the lysosomal system using enzymes such as cathepsin B_1, as has been described in liver. Another degradative process controlling the quantity of lung collagen involves the intracellular degradation of newly synthesized molecules before they ever leave the cell.[144] All of the mechanisms involved in this process have not been worked out, but it appears to be a way in which cells "monitor" the quality of newly synthesized collagen molecules and degrade those that are "defective."

C. Elastic Fibers

Elastin is very resistant to proteolysis; only one group of proteases, termed elastases, is capable of destroying this connective tissue component. Elastases attack elastin at several points along its component polypeptide chains, releasing fragments that are subsequently degraded by nonspecific proteases. The only known sources of elastase within the lung are alveolar macrophages and neutrophils.[145,146] Both enzymes are serine proteases, i.e., they have serine at their active site and are inhibited in vitro by a specific class of inhibitors, such as diisopropylfluorophosphate and phenylmethylsulfonyl fluoride. In the lung parenchyma, the major antielastase is α_1-antitrypsin. In the trachea and large airways, however, the so-called "bronchomucus inhibitor" is also present and likely protects these structures from elastase attack.

Compared to collagenase, elastase is relatively nonspecific. At neutral pH, it not only can degrade elastin, but other connective tissue components, such as the teleopeptides of collagen, fibronectin, and probably the protein moiety of the proteoglycans.[147]

There are no data available concerning the normal proteolysis of the microfibrillar component of elastic fibers. However, from what is known of their structure, they are likely susceptible to a variety of neutral proteases.

D. Proteoglycans and Other Connective Tissue Components

Very little attention has been directed toward the degradation of these macromolecules in lung, and nothing is known about the processes controlling destruction of laminin, anchoring fibrils, or the protein portion of proteoglycans. Enzymes such as β-glucuronidase and β-galactosidase are produced by alveolar macrophages and are likely important in the degradation of the glycosaminoglycan components of proteoglycans.

Fibronectin is very sensitive to proteolytic attack and can be destroyed by several enzymes that potentially could be present in lung, including neutrophil proteases[148] (including elastase), thrombin, and plasmin.[79] It is known that lung fibroblasts produce plasminogen activator,[149] an enzyme that can activate plasmin. Since production of plasminogen activator may be modulated by exogenous factors such as glucocorticoids, control of fibronectin destruction probably involves a number of complex physiologic systems.

V. RELATIONSHIP OF LUNG CONNECTIVE TISSUE TO LUNG STRUCTURE AND FUNCTION

The ability of the lung to serve as the organ of gas exchange is dependent upon its structure and mechanical properties. It is widely believed that connective tissue components play a critical role in maintaining lung structure and function, but the multiple types, distribution, interrelationships, and complex physical properties of each component have made it very difficult to define the contribution of each element. Thus, a number of methods have been developed to study lung connective tissue structure-function relationships. These include:

1. Morphologic — evaluation of the distribution and form of each class of macromolecules.[43,44,98,150-163]
2. Enzymatic — the in vivo, *in situ*, and in vitro exposure of lung tissue to connective tissue-specific enzymes allows inferences as to the role of those elements injured by the enzyme.[156,163-166]
3. Interactive studies of the purified components — in vitro mixing of connective tissue components permits study of factors controlling fiber size and the cooperation between elements.[167,168]
4. Mechanical — in vitro application of stress to purified components (e.g., stretching or centrifugal force applied by centrifugation techniques) allows inferences concerning the inherent static and dynamic properties of each component.[1,169]
5. Developmental approaches — the addition of purified components to developing lung buds has led to insights concerning the role of connective tissue in cell-matrix interactions during lung growth.[166,170]
6. Biochemical — covalent cross-links between connective tissue components can be reduced by the in vivo use of agents such as β-aminopropionitrile or penicillamine or by the induction of copper deficiency; covalent cross-links can be increased in vitro with agents such as formaldehyde.[16,31,37,161,171-177]
7. Genetic — morphologic, physiologic, and biochemical study of the lungs of individuals or animals with hereditary disorders of connective tissue (e.g., patients with Marfan's syndrome, osteogenesis imperfecta, Ehlers-Danlos syndrome,[178-182] or the so-called blotchy mouse and tight skin mouse[183-185]
8. Evaluation of acquired diseases including human fibrosis and emphysema and animal models of these disorders[186-189] From such studies we can make the following general statements concerning the relationships between lung connective tissue and lung structure and function. For further details, the reader should consult several recent reviews.[1,190-192]

A. Collagen

Most concepts concerning the intrinsic properties of collagen are derived from studies of purified Type I collagen; very little is known about the other collagen types. Type I collagen forms a stiff, rod-like molecule, and it has a high tensile strength and a low elastic modulus.[2,3] Collagen forms a "fibrous continuum" that travels down the airways and blood vessels (the "axial" component of the fibrous continuum), branches into the lung parenchyma (the "septal" component of the continuum), and meets with pleural and interlobular fibrous components (the "peripheral" component).[39,41,193] It is likely, therefore, that lung structure and function are significantly influenced not only by the inherent properties of collagen, but by its anatomic distribution.

Although collagen resists stretching, it is thought that collagen is not under tension at functional residual capacity,[43,192] thus allowing the meshwork of collagen to expand with lung inflation. However, with increasing lung volumes, the collagen within the fibrous continuum comes under increasing tension and, because of its high tensile strength, eventually limits lung expansion. However, it is likely that collagen plays a more complex role in modulating volume-pressure relationships than simply limiting maximal expansion. For example, basement membranes (of which collagen Types IV and V are major components) are placed under tension at most lung volumes. More importantly, collagen interacts with other connective tissue elements, such as glycosaminoglycans, fibronectin, and elastin, and thus influences the mechanical properties of other connective tissue components.

The relative proportion of collagen types present in the lung parenchyma seems to have a major effect on lung structure and function. In those fibrotic lung disorders studied, there is a shift to proportionally more Type I collagen, consistent with the concept that Type I collagen limits lung expansion.[29,43,194] Collagen cross-links also are important in lung mechanical properties. For example, when animals are treated with cross-link inhibitors, lung collagen is more readily extractable[16] and the lungs are more compliant.[37,171] Opposite changes are induced by treating normal alveolar walls with formaldehyde, an agent that induces artificial cross-links.[174] However, such studies must be interpreted with caution, as the same inhibitors and promoters also affect elastin cross-linking.

In addition to its role in mechanical structure-function relationships, collagen also influences cell growth patterns in the lung. Studies of developing buds have shown that collagen is a critical determinant of lung development.[166,170] In addition, in vitro studies of cell → fibronectin → collagen interactions suggest that the anatomic location of collagen within the lung matrix probably controls the site at which cells will "anchor".[195] Although the adhesion factors have not been identified, epithelial and endothelial basement membranes seem to control the location of epithelial and endothelial cells, particularly following lung injury.[176]

B. Elastic Fibers

Nothing is known about the mechanical properties of the microfibrillar component by itself. However, in contrast to collagen, elastic fibers have a high elastic modulus and relatively little tensile strength; this property is thought to stem from the elastin component of the fiber.[192] It is widely believed that elastic fibers are under stretch within the parenchyma at all lung volumes and thus have a major influence on lung mechanical properties in the mid-volume range.[192] However, it has also been suggested that, rather than being the primary determinant of lung elasticity, elastic fibers serve to orient collagen fibers so that increasing number of collagen units are placed under tension as lung volume increases.[197]

Technical problems complicate the assessment of the structural and functional role of elastic fibers in the lung. Most studies rely on the specificity of the enzyme elastase

Table 3
SUSCEPTIBILITY OF VARIOUS CONNECTIVE TISSUE COMPONENTS TO ELASTASE

Component	Susceptibility	Ref.
Elastic fibers		
Elastin	Yes	147
Microfibrillar component	Probable[a]	57
Collagen		
Type I	Yes (teleopeptide)	147,287
Type II	Yes (teleopeptide)	147,287
Type III	Yes (teleopeptide)	288
	? α Chain[b]	
Type IV	Probable	289
Type V	?	
Proteoglycans	Yes	290
Fibronectin	Yes	148
Other glycoproteins	Probable	

[a] The microfibrillar component of elastic fibers is sensitive to a variety of neutral proteases and is likely sensitive to elastase as well.

[b] Type III collagen is cleaved by trypsin at a site close to the collagenase-sensitive site;[291] it may also be sensitive to elastase.

to selectively disrupt lung elastin without influencing other connective tissue elements.[164,197] Unfortunately, elastase is a broad spectrum protease that attacks many connective tissue components of the alveolar structures (see Table 3). Thus, elastic fibers play a major role in defining the mechanical properties of the lung parenchyma over most lung volumes. However, an understanding of the role of elastin in lung and its interactions with other connective tissue components will require more definitive methods.

C. Proteoglycans and Other Connective Tissue Components

Evaluation of the structure-function relationships of proteoglycans and other lung connective tissue components is very difficult because these elements are heterogeneous, present in small quantities, and poorly defined morphologically and chemically.

It is thought that proteoglycans may contribute to lung mechanical properties by their interactions with other components as well as by their inherent properties. In regard to the latter, it is thought that these components exist as large aggregates within the intracellular matrix.[5,6] Proteoglycans occupy a much larger space than expected from their mass alone, e.g., cartilage proteoglycans occupy a solution volume of 30 to 50 times their dry weight and have radii of gyration of up to 600 Å.[5,6] However, these large volumes can be compressed by displacing solvent from the molecular domain. Thus, stress placed on lung structures by changes in volume likely causes alterations of lung proteoglycans, resulting in changes in their charge density and thus in their potential intramolecular interactions. In addition to these mechanical influences, proteoglycans are thought to strongly influence early lung development and thus seem to be important in defining overall lung structure.[72] The ability of proteoglycans to take up or release large quantities of water may also influence the permeability characteristics of the alveolar structures as may the alterations in proteoglycan charge density.[45,198]

The mechanical properties of fibronectin, laminin, and anchoring fibrils are unknown. However, fibronectin probably is important in defining lung mechanical properties because of its role in mediating cell-cell and cell-matrix interactions.

VI. LUNG CONNECTIVE TISSUE IN PATHOLOGIC STATES

A. Emphysema

Emphysema is defined as dilation of air spaces with accompanying destruction of alveolar walls. The current concept of the pathogenesis of emphysema is generally referred to as the "protease-antiprotease theory". This concept holds that the lung is constantly exposed to a variety of proteases which are balanced by an antiprotease screen, the most important of which is α_1-antitrypsin. While this antiprotease screen is sufficient in most individuals, in certain circumstances it is ineffective or the protease burden is too great and lung tissue destruction results.

The evidence favoring this theory is overwhelming. Its most important support derives from the association of panacinar emphysema with α_1-antitrypsin deficiency and from the induction of emphysema by proteases in experimental animals. For details, the reader is referred to the chapter by Kuhn in this text as well as several other reviews;[191,199] we will concentrate on the changes in lung connective tissue content and metabolism in human and experimental emphysema.

Most interest in connective tissue abnormalities in emphysema has focused on the elastic fiber. There are several reasons for this, including

1. The characteristic physiologic abnormality of emphysema is loss of elastic recoil throughout the volume range (i.e., the static deflation volume-pressure curve is shifted to the left); this is consistent with a loss or break in the elastic fibers of the alveolar structures.
2. Light microscopic evaluation of human emphysematous lung demonstrates fragmentation of elastic fibers.
3. The best animal model of human emphysema results from the intratracheal instillation of elastase;[191] this model can be mimicked with other enzymes which must be capable of digesting elastin.[200]

It is important to realize, however, that no matter how compelling the indirect evidence that abnormalities in elastic fibers are central to the pathogenesis of emphysema, there are few human data that directly support this concept. There have been very few morphologic studies of emphysematous lung connective tissue at the ultrastructural level;[154,201] those that have been carried out report changes in collagen, but not elastic fibers. Most biochemical studies have failed to find alterations in elastin content in emphysematous lung.[202-206] The one exception is the study by Mandl et al.[65] in which lung elastin was diminished in the parenchyma of individuals with emphysema. It has been suggested that the elastin present in emphysematous lung may differ from normal lung elastin in amino acid content,[207-209] but such changes may reflect technical problems in isolating intact, purified elastin that is representative of the bulk of the elastic fibers present.

Although biochemical methodologies have not yielded direct evidence to support the concept that abnormalities of elastic fibers are central to the pathogenesis of this disease, this does not mean that the overall concept is incorrect. For example, derangement of elastic fiber organization might have profound effects on lung mechanical properties, yet would be very difficult to detect using current biochemical techniques.

Interestingly, morphologic observations of human emphysematous lung have suggested that alveolar interstitial collagen may be disorganized.[154] In addition, it has been hypothesized that abnormalities of proteoglycans are critical to the pathogenesis of this disorder.[210,211] However, as in the case of elastic fibers, studies of lung collagen and glycosaminoglycans in human emphysematous lungs have been inconclusive.[212]

Sequential studies of animal lungs following intratracheal administration of protease with elastolytic activity have helped clarify some of the human data. After the initial proteolytic insult, lung elastin content seems to decrease.[33,145,214,215] After several months, however, the amounts of lung elastin return to normal, but morphological evaluation suggests that this elastin is abnormal in configuration and location.[36,145,215,216] It appears therefore that the early stages of pulmonary emphysema might start with elastin degradation; this is soon followed by elastin resynthesis, but in an abnormal fashion resulting in the disorganization observed morphologically.[67,156,163] Consistent with this concept are data showing that protease-induced experimental emphysema is associated with increased urinary excretion of elastin peptides,[214] increased rates of lung elastin synthesis,[33,213,214] and marked remodeling of lung parenchyma.

Elastin is not the only connective tissue component that varies in these animals; intratracheal administration of elastase also causes changes in lung collagen content and synthesis.[33,36] Interestingly, in several studies, the collagen content of lung became greater than normal following elastase injury.[33,36] This may be secondary to the lack of specificity of elastase in injuring lung connective tissue (see Table 3) and may also reflect the chronic inflammatory response following exposure of the lung to elastase.

B. Malignancy

There is increasing evidence that many forms of malignant cells do not produce connective tissue-related components in the same manner as do normal cells. Such studies have led to new biochemical "markers" for certain tumors and have suggested possible mechanisms leading to tumor growth, invasiveness, and metastatic potential.

Glycosaminoglycans are present in collections of pleural fluid. It is generally thought that at least some of these connective tissue components are produced locally, as their concentration in pleural fluid is manyfold that of plasma, and the distribution of glycosaminoglycan types in pleural fluid is very different from that of plasma. Several studies have suggested that hyaluronic acid may be a "marker" for malignant mesothelioma.[216-218] Whereas hyaluronic acid comprises less than 70% of the total glycosaminoglycans in most categories of pleural effusion, it represents greater than 90% in cases of mesothelioma. Confirmatory evidence for this concept comes from histological[219] and biochemical[220,221] studies that demonstrate large quantities of hyaluronic acid in these pleural tumors. However, oat-cell carcinoma of the lung has also been shown to have large amounts of hyaluronic acid.[222] Thus, before pleural fluid hyaluronic acid can be considered a specific "marker" for pleural mesothelioma, much broader clinical experience is needed, particularly with pleural effusions associated with other primary and secondary thoracic malignancies and infectious diseases.

In addition to tumor-related specificities of glycosaminoglycan types, it has also been shown that different tumors produce different collagen types. Most of these data do not relate to lung, but one case of bronchogenic carcinoma has been described in which the tumor contained Type II collagen, even though presumably no cartilage was evident.[223] Although such analyses may become important in the future, there is at present no role for collagen as a marker for malignant lung cells.

It is known that several malignant cell types are characterized by a reduced production of fibronectin, the connective tissue component that plays an important role in modulating cell-cell and cell-matrix interactions. In addition, certain tumor cells seem to be able to adhere spontaneously to basement membrane components.[224] The adhesion characteristics of tumor cells, mediated by fibronectin and by other, as yet, unidentified molecules, may determine how and where tumors grow. In addition, certain tumor cells with known metastatic potential are associated with the production of a collagenase specific for Type IV collagen.[225] Since this collagen type is a major component of epithelial and endothelial basement membranes, the production of such a

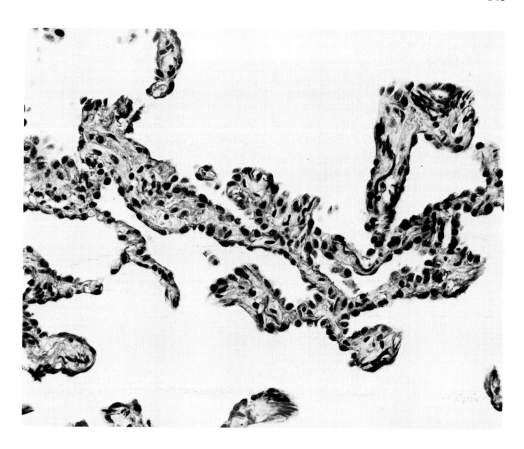

FIGURE 11. Alveolar septa in lung of patient with idiopathic pulmonary fibrosis show moderate degree of thickening by fibrous tissue. Hematoxylin and eosin stain. (Magnification × 250.)

collagenase may be important for such cells to metatasize to various organs. Although lung tumors have not as yet been studied, these concepts are universal and are likely also true for primary and secondary thoracic tumors.

C. Fibrotic Lung Disease

"Fibrosis" is a classical morphologic term used to describe the appearance of an increment in connective tissue fibers as seen with the light microscope (see Figure 11). In this regard, the "fibrotic lung diseases" are a group of heterogeneous, chronic disorders in which there is "fibrosis" of the alveolar structures. It is now known, however, that the connective tissue alterations in pulmonary fibrosis are much more complex than a simple buildup of "connective tissue fibers" and likely involve changes in the amounts, types, locations, and form of different connective tissue components. Several recent reviews[226] are available that discuss the clinical aspects of these disorders as well as the current concepts of their pathogenesis. For the present, we will summarize the overall concepts concerning lung connective tissue in these disorders.

One of the most studied human fibrotic diseases is idiopathic pulmonary fibrosis (IPF), a generally fatal disorder confined to lung in which there is chronic inflammation and progressive interstitial fibrosis.[227] Most interest in lung connective tissue in IPF has centered on collagen, as it is collagen fibers that appear to comprise the majority of what is morphologically assessed as "fibrosis". However, biochemical analyses of biopsies of human lung from patients with IPF have failed to demonstrate increases in collagen content.[194] This may be related to how biopsy data are expressed (e.g., amount of collagen/dry weight may give a false impression of collagen per alveolus). Alternatively, the fact that collagen content is normal may be a reflection of a rearrangement of collagen, analogous to the rearrangement of elastic fibers in emphysema. Consistent with the latter concept, transmission electron micrographs of IPF lung show collagen fibers that are randomly arrayed, twisted, frayed and in abnormal locations.[228] In addition, there is a difference in the types of collagen present in the IPF lung compared to the normal lung; in IPF, the normal 2:1 ratio of collagen Types I and III is increased to 4:1.[27] Since Type I collagen fibers are known to possess a high tensile strength, a proportional increase in Type I collagen is consistent with the decreased lung compliance found in these patients.

Recent studies have begun to shed light on the mechanism whereby lung collagen in IPF becomes deranged. Although lung collagen production is normal,[194] it is probably being laid down in abnormal locations as a result of topographic derangements in the collagen-producing cells. Most of the cells comprising the IPF lung appear to be intrinsically normal, but there is likely a change in the relative numbers of each cell type that are present. If so, the types of collagens produced may reflect the relative proportions of the different types of collagen-producing cells rather than changes in the properties of the cells themselves. In addition, the IPF lung contains an active collagenase.[229] Thus, some of the lung connective tissue abnormalities in this disease are likely mediated by destructive processes followed by resynthesis of collagens in the incorrect proportions and locations, resulting in the derangements in connective tissue that are characteristic of the disease.

In an effort to better understand what lung "fibrosis" is and how it occurs, a number of animal models of pulmonary fibrosis have been developed. The most widely used experimental models are induced by bleomycin (an antineoplastic agent in common clinical use),[22,37,158,159,187,188,230-237] paraquat (a powerful oxidant used as a herbicide),[40,94,106,160,161,240-246] and radiation (usually external X-ray).[13,20,29,30,35,150,247-255] Other experimental models in use include those induced in vivo by N-nitroso-N-methylurethane,[120,157,256,257] inhaled inorganic dusts (e.g., silica, asbestos, and beryllium),[173,258-263] toxic gases (ozone,[162] high concentrations of oxygen,[28,91-93,169,264-269] and nitrogen dioxide),[155,270-273] cigarette smoke,[274,275] and a variety of immunologic insults.[151,152,276-286] With these models, investigators have quantitated the amount, type, production and destruction of various lung connective tissue components as a function of time after insult, dose, and modification by different therapeutic agents. Similar approaches have been utilized in evaluating simplified in vitro models of pulmonary fibrosis. From such studies, the following generalizations can be made:

1. Collagen is not the only component of connective tissue that changes following such insults, e.g., elastin and glycosaminoglycan content may change as well.
2. Shifts in types of connective tissue within a certain class (e.g., proportionally more Type I collagen) may be missed if only total collagen is measured.
3. Measurements of rates of synthesis may be normal even when newly synthesized connective tissue is being laid down in a markedly deranged manner, i.e., biochemical methodologies are generally insensitive to anatomic changes.
4. Although theoretically possible, it is very difficult to inhibit the production of lung collagen without causing significant side effects in other collagen-producing organs, i.e., the known agents that interfere with collagen production are not selective for the organ that is becoming fibrotic.
5. Following an insult that results in pulmonary fibrosis, there seems to be an increase in collagen destruction as well as production.
6. Although some fibrosis-producing agents are directly toxic to lung cells (e.g., bleomycin), almost all forms of pulmonary fibrosis are biologically complex and are mediated through effector cells of the inflammatory and immune systems.

7. Once fibrosis occurs within a group of alveoli, it is very unlikely that those alveoli will ever return to normal, i.e., while the progression of fibrosis might be halted, the actual removal of the "fibrosis" is highly improbable.

8. Current methodologies to assess the extent of lung fibrosis are relatively insensitive and not very specific. Thus, routine physiologic parameters may be normal even in the presence of known fibrosis. Alternatively, routine physiologic tests may be abnormal when there is little fibrosis, but a great deal of inflammation.

VII. FUTURE APPROACHES

The basic knowledge of lung connective tissue has now been garnered, but there is much to be done. Over the next several years, more information will develop concerning the details of each class of connective tissue, particularly elastic fibers, proteoglycans, and other glycoproteins of the extracellular matrix. Along with cataloging the amount, type, form, and location of each component, it will be necessary to detail the contribution of each cell type in synthesizing, assembling, and destroing these macromolecules. It is only after such information is available that "breakthroughs" will be made in understanding the structure and function of lung in health and in important diseases, such as emphysema and pulmonary fibrosis.

REFERENCES

1. Hance, A. I. and Crystal, R. G., The connective tissue of lung, *Am. Rev. Respir. Dis.,* 112, 657, 1975.
2. Bornstein, P. and Traub, W., The chemistry and biology of collagen, in *The Proteins,* Vol. 4, Neurath, H. and Hiln, R. L., Eds., Academic Press, New York, 1979, 412.
3. Rucker, R. B. and Tinker, D., Structure and metabolism of arterial elastin, *Int. Rev. Exp. Pathol.,* 17, 1, 1977.
4. Gray, W. R. and Franzblau, C., Eds., *Elastin and Elastic Tissue,* Plenum Press, New York, 1977.
5. Hascall, V. C., Interaction of cartilage proteoglycans with hyaluronic acid, *J. Supramol. Struct.,* 7, 101, 1977.
6. Hascall, V. C. and Heinegard, D. K., Structure of cartilage proteoglycans, in *Glycoconjugate Research,* Vol. 1, Academic Press, New York, 1979, 341.
7. Green, H. and Goldberg, B., Collagen and cell protein synthesis by an established mammalian fibroblast line, *Nature (London),* 204, 347, 1964.
8. Reid, K. B. M. and Porter, R. R., Subunit structure and structure of subcomponent CIq of the first component of human complement, *Biochem. J.,* 155, 19, 1976.
9. Bhattacharyya, S. N., Passero, M. A., DiAugustine, R. P., and Lynn, W. S., Isolation and characterization of two hydroxyproline-containing glycoproteins from normal animal lung lavage and lamellar bodies, *J. Clin. Invest.,* 55, 914, 1975.
10. Bhattacharyya, S. N., Rose, M. C., Lynn, M. G., MacLeod, C., Alberts, M., and Lynn, W. S., Isolation and characterization of a unique glycoprotein from lavage of chicken lungs and lamellar organelles, *Am. Rev. Respir. Dis.,* 114, 843, 1976.
11. Rosenberry, T. and Richardson, J., Structure of 18S and 14S acetylcholinesterase, *Biochemistry,* 16, 3550, 1977.
12. Bradley, K. H., McConnell, S. D., and Crystal, R. G., Lung collagen composition and synthesis: characterization and changes with age, *J. Biol. Chem.,* 249, 2674, 1974.
13. Law, M. P., Hornsey, S., and Field, S. B., Collagen content of lungs of mice after X-ray irradiation, *Radiat. Res.,* 65, 60, 1976.
14. Bradley, K., Breul, S., and Crystal, R. G., Collagen in the human lung composition and quantitation of rates of synthesis, *J. Clin. Invest.,* 55, 543, 1975.

15. Pickrell, J. A. and Shafer, J., Lung connective tissue measurements. I. Amino acid analysis procedures for determination of canine lung connective tissue, *Arch. Intern. Med.*, 127, 891, 1971.
16. Hoffman, L., Blumenfeld, O. O., Mondshine, R. B., and Park, S. S., Effect of d-penicillamine on fibrous protein of rat lung, *J. Appl. Physiol.*, 33, 42, 1972.
17. Chrapil, M., Bartos, D., and Bartos, F., Effect of long-term stress on collagen growth in the lung, heart, and femur of young and adult rats, *Gerontologia*, 19, 263, 1973.
18. Juřicová, M. and Deyl, Z., Ageing processes in collagen from different tissues of rats, *Adv. Exp. Med. Biol.*, 53, 351, 1975.
19. Hurst, D. J., Kilburn, K. H., and Baker, W. M., Normal newborn and adult human lung collagen, *Connect. Tissue Res.*, 5, 117, 1977.
20. Collins, J. F., Jones, M. A., and Durnin, L. S., Collagen content and synthesis in the lungs of normal baboon and in baboon with experimental pulmonary fibrosis, *Tex. J. Sci.*, Spec. Publ. 3, 127, 1977.
21. Collins, J. F. and Jones, M. A., Connective tissue proteins of the baboon lung: concentration, content and synthesis of collagen in the normal lung, *Connect. Tissue Res.*, 5, 211, 1978.
22. Starcher, B. C., Kuhn, C., and Overton, J. E., Increased elastin and collagen content in the lungs of hamsters receiving an intratracheal injection of bleomycin, *Am. Rev. Respir. Dis.*, 117, 299, 1978.
23. Seethanathan, P., Radhakrishnamurthy, B., Dalferes, E. R., Jr., and Berenson, G. S., The composition of connective tissue macromolecules from bovine respiratory system, *Respir. Physiol.*, 24, 347, 1975.
24. Francis, G. and Thomas, J., Isolated and chemical characterization of collagen in bovine pulmonary tissues, *Biochem. J.*, 145, 287, 1975.
25. Seyer, J. M., Basement membrane associated collagens of human lung, *Fed. Proc. Fed. Am. Soc. Exp. Biol.*, 37, 1527, 1978.
26. Madri, J. A. and Furthmayr, H., Isolation and tissue localization of type AB_2 collagen from normal lung parenchyma, *Am. J. Pathol.*, 94, 323, 1979.
27. Seyer, J. M., Hutcheson, E. T., and Kang, A. H., Collagen polymorphism in idiopathic chronic pulmonary fibrosis, *J. Clin. Invest.*, 57, 1498, 1976.
28. Richmond, V. and D'Aoust, B. G., Effects of intermittent hyperbaric oxygen on guinea pig lung elastin and collagen, *J. Appl. Physiol.*, 41, 295, 1976.
29. Pickrell, J. A., Schnizlein, C. T., Hahn, F. F., Snipes, M. B., and Jones, R. K., Radiation-induced pulmonary fibrosis: study of changes in collagen constituents in different lung regions of beagle dogs after inhalation of beta-emitting radionuclides, *Radiat. Res.*, 74, 363, 1978.
30. Thyagarajan, P., Vakil, U. K., and Sreenivasan, A., Effects of wholebody X-irradiation on some aspects of collagen metabolism in the rat, *Radiat. Res.*, 66, 576, 1976.
31. Szemenyei, C. and Bálint, A., Studies on the ageing process of the rat lung, *Acta Morphol. Acad. Sci. Hung.*, 21, 295, 1973.
32. Goldstein, R. H., Faris, B., Hu, C-L., Snider, G. L., and Franzblau, C., The fate of newly synthesized lung collagen after endotracheal administration of ^{14}C-proline to hamsters, *Am. Rev. Respir. Dis.*, 117, 281, 1978.
33. Kuhn, C., Yu, S.-Y., Chraplyvy, M., Linder, H. E., and Senior, R. M., The induction of emphysema with elastase. II. Changes in connective tissue, *Lab. Invest.*, 34, 372, 1976.
34. Crystal, R. G., Lung collagen. Definition, diversity, and development, *Fed. Proc. Fed. Am. Soc. Exp. Biol.*, 33, 2248, 1974.
35. Pickrell, J. A., Harris, D. V., Pfleger, R. C., Benjamin, S. A., Belasich, J. J., Jones, R. K., and McClellan, R. O., Biological alterations resulting from chronic lung irradiation, *Radiat. Res.*, 63, 299, 1975.
36. Yu, S. Y. and Keller, N. R., Synthesis of lung collagen in hamsters with elastase-induced emphysema, *Exp. Mol. Pathol.*, 29, 37, 1978.
37. Fedullo, A. J., Karlinsky, J. B., Snider, G. L., and Goldstein, R. H., Biochemical and mechanical effects of penicillamine on normal and bleomycin fibrotic hamster lungs, *Am. Rev. Respir. Dis.* 119 (4, Part 2), 307, 1979.
38. Bradley, K., Breul, S., and Crystal, R. G., Lung collagen heterogeneity, *Proc. Natl. Acad. Sci. U.S.A.*, 71, 2828, 1974.
39. Madri, J. A. and Furthmayr, H., Collagen polymorphism in the lung: an immunochemical study during the early and late stages of pulmonary fibrosis, *Fed. Proc. Fed. Am. Soc. Exp. Biol.*, 38 (3, Part 2), 1407, 1979.
40. Reiser, K. M., Greenberg, D. B., and Last, J. A., Type I/Type III collagen ratios in lungs of rats with experimental pulmonary fibrosis, *Fed. Proc. Fed. Am. Soc. Exp. Biol.*, 38 (3, Part 1), 817, 1979.
41. Huang, T. W., Carlson, J. R., Bray, T. M., and Bradley, B. J., 3-Methyl-indole-induced pulmonary injury in goats, *Am. J. Pathol.*, 87, 647, 1977.
42. Fullmer, H. M., The histochemistry of the connective tissues, *Int. Rev. Connect. Tissue Res.*, 3, 1, 1965.

43. Pierce, J. A., The elastic tissue of the lung, in *The Lung*, Liebow, A. A. and Smith, D. E., Eds., Williams & Wilkins, Baltimore, 1968, 41.

44. Fung, Y. C. B., Sobin, S. S., Lindal, R. G., Tremer, H. M., Bernick, S., Wall, R., and Karspick, M., The connective tissue of the interalveolar wall, *Fed. Proc. Fed. Am. Soc. Exp. Biol.*, 38, (3, Part 2), 1235, 1979.

45. Low, F. N., Lung interstitium: development, morphology, fluid content, in *Lung Water and Solute Exchange*, Vol. 7, Staub, N. C., Ed., Marcel Dekker, New York, 1978, 17.

46. Strawich, E. and Nimni, M. E., Properties of a collagen molecule containing three identical components extracted from bovine articular cartilage, *Biochemistry*, 10, 3905, 1971.

47. McLees, B. D., Schleiter, G., and Pinnell, S. R., Isolation of Type III collagen from human adult parenchymal lung tissue, *Biochemistry*, 16, 185, 1977.

48. Nowack, H., Gay, S., Wick, G., Becker, V., and Timpl, R., Preparation and use in immunohistology of antibodies specific for type I and II collagen and procollagen, *J. Immunol. Methods*, 12, 117, 1976.

49. Glanville, R. W., Ranter, A., and Fietzek, P. P., Isolation and characterization of a native placental basement membrane collagen and its component α-chains, *Eur. J. Biochem.*, 95, 383, 1979.

50. Crouch, E. and Bornstein, P., Characterization of a type IV procollagen synthesized by human amniotic fluid cells in culture, *J. Biol. Chem.*, 254, 4197, 1979.

51. Burgeson, R. E., El Adli, F. A., Kaitila, I. I., and Hollister, D. W., Fetal membrane collagens: identification of two new collagen alpha chains, *Proc. Natl. Acad. Sci. U.S.A.*, 73, 2579, 1976.

52. Kefalides, N. A., Structure and biosynthesis of basement membranes, *Int. Rev. Connect. Tissue Res.*, 6, 63, 1973.

53. Seyer, J., Isolation and Characterization of Type I, III, IV, V Collagens of Porcine Lung, personal communication.

54. Davison, P. F. and Cannon, D. J., Heterogeneity of collagens from basement membranes of lens and cornea, *Exp. Eye Res.*, 25, 129, 1977.

55. Keith, D. A., Paz, M. A., and Gallop, P. M., Characterization of two types of elastin from bovine tissues, in 11th Int. Congr. Biochem., 1979, 215.

56. Paz, M. A., Keith, D. A., Traverso, H. P., and Gallop, P. M., Isolation, purification and crosslinking profiles of elastin from lung and aorta, *Biochemistry*, 15, 4912, 1976.

57. Ross, R. and Bornstein, P., The elastic fiber, *J. Cell Biol.*, 40, 366, 1969.

58. Robert, B., Szigeti, M., Derouette, J.-C., Robert, L., Bouissom, H., and Fabre, M. T., Studies on the nature of the ''microfibrillar'' component of elastic fibers, *Eur. J. Biochem.*, 21, 507, 1971.

59. Albert, E. N. and Fleischer, E., A new electron-dense stain for elastic tissue, *J. Histochem. Cytochem.*, 18, 697, 1970.

60. Brissie, R. M., Spicer, S. S., Hall, B. J., and Thompson, N. T., Ultrastructural staining of thin sections with iron hematoxylin, *J. Histochem. Cytochem.*, 22, 895, 1974.

61. Adnet, J.-J., Pinteaux, A., Pousse, G., and Caulet, T., Caracterisation du tissu elastique normal et pathologique en microscopie electronique (Sur coupes semi-fines et coupes fines), *Pathol. Biol. (Paris)*, 24, 293, 1976.

62. Kajikawa, K., Yamaguchi, T., Katsuda, S., and Miwa, A., An improved electron stain for elastic fibers using tannic acid, *J. Electron Microcs. (Tokyo)*, 24, 287, 1975.

63. Lansing, A. I., Rosenthal, T. B., Alex, M., and Dempsey, E. W., The structure and chemical characterization of elastic fibers as revealed by elastase and by electron microscopy, *Anat. Rec.*, 114, 555, 1952.

64. O'Dell, B. L., Kilburn, K. H., McKenzie, W. N., and Thurston, R. J., The lung of the copper-deficient rat, *Am. J. Pathol.*, 91, 413, 1978.

65. Mandl, I., Darnule, T. V., Fierer, J. A., Keller, S., and Turino, G. M., Elastin degradation in human and experimental emphysema, in *Elastin and Elastic Tissue*, Sandberg, L. B., Gray, W. R., and Franzblau, C., Eds., Plenum Press, New York, 1977, 221.

66. Collins, J. F., Durnin, L. S., and Johanson, W. G., Jr., Papain-induced lung injury: alterations in connective tissue metabolism without emphysema, *Exp. Mol. Pathol.*, 29, 29, 1978.

67. Yu, S. Y., Sun, C. N., and Still, M. F., Ultrastructural changes of elastic tissue in hamster lung during elastase-emphysema, in *Elastin and Elastic Tissue*, Sandberg, L. B., Gray, W. R., and Franzblau, C., Eds., Plenum Press, New York, 1977, 39.

68. Jones, A. W. and Barson, A. J., Elastogenesis in the developing chick lung: a light and electron microscopical study, *J. Anat.*, 110, 1, 1971.

69. Keeley, F. W., Fagan, D. G., and Webster, S. I., Quantity and character of elastin in developing human lung parenchymal tissues of normal infants and infants with respiratory distress syndrome, *J. Lab. Clin. Med.*, 90, 981, 1977.

70. Luna, C. G., *Manual of Histologic Staining Methods of the Armed Forces Institute of Pathology*, McGraw-Hill, New York, 1968.

71. **Luft, J. H.,** Ruthenium red and violet. II. Fine structural localization in animal tissues, *Anat. Rec.,* 171, 369, 1971.
72. **Horwitz, A.** and **Crystal, R. G.,** Content and synthesis of glycosaminoglycans in the developing lung, *J. Clin. Invest.,* 56, 1312, 1975.
73. **Ehrlich, K., Seethanathan, P.,** and **Taylor, P.,** Isolation of proteoglycans from lung tissue, *Fed. Proc. Fed. Am. Soc. Exp. Biol.,* 38 (3, Part 1), 653, 1979.
74. **Breen, M., Weinstein, H. G.,** and **Blacik, L. J.,** Rat lung proteoglycans, *Fed. Proc. Fed. Am. Soc. Exp. Biol.,* 38 (3, Part 1), 652, 1979.
75. **Radhakrishnamurthy, B., Dalferes, E. R., Jr.,** and **Berenson, G. S.,** Isoalation of proteoglycans from bovine respiratory system, in 11th Int. Congr. Biochem., 170, 1979.
76. **Radhakrishnamurthy, B., Dalferes, E. R.,** and **Berenson, G. S.,** Isolation and characterization of proteoglycans from bovine lung, *Fed. Proc. Fed. Am. Soc. Exp. Biol.,* 38, (3, Part 1), 652, 1979.
77. **Sahu, S.** and **Lynn, W. S.,** Isolation and characterization of proteoglycans from porcine lung, *J. Biol. Chem.,* 254, 4262, 1979.
78. **Hassell, J., Gehron-Robey, P., Barrach, H. J., Wilczek, J., Rennard, S.,** and **Martin, G. R.,** Basement membrane proteoglycan, in *Proc. 5th Int. Symp. Glycoconjugates Kidney,* 1979.
79. **Yamada, K.** and **Olden, K.,** Fibronectins — adhesive glycoproteins of cell surface and blood, *Nature (London),* 275, 179, 1978.
80. **Vaheri, A.** and **Mosher, D. F.,** High molecular weight glycoprotein (fibronectin) lost in molecular transformation, *Biochim. Biophys. Acta,* 516, 1, 1978.
81. **Kleinman, H., Klebe, R. J.,** and **Martin, G. R.,** Role of Collagenous Matrices in the Adhesion and Growth of Cells, submitted.
82. **Bray, B. A.,** Cold insoluble globulin (Fibronectin) in connective tissues of adult human lung and in trophoblast basement membrane, *J. Clin. Invest.,* 62, 745, 1978.
83. **Stenman, S.** and **Vaheri, A.,** Distribution of a major connective tissue protein, fibronectin, in normal human tissues, *J. Exp. Med.,* 147, 1054, 1978.
84. **Chung, A. E., Jaffe, R., Freeman, I. L., Vergnes, J. P., Braginski, J. E.,** and **Carlin, B.,** Properties of a basement membrane related glycoprotein synthesized in culture by a mouse embryonal carcinoma derived cell line, *Cell,* 16, 277, 1979.
85. **Timpl, R., Rhode, H., Gehron-Robey, P., Rennard, S., Foidart, J-M.,** and **Martin, G. R.,** Laminin — a glycoprotein from basement membranes, *J. Biol. Chem.,* 254, 9933, 1979.
86. **Foidart, J-M., Bere, E. W., Yaar, M., Rennard, S., Gullino, M., Martin, G. R.,** and **Katz, S. I.,** Distribution and immunoelectron microscopic localization of laminin, a noncollagenous basement membrane glycoprotein, *Lab. Invest.,* in press.
87. **Kawanami, O., Ferrans, V. J.,** and **Crystal, R. G.,** Anchoring fibrils in normal canine respiratory system, *Am. Rev. Respir. Dis.,* 120, 595, 1979.
88. **Newman, R. A.** and **Langrer, R. O.,** Age related changes in the synthesis of connective tissues in the rabbit, *Connect. Tissue Res.,* 3, 231, 1975.
89. **Pierce, J. A., Resnick, H.,** and **Henry, P. H.,** Collagen and elastin metabolism in the lungs, skin, and bones of adult rats, *J. Lab. Clin. Med.,* 69, 485, 1967.
90. **Métivier, H., Legendre, N., Dewaele, J.,** and **Masse, R.,** Renouvellment du collagene pulmonaire insoluble chez le rat adulte, *C. R. Acad. Sci. (Paris),* 287, 1341, 1978.
91. **Bhatnagar, R. S., Hussain, M. Z., Streifel, J. A., Tolentino, M.,** and **Enriquez, B.,** Alteration of collagen synthesis in lung organ cultures by hyperoxic environments, *Biochem. Biophys. Res. Commun.,* 83, 392, 1978.
92. **Hussain, M. Z., Streifel, J. A., Tolentino, M., Enriquez, B.,** and **Bhatnagar, R. S.,** Macromolecular synthesis in lung organ cultures in high O_2 atmosphere, *Fed. Proc. Fed. Am. Soc. Exp. Biol.,* 37, 1529, 1978.
93. **Hussain, M. Z., Belton, J. C.,** and **Bhatnagar, R. S.,** Macromolecular synthesis in organ cultures of neonatal rat lung, *In Vitro,* 14, 740, 1978.
94. **Greenberg, D. B., Lyons, S. A.,** and **Last, J. A.,** Paraquat induced changes in the rate of collagen biosynthesis by rat lung explants, *J. Lab. Clin. Med.,* 92, 1033, 1978.
95. **Hance, A. J., Bradley, K.,** and **Crystal, R. G.,** Lung collagen heterogeneity. Synthesis of type I and III collagen by rabbit and human lung cells in culture, *J. Clin. Invest.,* 57, 102, 1976.
96. **Collins, J. F.** and **Crystal, R. G.,** Characterization of cell-free synthesis of collagen by lung polysomes in a heterologous system, *J. Biol. Chem.,* 250, 7332, 1975.
97. **Cowan, M. J.** and **Crystal, R. G.,** Lung growth after unilateral pneumonectomy: quantitation of collagen synthesis and content, *Am. Rev. Respir. Dis.,* 111, 267, 1975.
98. **Takeda, T., Suzuki, Y.,** and **Yao, C. S.,** Experimental studies on the effect of ageing and endocrine control on collagen formation in various organs, *Acta Pathol. Jpn.,* 25, 135, 1975.
99. **Morishige, W. K.** and **Uetake, C. A.,** Receptors for androgen and estrogen in the rat lung, *Endocrinology,* 102, 1827, 1978.

100. Hemberger, J. A. and Shanker, L. S., Effect of thyroxine on permeability of the neonatal rat lung to drugs, *Biol. Neonate*, 34, 299, 1978.

101. Ooshima, A., Fuller, G. C., Cardinale, G. J., Spector, S., and Udenfriend, S., Reduction of collagen biosynthesis in blood vessels and other tissues by reserpine and hypophysectomy, *Proc. Natl. Acad. Sci. U.S.A.*, 74, 777, 1977.

102. Moss, J., Berg, R. A., Baum, B. J., and Crystal, R. G., In vitro model for fibrosis induced by β-adrenergic blockers: propranolol inhibits β-adrenergic suppression of collagen production of human fibroblasts, *Clin. Res.*, 27, 445a, 1979.

103. Moss, J., Berg, R. A., Baum, B. J., and Crystal, R. G., Etiology of β-Adrenergic Blocker-Induced Fibrosis: Loss of Suppression of Collagen Production by β-Adrenergic Agents, submitted.

104. Baum, B. J., Moss, J., Breul, S. D., and Crystal, R. G., Association in normal human fibroblasts of elevated levels of adenosine 3′:4′-monophosphate with a selective decrease in collagen production, *J. Biol. Chem.*, 253, 3391, 1978.

105. Kulonen, E., Aalto, M., Aho, S., Lehtinen, P., and Potila, M., The excessive proliferation of the connective tissue as a medical problem, Int. Symp. on Biology of Collagen, Aarhus, 1978.

106. Last, J. A. and Greenberg, D. B., Synthesis of type IV collagen by rat lungs in vitro, in Int. Congr. Biochem., Toronto, Canada, 1979, 696.

107. Fulmer, J., Elson, N., Bradley, K., Ferrans, V., and Crystal, R. G., Comparison of type-specific collagens synthesized by lung epithelial and mesenchymal cells, *Clin. Res.*, 25, 503A, 1977.

108. Howard, B. V., Macarak, E. J., Gunson, D., and Kefalides, N. A., Characterization of the collagen synthesized by endothelial cells in culture, *Proc. Natl. Acad. Sci. U.S.A.*, 73, 2361, 1976.

109. Jaffe, E. A., Minick, R., Adelman, B., Becker, C. G., and Nachman, R., Synthesis of basement membrane collagen by cultured human endothelial cells, *J. Exp. Med.*, 144, 209, 1976.

110. Barnes, M. J., Morton, L. F., and Levene, C. I., Synthesis of interstitial collagens by pig aortic endothelial cells in culture, *Biochem. Biophys. Res. Commun.*, 84, 646, 1978.

111. Burke, J., Balian, G., Ross, R., and Bornstein, P., Synthesis of types I and III procollagen and collagen by monkey aortic smooth muscle cells in vitro, *Biochemistry*, 16, 3243, 1977.

112. Layman, D. L., Epstein, E. H., Jr., Dodson, R. F., and Titus, J. F., Biosynthesis of type I and III collagens by cultured smooth muscle cells from human aorta, *Proc. Natl. Acad. Sci. U.S.A.*, 74, 671, 1977.

113. Mayne, R., Schlitz, J. R., and Holtzer, H., Some overt and covert properties of chondrogenic cells, in *Biology of Fibroblast*, Kulonen, E. and Pikkarainen, J., Eds., Academic Press, New York, 1973, 61.

114. Elson, N. A., Karlinsky, J. B., Kelman, J. A., Rhoades, R. A., and Crystal, R. G., Differentiated properties of the type 2 alveolar cell: partial characterization of protein content, synthesis and secretion, *Clin. Res.*, 24, 464A, 1976.

115. Davidson, J., personal communication.

116. Cantor, J. O., Parshley, M. S., Mandl, I., Keller, S., Darnule, T. V., Darnule, A. T., and Turino, G. M., Synthesis of elastin by a clone of rat lung endothelial cells, *J. Cell Biol.*, 79, 153a, 1978.

117. Ross R., The smooth muscle cell. II. Growth of smooth muscle in culture and formation of elastic fibers, *J. Cell Biol.*, 50, 172, 1971.

118. Ross, R. and Klebanoff, S. J., The smooth muscle cell. I. In vivo synthesis of connective tissue proteins, *J. Cell Biol.*, 50, 159, 1971.

119. De Luca, L. and Wolf, G., Effect of vitamin A on the mucopolysaccharides of lung tissue, *Arch. Biochem. Biophys.*, 123, 1, 1968.

120. Cantor, J. O., Bray, B., Ryan, S., Mandl, I., and Turino, G. M., Glycosaminoglycan and collagen synthesis in an animal model of pulmonary fibrosis, *Fed. Proc. Fed. Am. Soc. Exp. Biol.*, 38, 1373a, 1979.

121. Sampson, P., Parshley, M. S., Mandl, I., and Turino, G. M., Glycosaminoglycans produced in tissue culture by rat lung cells. Isolation from a mixed cell line and a derived endothelial clone, *Connect. Tissue Res.*, 4, 41, 1975.

122. Sjoberg, I. and Fransson, L., Synthesis of glycosaminoglycans by human embryonic lung fibroblasts, *Biochem. J.*, 167, 383, 1977.

123. Castor, C. W., Heiss, P. R., Gray, R. H., and Seidman, J. C., Connective tissue formation by lung fibroblasts in vitro, *Am. Rev. Respir. Dis.*, 120, 107, 1979.

124. Trelstad, R. L., Hayashi, K., and Toole, B. P., Epithelial collagens and glycosaminoglycans in the embryonic cornea, *J. Cell Biol.*, 62, 815, 1974.

125. Jarmolych, J., Daoud, A. S., Landan, J., Fritz, K. E., and McEluene, E., Aortic medial explants. Cell proliferation and production of mucopolysaccharides, collagen, and elastic tissue, *Exp. Mol. Pathol.*, 9, 171, 1968.

126. Castor, C. W., Wilson, S. M., Heiss, P. R., and Seidman, J. C., Activation of lung connective tissue cells in vitro, *Am. Rev. Respir. Dis.*, 120, 101, 1979.

127. Baum, B. J., McDonald, J. A., and Crystal, R. G., Metabolic fate of major cell surface protein of normal human fibroblasts, *Biochem. Biophys. Res. Commum.*, 79, 8, 1977.

128. Birdwell, C. R., Gospodarowicz, D., and Nicholson, G. L., Identification, localization and role of fibronectin in cultured bovine endothelial cells, *Proc. Natl. Acad. Sci. U.S.A.*, 75, 3273, 1978.

129. Chen, L. B., Maitland, N., Gallimore, P. H., and McDougal, J. K., Detection of the large external transformation sensitive protein on some epithelial cells, *Exp. Cell Res.*, 106, 39, 1977.

130. Burke, J. M. and Ross, R., Synthesis of connective tissue macromolecules by smooth muscle, *Int. Res. Connect. Tissue Res.*, 8, 119, 1979.

131. Sasse, J., Timpl, R., Dessan, W., Jilek, F., and von der Mark, K., Synthesis and secretion of fibronectin by chondrocytes in vitro, *J. Cell Biol.*, 79, 342, 1978.

132. Harris, E. D., Jr. and Cartwright, E. C., Mammalian collagenases, in *Proteases in Mammalian Cells and Tissues*, Barrett, A. J., Ed., North-Holland, Amsterdam, 1977, 249.

133. Kleinman, H. K., McGoodwin, E. B., Martin, G. R., Klebe, R. J., Fietzek, P. P., and Wooley, D. E., Localization of the binding site for cell attachment in the $\alpha 1(I)$ chain of collagen, *J. Biol. Chem.*, 253, 5642, 1978.

134. Horwitz, A. and Crystal, R. G., Collagenase from rabbit pulmonary alveolar macrophages, *Biochem. Biophys. Res. Commun.*, 69, 296, 1976.

135. Kelman, J., Brin, S., Horwitz, A., Bradley, K., Hance, A., Breul, S., Baum, B., and Crystal, R., Collagen synthesis and collagenase production by human lung fibroblasts, *Am. Rev. Respir. Dis.*, 115, 343, 1977.

136. Horwitz, A. L., Hance, A. J., and Crystal, R. G., Granulocyte collagenase: selective digestion of Type I over Type III collagen, *Proc. Natl. Acad. Sci. U.S.A.*, 74, 897, 1977.

137. Liotta, L., Abe, S., Robey, P. G., and Martin, G. R., Preferential digestion of basement membrane collagen by a metastatic tumor, *Proc. Natl. Acad. Sci. U.S.A.*, 76, 2268, 1979.

138. Wright, D. G., Kelman, J. A., Gallin, J. I., and Crystal, R. G., Extracellular release by human neutrophils (PMN's) of a latent collagenase stored in the specific (secondary) granules, *Clin. Res.*, 26, 387a, 1978.

139. Horwitz, A. L., Kelman, J. A., and Crystal, R. G., Activation of alveolar macrophage collagenase by a neutral protease secreted by the same cell, *Nature (London)*, 264, 772, 1976.

140. Jones, J. M., Creeth, J. M., and Kekwick, R. A., Third reduction of human α_2-macroglobulin, *Biochem. J.*, 127, 187, 1972.

141. Mosher, D., Saksela, O., and Vaheri, A., Synthesis and secretion of alpha-2-macroglobulin by cultured adherent lung cell, *J. Clin. Invest.*, 60, 1036, 1977.

142. Eisen, A. Z., Bloch, K. J., and Sakai, T., Inhibition of human skin collagenase by human serum, *J. Lab. Clin. Med.*, 75, 258, 1970.

143. Woolley, D. E., Roberts, D. R., and Evanson, J. M., Small molecular B_1 serum protein which specifically inhibits human collagenases, *Nature (London)*, 261, 325, 1976.

144. Bienkowski, R. S., Baum, B. J., and Crystal, R. B., Fibroblasts degrade significant proportions of newly synthesized collagen within the cell prior to secretion, *Nature (London)*, 276, 413, 1978.

145. Senior, R. M., Tegner, H., Kuhn, C., Ohlsson, K., Starcher, B. C., and Pierce, J. A., The induction of pulmonary emphysema with human leucocyte elastase, *Am. Rev. Respir. Dis.*, 116, 469, 1977.

146. Janoff, A., Sloan, B., Weinbaum, G., Damiano, V., Sandhaus, A., Elias, J., and Kimbel, P., Experimental emphysema induced with purified human neutrophil elastase: tissue localization of the instilled protease, *Am. Rev. Respir. Dis.*, 115, 461, 1977.

147. Starkey, P. M., Elastase and cathepsin G; the serine proteinases of human neutrophil leucocytes and spleen, in *Proteinases in Mammalian Cells and Tissues*, Barrett, A. J., Ed., North-Holland, Amsterdam, 1977, 57.

148. MacDonald, J., Baum, B., Rosenberg, D., Kelman, J. A., Brin, S. C., and Crystal, R. G., Destruction of a major extracellular adhesive glycoprotein (fibronectin) of human fibroblasts by neutral proteases from polymorphonuclear leucocyte granules, *Lab. Invest.*, 40, 350, 1979.

149. Rifkin, D. B., Plasminogen activator synthesis by cultured human embryonic lung cells: characterization of the suppressive effect of corticosteroids, *J. Cell. Physiol.*, 97, 421, 1978.

150. Phillips, T. L., An ultrastructural study of the development of radiation injury in the lung, *Radiology*, 87, 49, 1966.

151. Lavietes, M. H., Min, B., Hagstrom, J. W. C., and Rochester, D. F., Diffuse pulmonary granulomatous disease in the dog, *Am. Rev. Respir. Dis.*, 116, 907, 1977.

152. Burrell, R., Flaherty, D. K., DeNee, P. B., Abraham, J. L., and Gelderman, A. H., The effect of lung antibody on normal lung structure and function, *Am. Rev. Respir. Dis.*, 109, 106, 1974.

153. Huang, T. W., Composite epithelial and endothelial basal laminas in human lungs, *Am. J. Pathol.*, 93, 681, 1978.

154. Belton, J. C., Crise, N., McLaughlin, R. F., and Tueller, E. E., Ultrastructural alterations in collagen associated with microscopic foci of human emphysema, *Hum. Pathol.*, 8, 669, 1977.

155. Hugod, C., Ultrastructural changes of the rabbit lung after a 5 ppm nitric oxide exposure, *Arch. Environ. Health,* 34, 12, 1979.

155a. Hugod, C., Effect of exposure to 43 ppm nitric oxide and 3.6 ppm nitrogen dioxide on rabbit lung. A light and electromicroscopic study, *Int. Arch. Occup. Environ. Health,* 42, 159, 1979.

156. Kuhn, C., and Tavassoli, F., The scanning electron microscopy of elastase-induced emphysema. A comparison with emphysema in man, *Lab. Invest.,* 34, 2, 1976.

157. Barrett, C. R., Bell, A. L. L., Jr., and Ryan, S. F., Alveolar epithelial injury causing respiratory distress in dogs, *Chest,* 75, 705, 1979.

158. Jones, A. W., Bleomycin lung damage: the pathology and nature of the lesion, *Br. J. Dis. Chest,* 72, 321, 1978.

159. Aso, Y., Yoneda, K., and Kikkawa, Y., Morphologic and biochemical study of pulmonary changes induced by bleomycin in mice, *Lab. Invest.,* 35, 558, 1976.

160. Pepenoe, D. and Loosli, C. G., The morphological effects of a single exposure of paraquat on the mouse lung, *Proc. West. Pharmacol. Soc.,* 21, 151, 1978.

161. Niden, A. H. and Khurana, M., An animal model for diffuse interstitial pulmonary fibrosis — chronic low dose paraquat ingestion, *Fed. Proc. Fed. Am. Soc. Exp. Biol.,* 35, 631, 1976.

162. Plopper, C. G., Chow, C. K., Dungworth, D. L., Brummer, M., and Nemeth, T. J., Effect of low level ozone on rat lungs. II. Morphological responses during recovery and re-exposure, *Exp. Mol. Pathol.,* 29, 400, 1978.

163. Snider, G. L. and Korthy, A. L., Internal surface area and number of respiratory air spaces in elastase-induced emphysema in hamsters, *Am. Rev. Respir. Dis.,* 117, 685, 1978.

164. Karlinsky, J. B., Snider, G. L., Franzblau, C., Stone, P. J., and Hoppin, F. G., Jr., In vitro effects of elastase and collagenase on mechanical properties of hamster lungs, *Am. Rev. Respir. Dis.,* 113, 769, 1976.

165. Lieberman, J., Elastase, collagenase, emphysema, and alpha$_1$-antitrypsin deficiency, *Chest,* 70, 62, 1976.

166. Wessells, N. K. and Cohen, J. H., Effects of collagenase on developing epithelia in lung, ureteric bud, and pancreas, *Dev. Biol.,* 18, 294, 1968.

167. William, B. R., Gelman, R. A., and Peiz, K. A., Collagen fibril formation. Optimal in vitro conditions and preliminary kinetic results, *J. Biol. Chem.,* 253, 6578, 1978.

168. Lapiere, C. M., Nusgens, B., and Pierard, G. E., Interaction between collagen Type I and Type III in conditioning bundles organization, *Connect. Tissue Res.,* 5, 21, 1977.

169. Rigby, B. J., Mitchell, T. W., and Robinson, M. S., Oxygen participation in the in vivo and in vitro aging of collagen fibres, *Biochem. Biophys. Res. Commun.,* 79, 400, 1977.

170. Alescio, T., Effect of a proline analogue, azetidine-2-carboxylic acid, on the morphogenesis in vitro of mouse embryonic lung, *J. Embryol. Exp. Morphol.,* 29, 439, 1973.

171. Hoffman, L., Mondshine, R. B., and Park, S. S., Effect of dl-penicillamine on elastic properties of rat lung, *J. Appl. Physiol.,* 30, 508, 1971.

172. Jelenska, M. M., Dancewicz, A. M., and Przygoda, E., Radiation-induced aldehydes in collagen, *Acta Biochim. Pol.,* 22, 179, 1975.

173. Levene, C. I., Bye, I., and Saffiotti, V., The effect of beta-aminoproprionitrile on silicotic pulmonary fibrosis in the rat, *Br. J. Exp. Pathol.,* 49, 152, 1968.

174. Sugihara, T. and Martin, C. J., Simulation of lung tissue properties in age and irreversible obstructive syndromes using an aldehyde, *J. Clin. Invest.,* 56, 23, 1975.

175. Stanley, N. N., Alper, R., Cunningham, E. L., Cherniak, N. S., and Kefalides, N. A., Effects of a change in collagen on lung structure and mechanical function, *J. Clin. Invest.,* 55, 1195, 1975.

176. Caldwell, E. J. and Bland, J. H., The effect of penicillamine on the rabbit lung, *Am. Rev. Respir. Dis.,* 105, 75, 1972.

177. Boldstein, E. R., Haddad, R., and Hamosh, P., Effect of β-aminoproprionitrile on the elastic behavior of the rat lung, *Clin. Res.,* 18, 89a, 1970.

178. Reye, R. D. and Bale, P. M., Elastic tissue in pulmonary emphysema in Marfan syndrome, *Arch. Pathol.,* 96, 427, 1973.

179. Dwyer, E. M., Jr. and Troncale, F., Spontaneous pneumothorax and pulmonary disease in the Marfan syndrome, *Ann. Int. Med.,* 62, 1285, 1965.

180. Tueller, E. E., Crise, N. R., Belton, J. C., and McLaughlin, R. F., Idiopathic spontaneous pneumothorax, *Chest,* 71, 419, 1977.

181. Chisholm, J. C., Cherniak, N. S., and Carton, R. W., Results of pulmonary function testing in 5 persons with Marfan syndrome, *J. Lab. Clin. Med.,* 71, 25, 1968.

182. Fuleihan, F. J. D., Suh, S. K., and Shepard, R. H., Some aspects of pulmonary function in the Marfan syndrome, *Bull. J. Hopkins Hosp.,* 113, 320, 1963.

183. Starcher, B., Madaras, J., and Teppen, A., Lysyl oxidase deficiency in lung and fibroblasts from mice with hereditary emphysema, *Biochem. Biophys. Res. Commun.,* 78, 706, 1977.

184. Rowe, D. W., McGoodwin, E. B., Martin, G. R., and Grahn, D., Decreased lysyl oxidase activity in the aneurysm-prone mottled mouse, *J. Biol. Chem.*, 252, 939, 1977.

185. Fulmer, J., Elson, N., Szapiel, S., and Crystal, R. G., Structural and physiological characterics of lung in the tight-skin mouse, *Am. Rev., Respir. Dis.,* Suppl. 117, 339, 1978.

186. Snider, G. L., Shenter, C. G., Koo, K. W., Karlinsky, J. B., Hayes, J. A., and Franzblau, C., Respiratory mechanics in hamsters following treatment with endotracheal elastase or collagenase, *J. Appl. Physiol.*, 42, 206, 1977.

187. Snider, G. L., Celli, B. R., Goldstein, R. H., O'Brien, J. J., and Lucey, E. G., Chronic interstitial pulmonary fibrosis produced in hamsters by endotracheal bleomycin, *Am. Rev. Respir. Dis.*, 117, 789, 1978.

188. Goldstein, R. H., Lucey, E. C., Franzblau, C., and Snider, G. L., Failure of mechanical properties to parallel changes in lung connective tissue composition in bleomycin-induced pulmonary fibrosis in hamsters, *Am. Rev. Respir. Dis.*, 120, 67, 1979.

189. Fulmer, J. D., Roberts, W. C., von Gal, E. R., and Crystal, R. G., Morphologic-physiologic correlates of the severity of fibrosis and degree of cellularity in idiopathic pulmonary fibrosis, *J. Clin. Invest.*, 63, 665, 1979.

190. Crystal, R. G., Fulmer, J. D., Baum, B. J., Bernardo, J., Bradley, K. H., Breul, S. D., Elson, N. A., Fells, G. A., Ferrans, V. J., Gadek, J. E., Hunninghake, G. W., Kawanami, O., Kelman, J. A., Line, B. R., McDonald, J. A., McLees, B. D., Roberts, W. C., Rosenberg, D. M., Tolstoshev, P., von Gal, E., and Weinberger, S. W., Cells, collagen and idiopathic pulmonary fibrosis, *Lung*, 155, 199, 1978.

191. Karlinsky, J. B. and Snider, G. L., Animal models of emphysema, *Am. Rev. Respir. Dis.,* 117, 1109, 1978.

192. Snider, G. L. and Karlinsky, J. B., Relation between elastic behavior and the connective tissues of the lung, in *Pathology Annual*, Vol. 7, Ioachim, H. L., Ed., Appleton-Century-Crofts, New York, 1977, 115.

193. Krahl, V. E., Anatomy of the mammalian lung, in *Handbook of Physiology, Section 3, Respiration*, Vol. 1, Fenn, W. O. and Rahn, H., Eds., American Physiological Society, Washington, D.C., 1964, 213.

194. Fulmer, J. D. and Crystal, R. G., The biochemical basis of pulmonary function, in *The Biochemical Basis of Pulmonary Function*, Crystal, R. G., Ed., Marcel Dekker, New York, 1976, 419.

195. Klebe, R., Isolation of a collagen-dependent cell attachment factor, *Nature (London)*, 250, 248, 1974.

196. Vracko, R., Significance of basal lamina for regeneration of injured lung, *Virchows Arch. Pathol. Anat.*, 355, 264, 1972.

197. Senior, R., Bielefeld, D. R., and Abensohn, M. K., The effect of proteolytic enzymes on the tensile strength of human lung, *Am. Rev. Respir. Dis.*, 111, 184, 1975.

198. Hogg, J. C., Staub, N. C., Bergofsky, E. H., and Vreim, C. E., Workshop on the pulmonary endothelial cell, *Am. Rev. Respir. Dis.*, 119, 165, 1979.

199. Kuhn, C. and Senior, R. M., The role of elastases in the development of emphysema, *Lung*, 155, 185, 1978.

200. Snider, G. L., Hayes, J. A., Franzblau, C., Kagan, H. M., Stone, P. S., and Korthy, A. L., Relationship between elastolytic activity and experimental emphysema-inducing properties of papain preparations, *Am. Rev. Respir. Dis.*, 110, 254, 1974.

201. Martin, H. B. and Boatman, E. S., Electron microscopy of human pulmonary emphysema, *Am. Rev. Respir. Dis.*, 91, 206, 1965.

202. Pierce, J. A., Hocott, J. B., and Ebert, R. V., The collagen and elastin content of the lung in emphysema, *Ann. Intern. Med.*, 55, 210, 1961.

203. Wright, G. W., Kleinerman, J., and Zorn, E. M., The elastin and collagen content of normal and emphysematous human lungs, *Am. Rev. Respir. Dis.*, 81, 938, 1960.

204. Pierce, J. A., Age related changes in the fibrous proteins of the lungs, *Arch. Environ. Health*, 6, 56, 1963.

205. Keller, S. and Mandl, I., Qualitative differences between normal and emphysematous human lung elastin, in *Pulmonary Emphysema and Proteolysis*, Mittman, C., Ed., Academic Press, New York, 1972, 251.

206. Bruce, R. M., Adamson, J. S., and Pierce, J. A., Collagen and elastin content of the lung in antitrypsin deficiency, *Clin. Res.*, 18, 89a, 1970.

207. Fitzpatrick, M., Studies of human pulmonary connective tissue. III. Chemical changes in structural proteins with emphysema, *Am. Rev. Respir. Dis.*, 96, 254, 1967.

208. Fitzpatrick, M., Studies of human pulmonary connective tissue. IV. Some differences in polypeptides derived from elastic protein, *Am. Rev. Respir. Dis.*, 97, 248, 1968.

209. Keller, S. and Mandl, I., Qualitative differences between normal and emphysematous human lung elastin, in *Pulmonary Emphysema and Proteolysis*, Mittman, C., Ed., Academic Press, New York, 1972, 251.

210. Laros, C. D., The pathogenesis of emphysema, *Respiration*, 29, 442, 1972.
211. Laros, C. D., Kuyper, C. M. A., and Janssen, H. M. I., The chemical composition of fresh human lung parenchma, *Respiration*, 29, 458, 1972.
212. Saltzman, H. A., Schanble, M. K., and Sieker, M. K., Hexosamine content of aged and chronically diseased lung, *J. Lab. Clin. Med.*, 58, 115, 1961.
213. Yu, S. Y., Keller, N. R., and Yoshida, A., Biosynthesis of insoluble elastin in hamster lungs during elastase-emphysema, *Proc. Soc. Exp. Biol. Med.*, 157, 369, 1978.
214. Goldstein, R. A. and Starcher, B. C., Urinary excretion of elastin peptides containing desmosine after intratracheal injection of elastase in hamsters, *J. Clin. Invest.*, 61, 1286, 1978.
215. Kilburn, K. H., Dowell, A. R., and Pratt, P. C., Morphological and biochemical assessment of papain induced emphysema, *Arch. Intern. Med.*, 127, 884, 1971.
216. Arai, H., Endo, M., Yokosawa, A., Sato, H., Motomiya,, M., and Konno, K., On acid glycosaminoglycans (mucopolysaccharides) in pleural effusion, *Am. Rev. Respir. Dis.*, 111, 37, 1975.
217. Friman, C., Hellström, P. E., Juvani, M., and Riska, H., Acid glycosaminoglycans (mucopolysaccharides) in the differential diagnosis of pleural effusion, *Clin. Chim. Acta*, 76, 357, 1977.
218. Waxler, B., Eisenstein, R., and Battiforda, H., Electrophoresis of tissue glycosaminoglycans as an aid in the diagnosis of mesotheliomas, *Cancer*, 44, 221, 1979.
219. Arai, H., Endo, M., Sasai, Y., Yokorawa, A., Sato, H., Motomiya, M., and Konno, K., Histochemical demonstration of hyaluronic acid in a case of pleural mesothelioma, *Am. Rev. Respir. Dis.*, 111, 699, 1975.
220. Hatae, Y., Atsuta, T., and Makita, A., Glycosaminoglycans in human lung carcinoma, *Gann*, 68, 59, 1977.
221. Motomiya, M., Endo, M., Arai, H., Yokosawa, A., Sato, H., and Konno, K., Biochemical characterization of hyaluronic acid from a case of benign, localized, pleural mesothelioma, *Am. Rev. Respir. Dis.*, 111, 775, 1975.
222. Hatae, Y., Yoda, Y., and Makita, A., Glycosaminoglycans in a small cell carcinoma of human lung: histologically characteristic pattern, *Gann*, 70, 389, 1979.
223. Svojtkova, E., Deyl, Z., Smid, A., and Adam, M., The occurrence of collagen type II in bronchogenic carcinoma, *Neoplasma*, 24, 437, 1977.
224. Murray, J. C., Liotta, L., Rennard, S. I., and Martin, G. R., Adhesion characteristics of murine metastatic and nonmetastatic tumor cells in vitro, *Cancer Res.*, in press.
225. Liotta, L., Tryggvasson, K., Garbisa, S., Robey, P. G., and Murray, J. C., Interaction of metastatic tumor cells with basement membrane collagen, in *Metastatic Tumor Growth*, Grundman, E. and Fischer, G., Eds., Springer-Verlag, New York, 1979.
226. Fulmer, J. D. and Crystal, R. G., Interstitial lung disease, in *Current Pulmonology*, Vol. 1, Simmons, D. H., Ed., Houghton Mifflin, Boston, 1979, 1.
227. Crystal, R. G., Idiopathic pulmonary fibrosis, *Ann. Intern. Med.*, 85, 769, 1976.
228. Basset, F., Soler, P., and Bernaudin, J. F., Contributions of electron microscopy to the study of interstitial pneumonias, *Progr. Respir. Dis.*, 8, 45, 1975.
229. Gadek, J. E., Kelman, J. A., Fells, G. A., Weinberger, S. E., Horwitz, A. L., Reynolds, H. Y., Fulmer, J. A., and Crystal, R. G., Collagenase in the lower respiratory tract of patients with idiopathic pulmonary fibrosis, *N. Engl. J. Med.*, 301, 737, 1979.
230. McCullough, B., Collins, J. F., Johanson, W. G., Jr., and Grover, F. L., Bleomucin-induced diffuse interstitial pulmonary fibrosis in baboons, *J. Clin. Invest.*, 61, 79, 1978.
231. Pozzi, E. and Zanon, P., On the pathogenesis of bleomycin lung toxicity, *Int. J. Pharmacol. Biopharm.*, 16, 575, 1978.
232. Sikic, B. I., Young, D., Mimnaugh, E. G., and Gram, T. E., Quantification of bleomycin pulmonary toxicity in mice by changes in lung hydroxyproline content and morphometric histopathology, *Cancer Res.*, 38, 787, 1978.
233. Jones, A. W. and Reeve, N. L., Ultrastructure study of bleomycin-induced pulmonary changes in mice, *J. Pathol.*, 124, 227, 1978.
234. Maron, Z., Weinberg, K. S., and Fanburg, B. L., Effect of bleomycin on collagenolytic activity of the rat pulmonary macrophage, *Am. Rev. Respir. Dis.*, 119 (4, Part 2), 334, 1979.
235. McCullough, B., Schneider, S., Greene, N. D., and Johanson, W. G., Bleomycin-induced lung injury in baboons: alteration of cells and immunoglobulins recoverable by bronchoalveolar lavage, *Lung*, 155, 337, 1978.
236. Collins, J. F., Strong, G. L., Johanson, W. G., Jr., and McCullough, B., Collagen and elastin metabolism in bleomycin-induced pulmonary fibrosis in the baboon, *Am. Rev. Respir. Dis.*, 117 (4, Part 2), 323, 1978.
237. Szapiel, S. V., Elson, N. A., Fulmer, J. D., Hunninghake, G. W., and Crystal, R. G., Bleomycin-induced interstitial pulmonary disease in the nude, athymic mouse, *Am. Rev. Respir. Dis.*, 120, 893, 1979.

238. Thrall, R. S., McCormick, J. R., Jack, R. M., McReynolds, R. A., and Ward, P. A., Bleomycin-induced pulmonary fibrosis in the rat: inhibition by indomethacin, *Am. J. Pathol.*, 95, 117, 1979.

239. Snider, G. L., Hayes, J. A., and Korthy, A. L., Chronic interstitial pulmonary fibrosis produced in hamsters by endotracheal bleomycin: pathology and stereology, *Am. Rev. Respir. Dis.*, 117, 1099, 1978.

240. Lam, H. F., Takezaun, J., and Van Stee, E. W., The effect of paraquat and diquat on lung function measurements in rats, *Am. Rev. Respir. Dis.*, 119, (4, Part 2), 327, 1979.

241. Hussain, M. Z. and Bhatnagar, R. S., Involvement of superoxide in the paraquat-induced enhancement of lung collagen synthesis in organ culture, *Biochem. Biophys. Res. Commun.*, 89, 71, 1979.

242. Thompson, W. D. and Patrick, R. S., Collagen prolyl hydroxylase levels in experimental paraquat poisoning, *Br. J. Exp. Pathol.*, 59, 288, 1978.

243. Hollinger, M. A., Zuckermann, J. E., and Giri, S. N., Effect of acute and chronic paraquat on rat lung collagen content, *Res. Commun. Chem. Pathol. Pharm.*, 21, 295, 1978.

244. Hollinger, M. A. and Chvapil, M., Effect of paraquat on rat lung prolyl hydroxylase, *Res. Commun. Chem. Pathol. Pharm.*, 16, 159, 1977.

245. Greenberg, D. B., Reiser, K. M., and Last, J. A., Correlation of biochemical and morphologic manifestations of acute pulmonary fibrosis in rats administered paraquat, *Chest*, 74, 421, 1978.

246. Khurana, M. and Niden, A. H., The effect of penicillamine on pulmonary collagen synthesis in vivo, *Am. Rev. Respir. Dis.*, 119 (4, Part 2), 324, 1979.

247. Pickrell, J. A., Harris, D. V., Hahn, F. F., Belasich, J. J., and Jones, R. K., Biological alterations resulting from chronic lung irradiation. III. Effect of partial ⁶⁰Co thoracic irradiation upon pulmonary collagen metabolism and fractionation in Syrian hamsters, *Radiat. Res.*, 62, 133, 1975.

248. Pickrell, J. A., Harris, D. V., Mauderly, J. L., and Hahn, F. F., Altered collagen metabolism in radiation-induced interstitial pulmonary fibrosis, *Chest*, 69, 311, 1976.

249. Gerber, G. B., Dancewicz, A. M., Bessemans, B., and Casale, G., Biochemistry of late effects in rat lung after hemithoracic irradiation, *Acta Radiat. Ther. Phys. Biol.*, 16, 447, 1977.

250. Metivier, H., Masse, R., Legendre, N., and Lafuma, J., Pulmonary connective tissue modifications induced by internal α irradiation, *Radiat. Res.*, 75, 385, 1978.

251. Jennings, F. L. and Arden, A., Development of experimental radiation pneumonitis, *Arch. Pathol.*, 71, 437, 1961.

252. Collins, J. F., Johanson, W. G., Jr., McCullough, B., Jones, M. A., and Waugh, H. J., Jr., Effects of compensatory lung growth in irradiation-induced regional pulmonary fibrosis in the baboon, *Am. Rev. Respir. Dis.*, 117, 1079, 1978.

253. Tombropoulos, E. G. and Thomas, J. M., Effect of 800 R thoracic X-irradiation on lung tissue biochemistry, *Radiat. Res.*, 44, 76, 1970.

254. Pickrell, J. A., Harris, D. V., Benjamin, S. A., Cuddihy, R. G., Pfleger, R. C., and Mauderly, J. L., Pulmonary collagen metabolism after lung injury from inhaled ⁹⁰Y in fused clay particles, *Exp. Mol. Pathol.*, 25, 70, 1976.

255. Dubrawsky, C., Dubravsky, N. B., and Withers, H. R., The effect of colchicine on the accumulation of hydroxyproline and on lung compliance after irradiation, *Radiat. Res.*, 73, 111, 1978.

256. Ryan, S. F., Barrett, C. R., Lavietes, M. H., Bell, A. L. L., and Rochester, D. F., Volume-pressure and morphometric observations after acute alveolar injury in the dog from N-nitroso-N-methylurethane, *Am. Rev. Respir. Dis.*, 118, 735, 1978.

257. Ryan, S. F., Experimental fibrosing alveolitis, *Am. Rev. Respir. Dis.*, 105, 776, 1972.

258. Gross, P., Kociba, R. J., Sparschu, G. L., and Norris, J. M., The biologic response to titanium phosphate, *Arch. Pathol. Lab. Med.*, 101, 550, 1977.

259. Richards, R. J. and Jacoby, F., Light microscopic studies on the effects of chrysotile asbestos and fiber glass on the morphology and reticulin formation of cultured lung fibroblasts, *Environ. Res.*, 11, 112, 1976.

260. Singh, J., Kau, J. L., Pandey, S. D., Viswanathan, P. N., and Zaidi, S. H., Amino acid changes and pulmonary response of rats to silica dust, *Environ. Res.*, 14, 452, 1977.

261. Halme, J., Uitto, J., Kahanpaä, K., Karhunen, P., and Lindy, S., Protocollagen proline hydroxylase activity in experimental fibrosis of rats, *J. Lab. Clin. Med.*, 75, 535, 1970.

262. Stacy, B. D. and King, E. J., Silica and collagen in the lungs of silicotic rats treated with cortisone, *Br. J. Ind. Med.*, 11, 192, 1954.

263. Davis, J. M., Beckett, S. T., Bolton, R. E., Collings, P., and Middleton, A. P., Mass and number of fibers in the pathogenesis of asbestos-related lung disease in rats, *Br. J. Cancer*, 37, 673, 1978.

264. Frank, L., Bucher, J. R., and Roberts, R. J., Oxygen toxicity in neonatal and adult animals of various species, *J. Appl. Phys.*, 45, 699, 1978.

265. Välimäki, M., Juva, K., Rantanen, J., Ekfors, T., and Niinikosko, J., Collagen metabolism in rat lungs during chronic intermittent exposure to oxygen, *Aviat. Space Environ. Med.*, 46, 684, 1975.

266. Haschek, W. M., Meyer, K. R., Ullrich, R. L., and Witschi, H. P., Pulmonary fibrosis — a possible mechanism, *Fed. Proc. Fed. Am. Soc. Exp. Biol.*, 38 (3, Part 2), 1155, 1979.

267. Chvapil, M. and Peng, Y. M., Oxygen and lung fibrosis, *Arch. Environ. Health*, 30, 528, 1975.
268. Riley, D. J., Edelman, N. H., Berg, R. A., and Prockop, D. J., Use of a proline analogue to prevent lung injury following oxygen toxicity in rats, *Am. Rev. Respir. Dis.*, 119 (4, Part 2), 353, 1979.
269. Autor, A. P. and Stevens, J. B., Mechanism of oxygen detoxicification in neonatal rat lung tissues, *Photochem. Photobiol.*, 28, 775, 1978.
270. Ayaz, K. L. and Csallany, A. S., Long-term NO_2 exposure of mice in the presence and absence of vitamin E. Effect of glutathione peroxidase, *Arch. Environ. Health*, 33, 292, 1978.
271. Drozdz, M., Kucharz, E., and Szyja, J., Effect of chronic exposure to nitrogen dioxide on collagen content in lung and skin of guinea pigs, *Environ. Res.*, 13, 369, 1977.
272. Orthoefer, J. G., Bhatnagar, R. S., Rahman, A., Yang, Y. V., Lee, S. D., and Stara, J. F., Collagen and prolyl hydroxylase levels in lungs of beagles exposed to air pollutants, *Environ. Res.*, 12, 299, 1976.
273. Hussain, M. Z., Mustafa, M. G., Chow, C. K., and Cross, C. E., Ozone-induced increase of lung proline hydroxylase and hydroxyproline content, *Chest*, 69, 273, 1976.
274. Rosenkrantz, H., Esber, H. J., and Sprague, R., Lung hydroxyproline levels in mice exposed to cigarette smoke, *Life Sci.*, 8, 571, 1969.
275. Hurst, D. J., Gilbert, G. L., and McKenzie, W. N., Effect of cigarette smoke on lung collagen synthesis, *Clin. Res.*, 25, 590a, 1977.
276. Johnson, K. J. and Ward, P. A., Acute immunological pulmonary alveolitis, *J. Clin. Invest.*, 54, 349, 1974.
277. Richerson, H. B., Cheng, F. H. F., and Bauserman, S. C., Acute experimental hypersensitivity pneumonitis in rabbits, *Am. Rev. Respir. Dis.*, 104, 568, 1971.
278. Read, J., The pathological changes produced by anti-lung serum, *J. Pathol. Bacteriol.*, 76, 403, 1958.
279. Moore, V. L., Hensley, G. T., and Fink, J. N., An animal model of hypersensitivity pneumonitis in the rabbit, *J. Clin. Invest.*, 56, 937, 1975.
280. Joubert, J. R., Ascah, K., Moroz, L. A., and Hogg, J. C., Acute hypersensitivity pneumonitis in the rabbit. I. An animal model with horseradish peroxidase as antigen, *Am. Rev. Respir. Dis.*, 113, 503, 1976.
281. Brentjens, J. R., O'Connell, D. W., Pawlowski, I. B., Hsu, K. C., and Andres, G. A., Experimental immune complex disease of the lung, *J. Exp. Med.*, 140, 105, 1974.
282. Braley, J. F., Peterson, L. B., Dawson, C. A., and Moore, V. L., Effect of hypersensitivity on protein uptake across the air-blood barrier of isolated rabbit lungs, *J. Clin. Invest.*, 63, 1103, 1979.
283. Cate, C. C. and Burrell, R., Lung antigen induced cell-mediated immune injury in chronic respiratory diseases, *Am. Rev. Respir. Dis.*, 109, 114, 1974.
284. Ueda, E., Nishimura, K., Nagasaka, Y., Kokubu, T., and Yamamura, Y., Metabolism of vasoactive substances in the lung: change of metabolism and its significance in rabbits with experimental pneumonitis, *Jpn. Circ. J.*, 39, 559, 1975.
285. Van Toorn, D. W., Experimental interstitial pulmonary fibrosis, *Pathol. Eur.*, 5, 97, 1970.
286. Shannon, B. T., Love, S. H., and Myrvik, Q. N., Hyaluronic acid content of lungs of rabbits during a cell-mediated response to Bacillus Calmette-Guerin (BCG), *Fed. Proc. Fed. Am. Soc. Exp. Biol.*, 38, (3, Part 2), 1204, 1979.
287. Burleigh, M. C., Degradation of collagen by non-specific proteinases, in *Proteinases in Mammalian Cells and Tissues*, Barrett, A. J., Ed., North-Holland, Amsterdam, 1977, 285.
288. Gadek, J., work in progress.
289. Liotta, L. and Abe, S., work in progress.
290. Keiser, H., Greenwald, R. A., Feinstein, G., and Janoff, A., Degradation of cartilage proteoglycan by human leucocyte granule neutral proteases — a model of joint injury. II. Degradation of isolated bovine nasal cartilage proteoglycan, *J. Clin. Invest.*, 57, 625, 1976.
291. Miller, E. J., Finch, J. E., Jr., Chung, E., and Butler, W. T., Specific cleavage of the native type III collagen molecule with trypsin, *Arch. Biochem. Biophys.*, 173, 631, 1976.

Chapter 6

THE PATHOGENESIS OF EMPHYSEMA*

Charles Kuhn, Robert M. Senior, and John A. Pierce

TABLE OF CONTENTS

* The authors' work covered in this review was supported by a USPHS research grant HL16118.

I. INTRODUCTION

Emphysema is usually seen as a result of low-level, chronic exposure to toxic inhalants continued for many years. At present it is not possible to specify the properties of toxic inhalants which are essential to the production of emphysema since the clinically important inhalants are complex mixtures, and there are few reliable and uniformly accepted experimental models of emphysema using toxic inhalants. Some host factors which predispose to emphysema have been identified, but these do not account for all the variability in response. At least one mechanism of producing emphysema is known, enzymatic destruction of elastic tissue. This mechanism dominates current thinking about the production of emphysema and provides the basis for current theories of the sites where toxic agents may act. Admittedly, however, other mechanisms are possible,[1] and the occurrence of elastolysis has not yet been rigorously documented in human emphysema.

II. EMPHYSEMA IN MAN

Clinically, emphysema presents as one cause of the syndrome of "chronic airflow obstruction" or "obstructive pulmonary disease". The conditions associated with this syndrome consist of asthma, chronic bronchitis, bronchiolitis, and bronchiectasis, as well as emphysema. Any of these conditions may occur together, in particular chronic bronchitis, bronchiolitis, and emphysema do so commonly. However, each may be a cause of disability or even death in the absence of the other. Bronchitis is defined symptomatically by cough and sputum production; emphysema is defined anatomically and may be present without symptoms. Indeed, autopsy studies indicate that in most patients with symptomatic emphysema, a minimum of one fifth of the lung is involved.[2-4] Lesser amounts of disease are clinically silent.

A. Anatomic Features

Emphysema has been defined as an anatomic alteration of the lung characterized by an abnormal enlargement of air spaces distal to the terminal nonrespiratory bronchiole accompanied by destructive changes in the alveolar walls.[5] To this definition one should probably add that there is relatively little fibrosis in the emphysematous lung. When enlargement and destruction of air spaces occurs with severe fibrosis, it produces the condition termed honeycomb lung. Honeycomb lung is the end-result of a wide variety of insults ranging from granulomas to pneumoconioses to "collagen-vascular disease".[6] The clinical and physiological properties of honeycomb lung differ markedly from the large lungs typical of emphysema. Honeycomb lungs may be considered as small emphysematous lungs, since the air spaces are larger than normal. Total lung capacity is decreased, however, whereas a normal or increased total lung capacity is typical of emphysema.

The pathology of human emphysema has been described in a number of excellent monographs[7-9] and reviews.[10,11] Emphysema can involve different portions of the acinus and is ordinarily classified according to the portion of the acinus affected.

By looking at a slice of lung that has been inflated, one can recognize macroscopic units of lung parenchyma roughly 1.5 to 2 cm in diameter which are partially or completely outlined by connective tissue septa. Such units are termed secondary lobules and contain two to five acini.

Each acinus or gas-exchanging unit of lung is the unit supplied by a single terminal bronchiole. It consists of three generations of respiratory bronchioles, two to five generations of alveolar ducts, and alveolar sacs, all with their alveoli.[12,13]

Emphysema may involve the respiratory bronchioles selectively (centriacinar emphysema), the alveolar sacs as they abut the pleura and inter-lobular septa (distal acinar, or paraseptal emphysema), or the entire acinus (panacinar emphysema).

1. Centriacinar Emphysema

Emphysema that initially involves the respiratory bronchioles is termed centriacinar or centrilobular emphysema (CLE). CLE is recognizable as enlarged, roughly spherical spaces 1 to 5 mm in diameter on the sectioned surface of the lung usually located in the center of secondary lobules, although some lesions may be eccentric within the lobules (see Figure 1). Characteristically, a rim of normal parenchyma separates the emphysematous spaces from the perilobular septa, except in the most advanced instances. There is usually dark pigment associated with the emphysematous lesions, although this is not invariable.[14] Involvement of the upper lobes is usually more severe than of the lower lobes, and the apical segments have more severe involvement than the basal segments. Often inflammation is present in the bronchioles supplying the emphysematous foci, and this may result in stenosis of the bronchus.[6,15-17] Most patients with CLE are cigarette smokers with chronic cough and sputum production (chronic bronchitis).

2. Panacinar Emphysema

Panacinar emphysema (panlobular emphysema, PLE) (see Figure 2) affects the acinus diffusely. On the sectioned surface of the lung, the individual lobules vary in severity of involvement, but even in mildly involved lobules, the abnormally enlarged airspaces reach the perilobular septa. This process usually involves alveolar ducts more severely than respiratory bronchioles. At early stages, the alveolar ducts are dilated and the alveoli are wide and shallow with shortening or loss of alveolar septa.[6] All portions of the lung are affected in PLE, but the lower zones tend to have more severe disease. Inflammation in the bronchioles is less frequent than with CLE. Familial emphysema and emphysema in young people is usually of the panacinar type whether

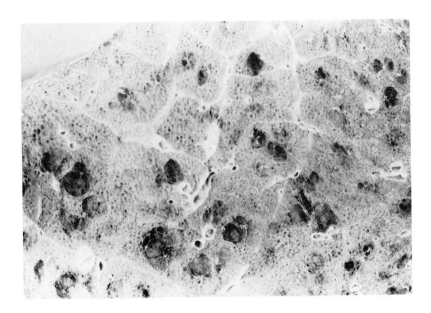

FIGURE 1. Centriacinar emphysema. The emphysematous spaces appear as relatively large pigmented spaces usually near the center of the secondary lobules which are partially outline by connective tissue septa. Delicate strands of tissue cross many of the emphysematous spaces. Barium sulfate impregnated lung. (Magnification × 1.4.)

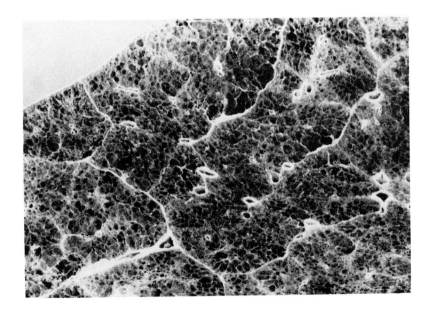

FIGURE 2. Panacinar emphysema. There is a generalized coarsening of the lung architecture. The airspace enlargement is present uniformly throughout the secondary lobules. Barium sulfate impregnated lung. (Magnification × 1.4.)

associated with deficiency of α_1-antitrypsin[18,19] or with normal levels of α_1-antitrypsin.[20] However, many cases also occur in middle-aged cigarette smokers.[2]

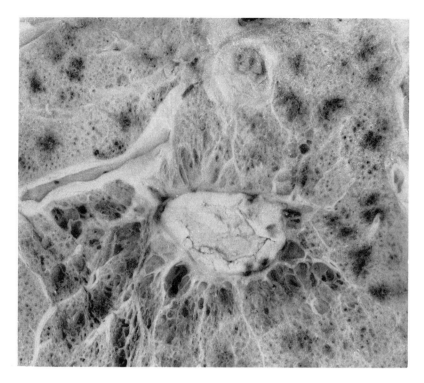

FIGURE 3.   Irregular emphysema. Abnormal airspaces surrounding a caseous granuloma
in a case of tuberculosis. Barium sulfate-impregnated lung. (Magnification × 1.85.)

3. Irregular Emphysema
Emphysema is often seen surrounding scars resulting from any cause (see Figure 3).
Since such emphysema may result from a process which does not respect acinar archi-
tecture, it is termed irregular emphysema.

4. Distal Acinar Emphysema
Distal acinar or paraseptal emphysema refers to emphysema localized subpleurally
or along perilobular septa. As an isolated finding, it may be a cause of pneumothorax,
but otherwise produces little pulmonary dysfunction.

5. Emphysema in Coal Workers Pneumoconiosis
Coal workers and workers exposed to certain other dusts, such as hematite, graphite,
or carbon black, develop a form of emphysema which initially involves the respiratory
bronchioles.[21,22] Pathologists in the U.K. believe it has features which justify its separation from CLE of the usual type,[2,11,23] but many in this country do not make the
distinction.[24,25] The lesions develop as dust accumulates in macrophages in the alveoli
along the respiratory bronchioles. The alveoli become obliterated, and the dust-laden
macrophages become incorporated into the wall of the respiratory bronchiole accompanied by mild reticulin fibrosis and atrophy of the muscle. Initially simple dilation
of the respiratory bronchioles occurs, but in advanced cases, there is disruption of air
space walls (see Figure 4).

6. Mixed Forms of Emphysema and Problems in Classification
Since one type of emphysema does not protect against development of another, mixtures of the different types of emphysema are to be expected. Often, cases of emphy-

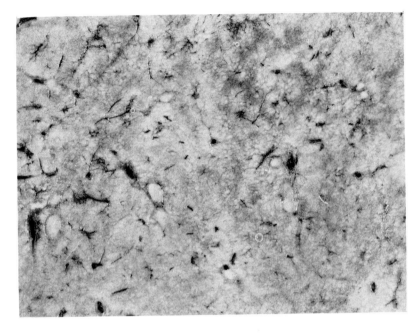

A

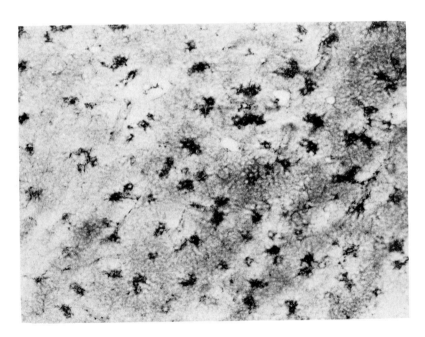

B

FIGURE 4. Coal workers pneumoconiosis. (A) Normal lung; (B) minimal coal workers pneumoconiosis; the small bronchioles and respiratory bronchioles are now visible, outlined by coal dust; (C) moderately severe coal workers pneumoconiosis; the respiratory bronchioles are distinctly more dilated than in (B); (D) destructive emphysema developing in coal workers pneumoconiosis. Paper-mounted lung sections. (Magnification × 1.85.) (Courtesy Professor Jethro Gough).

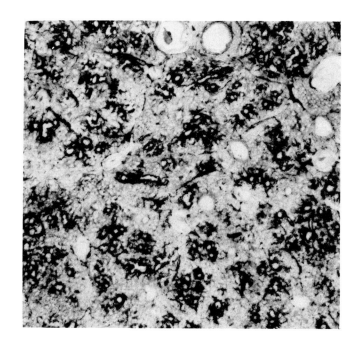

FIGURE 4C

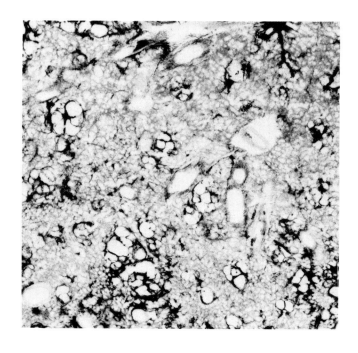

FIGURE 4D

sema do not fit unambiguously into one of the above categories. In one study of 122 emphysematous lungs examined by 3 expert pulmonary pathologists, only 27 cases were unequivocally CLE or PLE, the remaining cases being either mixed or unclassifiable.[26] There is agreement that CLE affects the upper lobes predominantly, while PLE affects the lung more evenly, but with accentuation in the lower lobes,[26-28] but no other clinical or pathological feature consistently separates them. Thus, while there are observations which suggest that CLE and PLE are separate processes each with a different pathogenesis, it is not clearly established that this is the case.

B. Physiological Properties of Emphysematous Lungs

The clinical physiology of emphysema is well described in standard textbooks and will not be repeated here. While many of the derangements of clinical concern are late effects and do not help in clarifying events in the tissue, certain features can be related to the tissue changes.

Slowing of airflow during forced expiration is a prominent clinical feature of emphysematous patients. This can be quantiated by spirograms or flow-volume curves, but does not distinguish emphysema from other forms of obstructive lung disease, such as chronic bronchitis, bronchiolitis, asthma, or bronchiectasis, which may coexist with emphysema. Consequently measurements of expiratory airflow do not by themselves establish either the presence or severity of emphysema.

In the emphysematous lung, the diffusing capacity for carbon monoxide is reduced due to the loss of respiratory surface area[29] and capillary bed which are part of the emphysema itself and due to the abnormal distribution of ventilation and perfusion which are its consequence. Diffusing capacity can also be reduced by a variety of other diseases involving the pulmonary acinus, but in a patient with the clinical syndrome of chronic airway obstruction, loss of diffusing capacity provides a reasonable measure of emphysema.[30-32]

The most specific physiologic features of emphysema are reduced elastic recoil and increased compliance.[30,31,33,34]

Although elastic recoil normally decreases with age,[35,36] the decrease in emphysema is excessive when normalized for age.[36] Clinically, measurements of elastic recoil may not reflect minimal emphysema,[32] but when the pressure-volume characteristics of excised lungs obtained at autopsy are studied, even involvement of less than 10% of the lung by emphysema is associated with decreased elastic recoil and increased compliance.[36]

Decreased elastic recoil can account for the abnormal expiratory airflow in some patients with emphysema.[37,38] This can be demonstrated by measurements of airway conductance, the reciprocal of airway resistance. In selected patients with emphysema, uncomplicated by intrinsic airway disease, airway conductance is normal relative to static pleural pressure [P_{st}(L)] (a measure of elastic recoil),[39,40] although larger lung volumes than normal are required to achieve every level of P_{st}(L). In contrast, with diseases causing anatomic obstruction of airways, such as asthma, conductance is low relative to P_{st}(L), while the relationship between lung volume and P_{st}(L) may remain normal.

The elastic recoil of the expanded lung derives in part from tension developed by stretching of the tissue and in part from surface tension generated at the air-fluid interfaces of the airspaces. The enlarged air spaces and decreased surface area associated with destruction of alveoli in the emphysematous lung lead to a decrease in the component of lung elastic recoil due to surface tension. Abnormalities of connective tissue may also contribute. Loss of elastin decreases elastic recoil and increases lung compliance.[41,42] Loss of collagen on the other hand has little effect on lung compliance at physiologic lung volumes,[41,42] although the tensile strength of the tissue depends on collagen.[43,44] Thus, abnormalities in elastin could contribute to the disturbed lung mechanical properties observed in emphysema.

Studies of the stress strain characteristics of tiny strips of tissue from emphysematous and normal lungs show that the length-tension properties of the emphysematous lung tissue itself are abnormal. The maximum extension ratio of the tissue, λ_{max}, is defined as the ratio of the maximum obtainable length (L_{max}) to the length of the tissue when under no tension (L_o):[45]

$$\lambda_{max} = L_{max}/L_o$$

λ_{max} decreases with age, but is lower at any age with emphysematous lungs.[43] In view of the increased residual volume and decreased elastic recoil of emphysematous lung, it is reasonable to attribute the decrease in λ_{max} to an increase in L_o rather than a decrease in the mechanical stop, L^{max}.

These changes point to abnormalities of the connective tissue of the lung in emphysema. Consequently, Martin and Sugihara assessed the effect of enzymatic degradation of specific connective tissue components on the length tension properties of lung strips.[43] Hyaluronidase produced little effect, while collagenase treatment caused the tissue to rupture at low forces. Elastase produced a fall in λ_{max}, resembling emphysema, but of lesser degree. On the other hand, the energy loss in stretching increased with elastase treatment, but was not increased in emphysema. Thus, elastolysis in vitro produces changes in the tissue which have some properties like emphysema, but which reproduce emphysema imperfectly.

C. Connective Tissue Composition of Emphysematous Lungs

The histologic observation of disruption and disorganization of the elastic fiber network of the lung in emphysema was made more than 100 years ago[46] and has been confirmed many times since.[47-49] Ultrastructural studies have shown clumping of elastic fibers[50] and disorganization of collagen fibrils as well.[51] The biochemical documentation of altered connective tissue components has been difficult, however.

A major difficulty in attempting to study connective tissue composition in diseased lung is the selection of the optimal unit to which to refer analyses. If an anatomic unit such as an entire lung or a lobe is selected as the reference, a change in composition limited to the acinar tissue may be missed, obscured by the large pleural, vascular, and bronchial contributions to the total. If parenchymal tissue is separated from pleura and bronchovascular structures, only relative concentrations can be measured. A decrease in one component cannot be distinguished from increases in other components.

Since elastin is the main tissue determinant of elastic recoil at physiologic lung volumes,[41,52,53] this component of connective tissue has received most attention.

Two changes in lung elastin have been associated with ageing.

1. The elastin content of the lung increases,[54-58] a change that occurs mainly in the pleura.[58,59]
2. The content of desmosine cross-links in the lung elastin decreases.[58]

The elastin content of emphysematous lungs has usually been found to be normal for age, whether as a fraction of dry weight[55,57,60,61] or as total elastin in a defined anatomic unit of lung, i.e., a lobe.[60] A few studies have described a decrease in elastin concentration in local areas of diseased lung, i.e., near bullae,[54] but such data are difficult to interpret because an increase in another tissue component rather than loss of elastin could explain the change.

Attempts to find qualitative abnormalities in lung elastin have been technically frustrating. John and Thomas point out that lung elastin becomes more difficult to purify with age,[58] a difficulty probably even greater in disease. Fitzpatrick found differences between normal lungs and emphysematous lungs in the peptides released by elastase from a crude elastic fiber preparation.[61] Peptides released from emphysematous lung contained appreciable quantities of polar amino acids, including cysteic acid, methionine, and histidine, amino acids not found in typical elastin.

Keller and Mandl in preliminary analyses also reported changes in the amino acid composition of elastin prepared by hot alkali extraction of emphysematous lungs.[63]

More recently, however, when their laboratory compared the elastin from eight patients with panacinar emphysema to six controls, the amino acid analyses of the elastin from the two groups were similar, with the elastin having the accepted composition for pure elastin. The number of desmosine and isodesmosine cross-links was similar in the two groups. It appears that the changes in amino acid composition reported in their earlier studies stemmed from contaminating proteins. One difference between the normal and emphysematous tissue was found, however. Calculated from the concentration of desmosines in a dry connective tissue fraction, emphysematous lung tissue had only half as much elastin as normal.[63]

D. The Etiology of Emphysema

1. Smoking

An abundance of evidence indicates that cigarette smoking is the major cause of emphysema in the U.S.[64,65] and abroad.[66,67] Autopsy studies of hospital populations,[68-70] coroner's populations,[71] and mixed populations[67,72] show the same association. Severity of emphysema is dose related: heavy smokers have more severe and extensive disease than light smokers. Emphysema is infrequent in nonsmokers, and high grades are almost never found. At autopsy, normal lungs are the exception in smokers, and 20 to 40% of those who smoke in excess of a pack per day have disease of relatively high grade (Grade 20 or above on a scale of 0 to 100).[67,70,71] Emphysema of a given grade occurs at a younger age in smokers. Prospective clinical studies show a markedly increased risk of obstructive lung disease including emphysema in smokers. The relative risk of death due to bronchitis and emphysema for smokers compared to nonsmokers' is 16, even greater than that for lung cancer, 8.[73]

2. Community Air Pollution

Community air pollution influences cough, frequency of lower respiratory infections, and ventilatory function as measured by spirometry.[74] There is very little information concerning its association with the anatomic lesions of emphysema. Ishikawa et al. compared whole paper-mounted lung sections obtained at autopsy in St. Louis, Mo. and Winnipeg Manitoba. St. Louis is more heavily industrialized and has higher air pollution levels. When matched for age, sex, and smoking history, St. Louis residents had more severe emphysema.[75]

3. Industrial Pollutants

The association of emphysema with exposure to coal and carbonaceous dusts has been discussed above.

Emphysema has been reported in workers exposed to cadmium oxide (CdO_2) fumes.[76] The emphysema can be rapid in its evolution, leading to death within a few years of starting foundry work. The importance of low level exposure to Cd is unclear. Some chronically exposed workers have had increased rates of deterioration of pulmonary function,[77,78] but in one study, pulmonary function tests and chest radiographs were more suggestive of pulmonary fibrosis than emphysema.[78]

In the general population, the Cd content of emphysematous lungs is elevated,[79] and patients with emphysema also have higher hepatic Cd levels than patients with no emphysema,[80,81] Cigarette smoke is a significant source of inhaled Cd.[82] It cannot therefore be assumed that Cd is the cause of the emphysema in nonindustrial populations. It may simply be a marker for cigarette exposure.

4. Familial Factors in Emphysema

A familial factor operates in the prevalence of chronic airflow obstruction independently of cigarette smoking, α_1-antitrypsin concentration or the cystic fibrosis gene.[83,84] The basis for this familial influence has not been defined. In addition, three hereditary diseases are associated with emphysema: Marfan syndrome, cutis laxa, and α_1-antitrypsin deficiency. Although rare, these diseases provide clues to the pathogenesis of emphysema.

The Marfan syndrome is a disease affecting connective tissues throughout the body. Skeletal, cardiovascular, and occular manifestations usually dominate the clinical picture.[85] The condition is inherited in an autosomal dominant fashion, but the biochemical defect has not been defined.[80]

Lung involvement is not severe in the typical patient, and only minimal pulmonary dysfunction is usually found.[87,88] However, a number of patients have been described with severe bullous emphysema, in the first weeks of life[89,90] as well as in adulthood.[91,92] Pneumothorax may occur.[89,92] In emphysematous areas, the elastic fibers are thickened,[89] fragmented, and irregularly clumped.[90,91] Ultrastructurally they show cystic foci, increased osmiophilia, and appear to be separating into small filaments.[91]

Cutis laxa, also known as generalized elastolysis, occurs in several forms. In the congenital form, the commonest mode of inheritance is autosomal recessive, but cases with autosomal dominant and X-linked recessive inheritance have also been described.[85] Sporadic cases diagnosed in adulthood are apparently acquired. The characteristic clinical feature is inelastic, loose pendulous skin giving the affected individual a prematurely aged appearance. The lung is the most frequently involved of the viscera. Diverticula of the GI tract and cardiovascular lesions are less common. Progressive emphysema is the usual pulmonary lesion, present in approximately half the patients. Pulmonary fibrosis and tracheobronchiomegaly occur rarely.[93]

The basic biochemical lesion of cutis laxa has not been defined. The possibility of a biosynthetic defect involving decreased lysyl oxidase activity has been reported,[94] but needs confirmation.[86,93] There is a marked reduction in the size and number of elastic fibers. By electron microscopy, the normal amorphous component of the elastic fiber (elastin) is reduced in amount, and abnormal electron-dense deposits surround the fiber.[91,93] Although the histologic appearances suggest destruction of elastin, there is no evidence of decreased serum elastase-inhibitory activity.

Serum elastase-inhibitory activity is decreased in α_1-antitrypsin deficiency.[95]

The discovery of antitrypsin deficiency resulted from the observation of an absent α_{-1} globulin band on the protein electrophoretogram of plasma, and knowledge that the principal stainable compent of the band was a-[1] antitrypsin.[18] A total of 27 of the initial 36 patients with the deficiency had obstructive airways disease, primarily emphysema.[19] The original description by Eriksson stands as a model of thoroughness and lucid presentation.

The emphysema of α_1-antitrypsin deficiency (Pi ZZ) is frequently symptomatic at early age. The lesions which are typically panacinar emphysema,[96-98] predominantly in the basilar portions of the lungs,[98,99] occur with almost equal frequency in men and women. The insidious onset of exertional dyspnea occurs 15 years earlier in deficient subjects who smoke cigarettes than in those who do not.[100] Some deficient subjects live to advanced ages without clinical evidence of emphysema provided they do not smoke cigarettes. Perhaps 15 to 30% deficient subjects have recurrent respiratory tract infections prior to the development of clinical obstructive disease, and some have multiple allergies.[100]

Studies of antitrypsin deficiency have provided important insights about cellular mechanisms in the development of the emphysema. The plasma of deficient subjects contains about 10% of the normal plasma concentration of antitrypsin. The enzyme-inhibitory function of the deficient (Z-type) antitrypsin molecule is normal, however, so that the defect is one of inhibitor concentration. Eriksson proposed the deficiency of serum protease inhibitor might permit proteolysis in the extracellular connective tissues and result in remodeling the architecture of the normal lung into an emphysematous form.[19]

In 1969 Sharp recognized the occurrence of liver disease in infants and children with antitrypsin deficiency.[101] Characterized by jaundice, retarded growth, and prolonged liver-chemical abnormalities in the plasma, this complication of the deficiency occurs in approximately 10% of affected (PiZ) subjects early in life. The livers of affected children show cirrhosis which is sometimes accompanied by striking bile stasis, proliferation of perilobular bile ducts, and hypoplasia of extrahepatic bile ducts.[102,103] The characteristic morphologic feature of the livers is the presence of periodic acid-Schiff positive globules in the endoplasmic reticulum which react with antisera to α_1-antitrypsin.[102] In adults with the deficiency, mild portal fibrosis and PAS positive inclusions are usually found, but cirrhosis also occurs.[104] Eriksson and Hogerstrand reported an unusual frequency of hepatoma in older subjects with homozygous antitrypsin deficiency who had escaped emphysema.[105] This finding raises the question whether failure to release Pi type Z antitrypsin from the hepatocytes imposed some burden to these cells that ultimately resulted in their malignant transformation. Instances of α_1-antitrypsin deficiency have also been associated with rheumatoid arthritis, pancreatitis, glomerulonephritis,[103] and intestinal atrophy,[106] but it is not established that these are more than chance occurrences.

Among several protease inhibitors in plasma, α_1-antitrypsin is important because of its relatively high concentration and broad enzymatic-inhibitory spectrum. It inhibits several serine proteases in addition to trypsin, including chymotrypsin, plasmin, and both leukocyte and pancreatic elastases. It is inherited as a codominant trait; one antitrypsin (AT) allele produced from each parent is completely expressed in the offspring. The protein is a strong phase reactant, so that plasma levels rise during illnesses and pregnancy.

A glycoprotein with a mol wt of approximately 54,000 daltons, α_1-antitrypsin is synthesized in the liver and distributed widely throughout body fluids. Its amino acid composition (see Table 1) is distinctive for a large number of acidic residues (aspartic acid, glutamic acid, serine, and threonine), which accounts for its low isoelectric point (pH 4.95). The molecule has a single cysteine residue with an available reactive thiol group. In normal plasma, the protein circulates as a mixed disulfide with cysteine. The reactive thiol group provides a convenient functional site which has facilitated its purification by thiol interchange chromatography; initially with Bence-Jones kappa chains[107] and more recently with glutathione-Sepharose®.[108] The cysteine thiol group probably lies some distance from the reactive site for enzyme inhibition.

The normal antitrypsin molecule contains approximately 13% carbohydrate with four complex side chain structures that terminate in six sialic acid residues. Electrophoresis at acid pH (4.5 to 5.0) results in a characteristic polymorphic pattern consisting of eight or more protein bands. Differences in electrophoretic mobility of the entire band pattern constituted the earliest evidence for a system of inherited variants of the protein.[109] Fagerhol and Laurell devised a crossed immunoelectrophoretic system to identify several phenotypic variants and suggested the term proteinase inhibitor sys-

Table 1
AMINO ACID AND CARBOHYDRATE COMPOSITION, RESIDUES PER MOLECULE, OF α_1-ANTITRYPSIN FROM M-1 AND Z-PROTEIN, ASSUMING A MOL WT OF 56,000

Compound	M-protein	Z-protein
Amino Acid		
Lysine	36.8	37.0
Histidine	14.3	13.8
Arginine	6.9	7.2
Half-cystine	0.8	0.9
Aspartic acid	44.0	44.0
Threonine	28.4	28.9
Serine	22.6	23.1
Glutamic acid	47.9	48.3
Proline	17.9	18.2
Glycine	21.6	22.0
Alanine	24.9	25.9
Valine	24.2	23.6
Methionine	7.9	7.8
Isoleucine	18.2	18.7
Leucine	42.4	43.1
Tyrosine	8.6	8.5
Phenylalanine	22.3	22.7
Tryptophan	1.8	1.8
N terminals	Glu	Glu
Carbohydrate		
Glucosamine	12.2	12.5
Hexose	17.8	17.5
Sialic acid[a]	6.5	5.2

[a] Thiobarbituric acid method. Although thiobarbituric assay gives a difference of sialic acid residues between M- and Z-proteins, stepwise desialation with neuraminidase indicates an identical number of residues.[108]

tem, abbreviated as Pi.[110] Types were designated, F for fast, M for medium, S for slow, and Z for ultra slow mobility. The original classic deficiency represented the homozygous individual with two alleles for the severely abnormal protein — the genetic type now called Pi ZZ. More recent studies with isoelectric focusing at pH 4 to 5 in polyacrylamide gels have permitted the identification of more than 20 genotypic and over 50 phenotypic variants of antitrypsin. Of these, only the Pi Z, Pi SZ, and Pi Null are definitely associated with emphysema.[111-113]

There has been much controversy about the relationship of the MZ heterozygous deficiency state to emphysema. Typically MZ phenotype, which occurs in as many as

10% of the population, is associated with approximately one half of the normal antitrypsin concentration. In general, case control studies of patients with chronic airflow obstruction show an excess prevalence of MZ heterozygotes in patients compared to controls, but studies of small numbers of MZ individuals often have failed to show an excess prevalence of physiologic or radiographic abnormalities compared to normal MM individuals.[103] Explanations for this apparent discrepancy have been critically discussed by Mittman, who concluded that the evidence was inconclusive, but suggested small increased risk in MZ subjects.[114] Studies conducted in Sweden which avoid the major pitfalls of earlier studies indicate that in MZ individuals who smoke, there is an increased prevalence of emphysema at autopsy[115] and of physiological changes of emphysema during life.[116] Longitudinal studies of large cohorts of MZ individuals will be required to establish the clinical significance of these findings.

Studies with peptide fragments obtained from papain or cyanogen-bromide hydrolysis of pure, type-specific antitrypsins have revealed substitution of a glutamic acid residue in the normal Pi M protein with a valine residue in Pi type S,[117] and with a lysine residue in the Pi type Z[118,119] product. These findings explain the differences in electrophoretic mobility between the Pi M and Pi S proteins, which is one electron charge unit, and between the Pi M and Pi Z types, which is two charge units per molecule.

The hepatocytes of all subjects with a Pi Z allele contain the globules of antitrypsin within the endoplasmic reticulum which stain with the periodic acid-Schiff reaction after digestion with diastase. The globules have been isolated and characterized chemically.[120,121] The material isolated was extremely difficult to solubilize in aqueous media, but contained identical (or nearly identical) amino acids to those found in normal (Pi M) plasma antitrypsin. Although the inclusion material reacted with specific antitrypsin antibody, it did not inhibit trypsin. Most interesting, the carbohydrate composition of antitrypsin inclusion globules was much less than that found in normal (Pi M) plasma antitrypsin. The globules had no sialic acid and only a small percentage of the normal hexose concentrations.

Considerable debate ensued over the initial report of a decreased sialic acid concentration in the plasma antitrypsin of deficient (Pi Z) subjects.[122,123] The issue seems settled now. It appears that circulating antitrypsin in deficient subjects has a normal (six residues per molecule) complement of sialic acid;[108] only the hepatic antitrypsin is under-glycosylated. This strongly suggests that subjects who inherit the genetic code for type Z antitrypsin (whether hetero- or homozygotes), synthesize a species of antitrypsin in their hepatocytes that cannot be properly glycosylated. Without adequate glycosylation in the terminal endoplasmic reticulum and Golgi apparatus, the protein fails to be secreted from the hepatocytes into the circulation.

III. THE EXPERIMENTAL PRODUCTION OF EMPHYSEMA

A. Criteria of Emphysema

Since enlargement of air spaces can occur on a basis of distension of the lung alone, clear-cut proof of emphysema depends upon the demonstration of parenchymal destruction. To evaluate air space size or destruction, the lungs must be examined in the expanded state and for comparative purposes the degree of expansion must be controlled.[124] The lungs may be inflated to a consistent fraction of total lung volume or more commonly to a constant transpulmonary pressure.

Increased numbers of fenestrae and departition of alveoli also reflect destruction of lung tissue. With lungs from large animals, these changes can be seen with the dissecting microscope. For lungs from small animals, a scanning electron microscope is helpful.[125] In histologic sections, departition appears as alveolar septa which appear detached from the surrounding parenchyma (see Figure 5). The actual attachment sites, of course, would lie outside the plans of the section.

For illustrative purposes, gross specimens provide more convincing evidence than histology, especially since they indicate extent as well as severity of disease. Methods such as fume fixation,[126] barium sulfate impregnation,[127] and paper-mounted lung sections[128] are particularly effective.

Morphometric measurements on histologic sections can provide both proof of tissue destruction and quantitation for comparative purposes. The average distance between air space walls, the mean linear intercept (Lm), is a highly reproducible measurement of air space size.[129,130] Increased Lm indicates the presence of airspace enlargment, but may occur on a basis of overinflation alone. If lung volume and the mean linear intercept are known, the surface area of the gas-exchanging portion of the lung (ISA, internal surface area) can be calculated.[129,130] A decrease in ISA proves lung destruction; simple over-expansion would increase ISA. Enumeration of alveoli also can demonstrate lung destruction.[131] However, the recognition of alveoli in diseased tissue is not always easy.

Physiological measurements are useful in comparing experimental lesions to human emphysema and in quantitating severity of disease. They may permit sequential observations to be made in the same animal. As in man, changes in static lung compliance and elastic recoil are the most specific for emphysema. Diffusing capacity provides useful quantitation, but does not distinguish emphysema from other lung diseases. Measurements of airflow are useful for comparing the pathophysiology of the model to the human disease, but are less readily related to the defining characteristics of emphysema, air space size, and destruction.

B. Experimental Models

Two general approaches have been taken for the experimental production of emphysema in animals. One is to expose animals to agents implicated in the human disease; the other is to use manipulations which test theories of the pathogenesis of emphysema.

1. Exposure to Toxic Inhalants
a. Tobacco Smoke

As the major toxic inhalant implicated in human emphysema, cigarette smoke has been tested in animals. Hernandez et al. exposed greyhounds to cigarette smoke 30 to 45 min daily 5 days a week for varying periods.[132] Emphysema was evaluated from paper-mounted sections and quantitated by comparison with standard sections, a method thoroughly validated with human lungs.[133] Animals exposed for more than 12 months had emphysema, its severity increasing with duration of exposure. Microscopically the emphysema occurred in areas of chronic inflammation.

Auerbach et al. studied beagles exposed daily to cigarette smoke through a tracheostomy for more than 420 days.[134] They observed changes believed to be emphysema. The lungs were not fixed inflated to constant pressure, and morphometry was not performed. Subsequent electron microscopic study of the lungs showed fibrosis and loss of capillaries in emphysematous foci.[135]

Holland et al. described emphysema in rabbits exposed to cigarette smoke for 2-5½ years.[136] Rabbits are known to develop emphysema spontaneously.[137] Compared to controls, the exposed animals had a higher incidence, more widespread disease, and developed the lesions at an earlier age. The methods and criteria for emphysema were not detailed, and the lesions were not illustrated.

In the only study to combine pulmonary physiology and modern morphometric measurements, Park et al. found neither physiologic nor morphometric evidence of emphysema in beagles exposed to cigarette smoke for up to 1 year. Macrophage function was impaired in dogs exposed to smoke.[138]

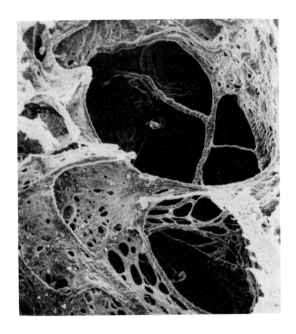

A

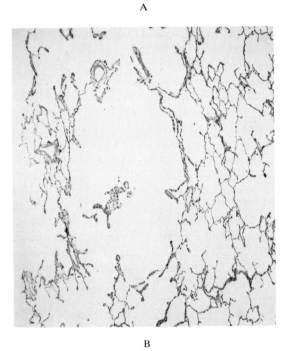

B

FIGURE 5.   Departition of airspaces. (A) Fenestrations in air space walls varying from numerous and small to few and large, suggesting coalescence. In the upper half of the photograph, only strands of tissue remain. (Scanning electron micrograph; magnification × 85.) (Reproduced from Kuhn, C. and Tavassoli, F., *Lab. Invest.*, 34, 2, 1976. With permission.) (B) The appearance of a similar area in a histologic section. Strands of tissue appear as detached "floating" segments of air space wall, near the center of an emphysematous space. The largest strand contains a blood vessel. (Hematoxylin-eosin; magnification × 85.)

It is difficult to compare these relatively few studies of chronic cigarette smoke exposure. Differences in exposure systems render dose comparisons difficult. In future studies, it would be useful to report on carboxyhemoglobin levels of animals after smoking as an indicator of the amount of gas phase delivered and on the deposition of a marker such as decachlorobiphenyl in the lung as a measure of particle deposition. In general, in reported experiments, exposures were short compared to the duration of smoking in human patients with emphysema whether in absolute time or fraction of life span. Taken together, the results discussed suggest that exposures in excess of one year can produce emphysema in animals, although the lesions illustrated have not been severe. As discussed elsewhere, tobacco smoke is known to have biologic effects on phagocytes and protease inhibitors which fit current hypotheses of the pathogenesis of emphysema.

b. Irritant Gases

The most extensively studied of the irritant gases is nitrogen dioxide, a compound of interest both as one of the ingredients of cigarette smoke and as an air pollutant. In cigarette smoke, the concentration is of the order of 250 ppm,[64] while in urban air, it is tenths of ppm. In addition, inhalation of NO_2 can occur in silofillers' disease and in a variety of industrial occupations.

The biologic effects of NO_2 have been reviewed elsewhere.[139-141] High concentrations can produce overt pulmonary edema, while chronic exposures to lesser concentrations (5 to 50 ppm) damage bronchiolar epithelium, impair the bactericidal activity of macrophage, decrease resistance to viral infections, and result in altered surfactant composition.

In terms of the development of emphysema, mice have been reported to be the most susceptible to NO_2. Exposure to 0.5 ppm produced bronchiolitis and overexpansion of air spaces which increased in severity with increasing duration of exposure up to 12 months.[142] Actual tissue destruction was not demonstrated morphometrically. It is likely from the microscopic description that the mice were infected with chronic murine pneumonia which may have contributed to the unusual susceptibility.

Rats exposed to 12 to 50 ppm of NO_2 also develop bronchiolitis, with ciliary loss, hyperplasia of bronchiolar epithelium, and Type II cells just distal to the terminal bronchiole. Air spaces are enlarged, and loss of surface area has been demonstrated after lifetime exposure.[143] At 2 ppm, emphysema does not develop.[144,145]

Studies in rabbits and hamsters have correlated physiological and anatomic changes and examined their reversibility. Exposure of rabbits to 10 ppm for 4 months produced bronchiolitis with enlargement of air spaces. Airway resistance and residual volume were increased, but static lung compliance $[C_{st}(L)]$ was normal. Recovery from exposure resulted in disappearance of the bronchiolitis and return of the physiological abnormalities to normal. Although airspace enlargement decreased, it did not return to normal.[146]

Kleinerman and co-workers conducted careful, detailed studies of NO_2 exposure at 20 ppm in hamsters. After 12 to 14 months exposure, the animals had increased airway resistance, but normal C_{st} (L) and C_{dyn} (L). Microscopically the animals showed a proliferative bronchiolitis and airspace enlargement. ISA was slightly but statistically significantly reduced. After 3 months, the airway resistance returned to normal. ISA was further reduced, although only mild and focal bronchiolar lesions remained. These consisted of mild epithelial proliferation and collections of macrophages. Thus, mild irreversible alveolar loss had occurred.[141]

During the first 2 days of exposure, the neutral protease activity in the lungs of exposed animals increased to twofold that of controls. The serum protease inhibitory activity also increased *pari passu*. By 50 days, both neutral protease activity and pro-

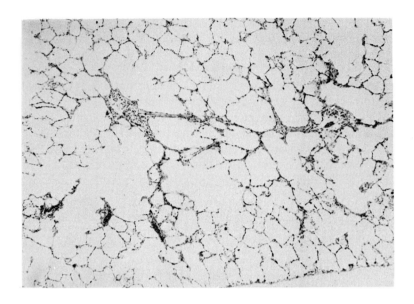

FIGURE 6.   Cadmium chloride-induced emphysema. Lung of a rat 15 days after the last of a series of 15 1-hr exposures to a 0.2% CaCl₂ aerosol. Delicate fibrous scars are surrounded by enlarged and distorted air spaces. (Hematoxylin-eosin; magnification × 85.) (Courtesy of Dr. Gordon Snider.)

tease inhibitory activity were normal.[147] Acid proteases, presumably cathepsins, in macrophages were increased in activity, but it is doubtful that these enzymes are active in the extracellular space where neutral pH prevails.[148] The transient nature of the rise in neutral protease activity and the compensating rise in protease inhibitory activity may account for the failure of NO₂ to produce more severe emphysema.

Boren failed to produce emphysema in mice with daily 30-min exposures to 25 ppm NO₂. In the expectation that adsorption of the gas onto an inert particulate carrier would permit greater deposition of the NO₂ in distal air spaces, he also exposed mice to a carbon aerosol saturated with NO₂. This resulted in enlargement of air spaces and loss of alveolar walls.[149] Other investigators found that simultaneous exposure of NO₂ and aerosols of NaCl[150] and fly ash[141] did not exaggerate the effects produced by NO₂ alone.

Other irritants have also been used to produce emphysema. Clay and Rossing used phosgene to produce emphysema in dogs. After 30 to 40 exposures to 24 to 40 ppm, the animals' lungs showed an obliterative bronchiolitis, enlarged air spaces, and fenestrations of up to 75 μm in alveolar walls.[151]

c. Cadmium Salts

Cadmium chloride administered by intratracheal injection[152] or aerosol[153,154] produces emphysema associated with foci of fibrosis. Initial acute damage to the proximal acinus with inflammation heals leaving fine scars surrounded by enlarged distorted alveoli (see Figure 6). The compliance of the lungs is reduced during the early inflammatory phase of the disease, but later increases to above normal.[155]

In summary, experiments using respiratory irritants have been only moderately successful in producing emphysema in animals. The emphysema which has been produced is of mild degree. The duration and intensity of exposure are the most obvious variables which influence the severity of disease. Physical properties of the irritant, such as the solubility of a gas or size of the particles in an aerosol, influence the extent of delivery to the alveolar level. Differences between species in airway anatomy, protease inhibitor levels, etc. may all be important. Further more, many human cigarette smokers deliberately inhale deeply; physical exertion may cause workers exposed to occupational irritants to do likewise. Comparable "cooperation" is rarely achieved in experimental animal exposures. Human subjects are exposed to complex mixtures, whereas animals are usually subjected to single chemically defined irritants. In light of all these variables, the failure of animal exposures to reproduce severe human emphysema is not surprising.

2. Experimental Studies of Pathogenesis
a. Early Studies

Early studies of the mechanism of production of experimental emphysema, reviewed elsewhere,[156,157] emphasized mechanical factors and alveolar atrophy. Repeated attempts to produce emphysema with valves or stenosis of the trachea have failed to produce the typical lesions of advanced destructive emphysema, although dilated airspaces have been found. Clinically, emphysema does not develop as a sequel to asthma.[158] Some patients with emphysema have no anatomic obstruction of airways. It is most unlikely that overdistension of the lung due to airway narrowing is sufficient to account for emphysema. Anderson et al. combined overdistension of the lungs produced with a venturi valve in the trachea with inflammation produced by injection of dilute nitric acid.[159] The combination produced emphysema while the valve alone did not. Unfortunately, there was no control group receiving the acid alone, so that the role of obstruction combined with tissue damage was not defined.

Another approach to enhancing the mechanical stress on the lung has been to stimulate ventilatory effort by exercise. Tura produced emphysema in rats by daily swimming to exhaustion for 90 days.[160] Emphysema judged from microdensitometry of chest X-rays and from histology was mild in most cases, but severe in a few. Cowdry et al. were unable to confirm Tura's results with less extreme swimming and suggested that Tura's results were the result of repeated aspiration.[161] The present authors have found that hamsters can be trained to swim for an hour per day or to run on a treadmill for 2 hr/day. Ten weeks of such exercise produces no change in the average distance between alveolar walls (Lm) or in the internal surface area of the lung.[162]

Besides the mechanical theory for the cause of emphysema, work has been done to test the idea that emphysema results from atrophy of alveolar walls due to ischemia. Strawbridge injected particles 10 to 25 μm in diameter of an inert dye caledon blue RC. Emphysema was observed after 3 to 6 months of weekly injections. The lesions were similar to those of spontaneous emphysema in the rabbit, but the incidence was significantly higher in animals receiving injections.

Wright and Kleinerman were unable to confirm that repeated i.v. injections of small particles produced emphysema. Neither glass beads 10 to 20 μm in diameter nor small silica particles were successful.[164] Boatman and Martin examined spontaneous emphysema in rabbits by electron microscopy and observed thin extensions of cytoplasm surrounding collagen and interpreted their observations as showing disrupted capillaries filled with collagen.[65] Since that publication, much more has been learned about the organization of the pulmonary interstitium. It now appears more likely that the cytoplasmic extensions which they observed were those of interstitial connective cells rather than endothelial cells and that the observations do not demonstrate vascular obliteration.

McLaughlin et al. injected chlorpromazine into the bronchial arteries of horses.[166] The chlorpromazine produced an acute necrotizing arteritis. Six horses died of the injections. Only 2 survived more than 12 weeks, and they had emphysema at autopsy.

However, the acute inflammation associated with the arteritis produced necrosis of bronchioles and even microinfarcts of alveolar walls. In these complicated lesions, it is not clear that ischemia can be blamed for the emphysema. In view of the presence of bronchial-pulmonary artery anastamoses at the bronchiolar level and a richly anastamotic pulmonary capillary bed, it is doubtful that ischemia plays a role in the development of human emphysema.

b. Injury to Connective Tissue

It is reasonable to assume that connective tissue plays the major role in the maintenance of an intact lung structure. Agents which damage connective tissue relatively selectively provide an approach to investigating the role of connective tissue in emphysema. Two approaches have been used: (1) experimental manipulations to interfere with the synthesis of normal connective tissue and (2) use of enzymes to destroy connective tissue elements once formed.

c. Abnormal Connective Tissue Synthesis
1. Dietary Lathyrism

The major connective tissue proteins, collagen and elastin, are discussed in detail elsewhere (see Chapter 5). Both collagen and elastin are stabilized by cross-links derived from the amino acid lysine. An essential first step in the formation of these cross-links is the oxidative deamination of certain lysines in the peptide chains of collagen and elastin to α adipic acid δ-semialdehyde (allysine) catalyzed by the copper-containing enzyme lysyl oxidase.[167,168] Interference in this cross-linking process in growing animals produces lathyrism, a syndrome dominated by aortic aneurysms and osseous deformities.[169]

The effect of feeding several lathyrogens on lung has been studied. Usually the lathyrogens have been fed for several weeks. Similar effects were produced by penicillamine ($\beta\beta$ dimethyl cysteine), a compound which prevents the participation of allysine in cross-linking and β-amino proprionitrile (βAPN), an inhibitor of lysyl oxidase which prevents formation of allysine. Lung compliance was increased, elastic recoil decreased, but only minimal if any morphologic abnormalities were produced.[170-172] Semicarbazide, a third lathyrogen, seemed to have a selective effect on collagen. Lung compliance was increased only at high transpulmonary pressure. Lungs ruptured easily, and mild airspace enlargement was observed morphologically in lungs fixed at 30 cm of water pressure, but lungs fixed at 20 cm of water pressure appeared normal.[173]

2. Congenital Lathyrism

Lathyrogens exert their effect only upon collagen and elastin molecules which are being synthesized during the period of feeding. Since connective tissue protein synthesis and degradation are slow in mature animals,[174,175] only a fraction of the total collagen and elastin are abnormal when the lathyrogen is applied late in life. Accordingly feeding lathyrogens has produced only small effects. In two models, the Blotchy mouse and the congenitally copper-deficient rat, deficient cross-linking of connective tissue proteins is present throughout development, so that the biochemical defect can be more widespread than with dietary lathyrism. Furthermore, elastin is believed to play an important developmental role in the formation of alveoli along alveolar ducts.[176-178] Thus, structural abnormalities in these congenital models of lathyrism may result from the impaired elastogenesis occuring at a critical time in development, as well as from the more widespread defect in cross-linking in comparison with late dietary lathyrism.

''Blotchy'' is one of several alleles at the ''mottled'' locus on the X-chromosome in the mouse. The mottled locus controls several copper-requiring enzymes, including those concerned with skin pigmentation and lysyl oxidase. Male mice hemizygous for the blotchy allele are deficient in lysyl oxidase.[179,180] They have an increased proportion of soluble collagen in their skin and have only 60 to 80% as much desmosine as normal mice per milligram of lung protein.[180] The lungs of blotchy mice are voluminous, air spaces are enlarged, and the surface area per unit lung volume is low compared to normal mice. Lung compliance with air and saline is increased, and elastic recoil is decreased. The architecture of the lung is markedly abnormal in some mice, but in others there is only dilation of alveolar ducts with shallow alveoli (see Figure 7).[181]

Deficiency of lysyl oxidase is also seen in copper deficiency. O'Dell et al. maintained female rats on a copper deficient diet throughout pregnancy and during the period of suckling and continued their offspring on the deficient diet after weaning.[182] The alkali-insoluble elastin content of the lungs of the offspring was reduced, and the lungs were large with dilated alveolar ducts and alveolar effacement very similar to that observed in the Blotchy mice. The lungs were abnormally fragile, and their pressure-volume characteristics could not be studied.

d. Enzyme-Induced Emphysema

In 1964 Gross et al. described the experimental production of emphysema with the intratracheal administration of papain, a broad spectrum protease.[183,184] This result was soon confirmed in other laboratories.[185-189] Currently, the use of proteases with appropriate specificity is the only reproducible model for producing severe emphysema in experimental animals. Together with the recognition of emphysema associated with α_1-antitrypsin deficiency, the capacity of proteases to produce emphysema has led to the hypothesis that an imbalance of proteases and their inhibitors is the mechanism of emphysema in man.

1. Proteolytic Specificity

A variety of enzymes, both pure and in crude mixtures, will produce emphysema. Included among the preparations used successfully are papain, bacterial and plant proteases,[190] leukocyte homogenates,[191] pancreatic elastase,[192,193] and granulocyte elastase.[194,195]

Not all proteases are effective, however, in causing emphysema. It appears that the capacity to destroy elastin is the essential property for the production of emphysema with proteolytic enzymes. For example, the ability of crude papain solutions to produce emphysema is closely related to their ability to degrade insoluble elastin.[196] Similarly, when a series of bacterial enzymes were tested, there was a close relationship between elastolytic activity and ability to produce emphysema.[190] Nonspecific protease activity correlated with ability to produce hemorrhage, but not emphysema. The severity of the emphysema produced by two different elastases of equal elastolytic activity in vitro was related to the amount of elastin destroyed in vivo and not to other signs of tissue injury, such as change in lung weight or mortality.[195] It has not been possible to produce emphysema with proteases lacking elastolytic activity. Notably bacterial collagenase does not produce emphysema, even at a dose acutely fatal to many of the experimental animals.[197]

Two points concerning elastases in the causation of emphysema merit comment:

1. Nonelastolytic enzymes may contribute to the breakdown of lung tissue that has been initiated by an elastase, so enzymes released in tissues along with elastases may enhance the effects of the elastolytic enzymes.[198]
2. The action of elastases upon lung constituents other than insoluble elastin may be important in producing the lung injury caused by elastase.

Two constituents of the lung's interstitial matrix, fibronectin and proteoglycans, are readily digested by some elastases.

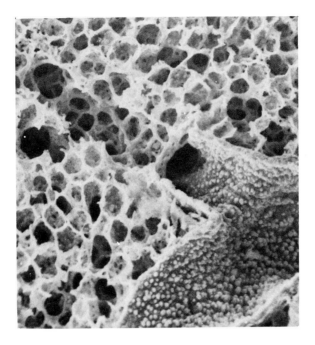

A

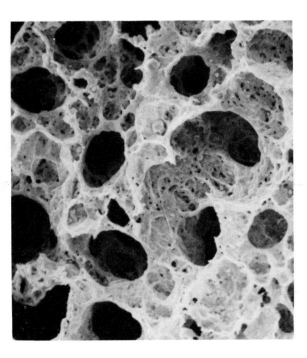

B

FIGURE 7. (A) A scanning electron micrograph of a normal lung from a $C_{57}B1$ mouse. (Magnification × 180.) (B) Lung from a male hemizygous Blotchy mouse showing enlarged and abnormal air spaces. (Magnification × 180.)

2. Route of Enzyme Exposure

Direct contact between lung tissue and protease is required to produce emphysema. Instillation of papain or leukocyte homogenates into one lung results in emphysema only in that lung.[199,200] The opposite lung is unaffected. Such observations do not, however, rule out the possibility that emphysema in these experiments occurs as a result of elastolytic activity released from cells brought to the lung by inflammatory contact between the protease and the lung tissue. Against this possibility is the fact that nonelastolytic proteases also elicit inflammation, but without causing emphysema.

While severe emphysema can be produced by introducing elastolytic enzymes into the air spaces, it is not clear whether emphysema can result from similar enzymes that enter the lungs through the pulmonary circulation under experimental conditions. Several studies have examined this issue with conflicting results.[200-203] There is agreement that if emphysema is to be produced by a single i.v. injection of enzyme, a large amount of elastolytic activity is needed. Schuyler et al. found that approximately 120 units of pancreatic elastase given i.v. to hamsters produced only minimal changes in lung elastic recoil without affecting the histology of the lungs or dimensions of air spaces.[203] This dose contrasts with a requirement for only five units to produce easily detectable emphysema when the enzyme is introduced through the airways.

One obvious explanation for the ineffectiveness of the intravenous route is the abundance of protease inhibitors in serum. Using the ability of enzymes to produce airspace enlargement in vitro in a perfused blood-free lung as an assay of emphysema production, Weinbaum et al.[200] found that the alveolar route was more effective than the vascular route even when serum was absent. Since the endothelium is more permeable to macromolecules than the alveolar epithelium,[204-206] the explanation cannot be differential permeability. Membrane bound protease inhibitors on endothelial cells[207] may reinforce the protection offered by circulating protease-inhibitors.

3. Properties of Enzyme-Induced Emphysema

The emphysema produced by papain and by pancreatic elastase are generally similar morphologically and physiologically. Emphysema produced by other enzymes has not been studied in comparable depth.

Morphologically, fully developed enzyme-induced emphysema is characterized by enlarged, abnormal air spaces with diminished alveolar surface area[131,189,192,208] and decreased alveolar number.[131] There is little evidence of fibrosis or inflammation by light microscopy. Focal goblet cell metaplasia occurs in large noncartilaginous airways.[209] In late stages of disease, the right ventricle is hypertrophic.[210]

Physiologically, the lungs have the major features of emphysema in man: total lung capacity (TLC), residual volume (RV), and RV/TLC are all increased; the lungs are abnormally compliant; elastic recoil is reduced; and carbon monoxide diffusing capacity is decreased.[187,189,208,211-213] Studies of airway resistance have given somewhat conflicting results, however. Comparing normal rats to rats with papain-induced emphysema, Park et al. found that expiratory airflow was normal for comparable degrees of elastic recoil. The mild expiratory airflow limitation they observed was entirely explicable by reduced elastic recoil.[211] Caldwell found decreased expiratory flow in rabbits with papain-induced emphysema, although he was unable to demonstrate altered compliance or decreased recoil.[188] He attributed flow limitation to loss of the tethering of small airways by the surrounding lung because he found decreased numbers of alveolar attachments to membranous bronchioles.

4. The Natural History of Enzyme-Induced Emphysema

The evolution of emphysema induced by intratracheal injection of pancreatic elastase in the hamsters has been studied in most detail. The natural history of papain-induced emphysema in the rat is generally similar and both enzymes produce similar morphologic and physiologic changes. Some of the biochemical details may differ, however.

Following a single intratracheal injection of 25 units of pancreatic elastase, there is very little recognizeable change in the first hour. In the second hour, the lung begins to increase in weight. Edema focal hemorrhages and infiltration with inflammatory cells appear and progressively increase for the first 24 hr.[192,193] Ultrastructurally there is evidence of injury to the alveolar epithelium. Intracellular edema, swelling of mitochondria and endoplasmic reticulum, and other nonspecific changes occur. Frank necrosis is extremely rare; denudation of the basal lamina is almost never seen. Elastic fibers begin to look smudged by light microscopy and acquire a granular ragged appearance by electron microscopy within the second hour.[162] The initial destruction of elastin is very rapid. Although damaged elastic fibers can be recognized up to day four by electron microscopy, the elastin content of the lung reaches its nadir approximately 4 hr after injection.[214,215] By light microscopy, many fibers have disappeared. Most of the destroyed elastin is rapidly cleared from the lung. The majority can be recovered in the first two days in the urine as peptides containing the desmosine cross-links characteristic of elastin.[215] The inflammatory response peaks within 1 to 2 days and subsides by 4 days. Neutrophils peak in lung lavage fluid in 24 hr and subsequently disappear. Macrophages begin to increase a day later and remain increased for several weeks.[216-218]

Despite the subsidence of the overt inflammation, the emphysema continues to evolve. Airspace enlargement, detectable within hours, progresses for 1 to 2 months (see Figures 8 and 9), accompanied by loss of surface area (see Figure 10).[192,208] The enlargement occurs mainly by dilation of alveolar ducts with shortening and effacement of alveolar walls.[125] Although morphologic changes stabilize,[189,208] physiologic deterioration continues. Static compliance increases for 6 weeks, correlating well with the anatomic changes. Residual volume, total lung capacity, and RV/TLC continue to increase for approximately 6 months.[208]

The elastin content of the lungs returns to normal or slightly above normal during the first 2 months after injection.[214] The elastic fibers synthesized under these conditions, however, are disorganized and do not reform a complete elastic network (see Figure 11). Collagen synthesis is also stimulated.[214]

Animals with elastase-induced emphysema suffer surprisingly little disability. Normal weight gain may be somewhat impaired, but hamsters can survive for at least 1 year, and rats can survive for at least 18 months (half the normal lifespan) and perhaps longer. They are able to exercise[219] and to withstand extended exposure to relatively high levels of air pollutants.[220]

5. The Mechanisms of Progression

Although the events involved in the progression of enzyme-induced emphysema are under active investigation, the mechanisms are far from clear. The duration of action of the injected enzyme has not been established. Kaplan and co-workers noted that after a single injection of elastase, active enzyme could be recovered in lung homogenates for several hours. A marked decrease in enzyme activity occurred at 2 to 4 hr, concurrent with the development of pulmonary edema.[192] They concluded that the influx of edema fluid containing serum protease inhibitors inactivated the enzyme. While it is now evident that the majority of the injected enzyme does become bound to inhibitors[221] and is cleared from the lung, a small amount may remain in the tissue. Stone et al. prepared ^{14}C-labeled elastase which retained full biological activity.[222] Although 90% of the injected elastase disappeared from the lung in the first 24 hr, 1% remained at 96 hr and later. Most of the label was associated with the tissue. It has

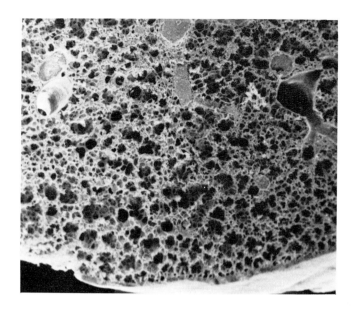

A

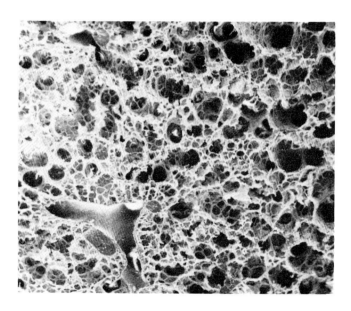

B

FIGURE 8.   Scanning electron micrographs showing the progression of the emphysema induced by a single intratracheal injection of pancreatic elastase. (A) In 2 days after the injection. (B) 2 weeks; (C) 2 months; (D) 12 months. (Magnification × 24.) (From Kuhn, C. and Tavassoli, F., *Lab. Invest.*, 34, 2, 1976. With permission.)

not been shown, however, whether this label is associated with enzymatically active elastase so long after injection. Consequently its importance in the progression of the lesion remains a matter for speculation.

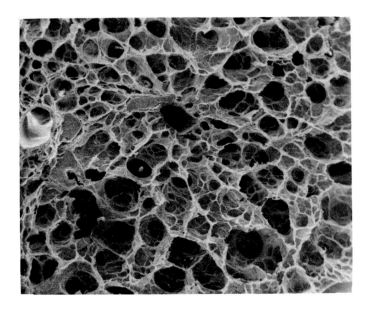

FIGURE 8C

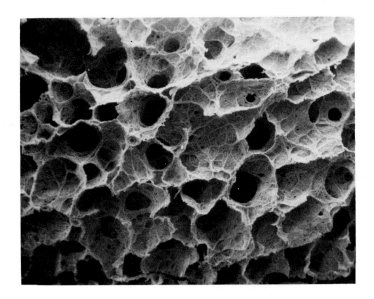

FIGURE 8D

Since inflammatory cells are recruited into the lung in response to enzyme injections, it is possible that products released from the inflammatory cells contribute to the progression. The influx of inflammatory cells can be diminished by treatment of the animals with cyclophosphamide[217] or antigranulocyte serum,[218] but the emphysema is no less severe. These experiments do not support a role for inflammatory cells in the progression of the emphysema.

Several lines of evidence support the idea that the ability of the lung to synthesize new connective tissue in response to the injury caused by enzyme injection prevents the progression of the disease. The anatomic progression slows or ceases at approxi-

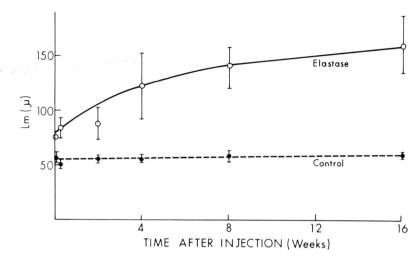

FIGURE 9. Changes in the average distance between air space walls (Lm) at intervals after a single injection of 25 units of pancreatic elastase.

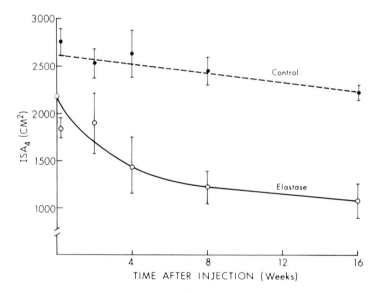

FIGURE 10. Changes in the internal surface area at intervals after a single injection of 25 units of pancreatic elastase. The surface area has been corrected to a standard lung volume of 4 cc (ISA_4).[130] The decrease in surface area is a measure of lung destruction.

mately 2 months after a single injection of 25 units of pancreatic elastase, a point that corresponds approximately to the time when the elastin content of the lung returns to normal. Doses of papain too low to produce emphysema do stimulate connective tissue synthesis.[223] This finding suggests that the lungs can repair low levels of damage and prevent the development of emphysema if the proteolytic insult is not harsh. If lathyrogens, BAPN or penicillamine, are fed to animals treated with elastase, the resultant emphysema is much more severe than that produced by the same dose of elastase in animals on a diet without lathyrogens.[224] Large bullae (see Figure 12) are common after as little as five units of elastase, a dose that otherwise leads to only minor emphysema. Since these lathyrogens do not produce structural changes in the lungs of saline injected animals, it is likely that their effect is due to their prevention of the synthesis of normal, cross-linked elastin and collagen following elastase injection.

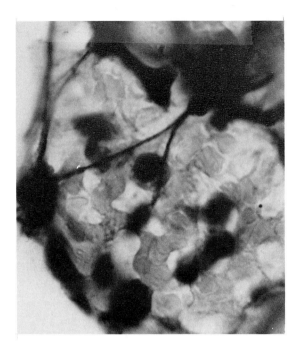

A

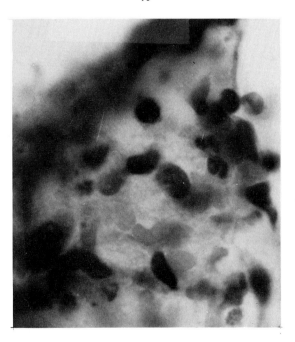

B

FIGURE 11.   Elastic fibers in thick sections (25 μm) of hamster lung. The alveolar walls are viewed *en face.* (A) In the normal lung the elastic fibers are smooth and straight; (B) 1 day after injection of pancreatic elastase the elastic fibers have disappeared; (C) and (D) 2 months after the injection. Disorganized, serpiginous elastic fibers. (Acid orcein-Verhoeff stain. Magnification × 1200.) (From Kuhn, C., Yu, S-Y., Chraplyvy, M., Linder, H. E., and Senior, R. M., *Lab Invest.,* 34, 372, 1976. With permission.)

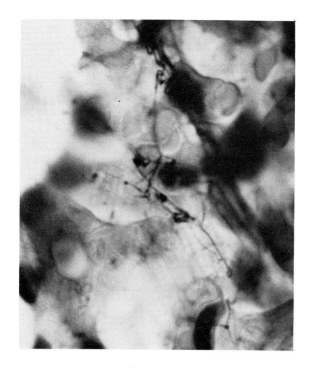

FIGURE 11C

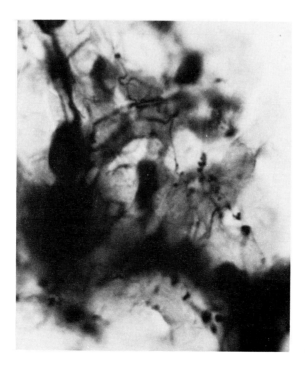

FIGURE 11D

An important function of lung connective tissue, especially elastic fibers, is to resist the mechanical stress accompanying normal respiratory movements. When the elastic

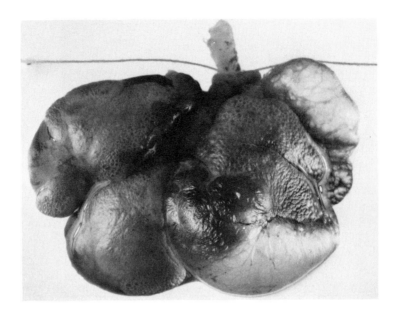

FIGURE 12.   Lung from a hamster fed a diet containing β-amino-proprionitrile (βAPN) and injected with 20 units of pancreatic elastase 6 weeks before sacrifice. This diet interferes with the cross-linking of connective tissue proteins and thus interferes with repair of elastase-induced damage. Severe emphysema with large bullae. Bullous emphysema, which is very rare following elastase injection alone, was seen in roughly half the animals injected while receiving the βAPN diet.

network is destroyed, the stress of breathing may produce progressive tissue deformity. Sahebjami and Vassallo have presented some evidence for this view.[219] They found larger shifts from the normal in the pressure volume curves of the lungs of papain-injected rats that were subjected to treadmill exercises than in animals not forced to exercise. Their findings suggested that the greater transpulmonary pressure changes associated with exercise-induced hyperpnea influenced the ultimate severity of the disease. Unfortunately, morphological measurements of the emphysema were not reported so that the quantitative difference between the two groups could not be stated. The ability of the lung to replace the destroyed elastin, even in the form of disorganized fibers, may improve its ability to resist mechanical stress.

The role of protease inhibitors in emphysema needs further study in experimental systems. Kaplan et al. observed that mixing pancreatic elastase with normal serum before injection prevented the development of emphysema, whereas α_1-antitrypsin deficient (Pi Z) serum was ineffective. They interpreted this result as demonstrating the requirement for uninhibited enzyme.[192] It has since been suggested that complexes formed between α_2-macroglobulin and elastase remain active against elastin and its soluble precursors.[225] Such complexes may have been operative when the elastase was mixed with Pi Z serum. Since α_2-macroglobulin complexes with proteases are rapidly taken up by macrophages, however, they may be less important in lung destruction than in vitro experiments would suggest.

Martorana and Share found that treatment of hamsters by the intratracheal instillation of α_1-antitrypsin 40 min before exposure to papain protects against the development of emphysema. I.v. injection of α_1-antitrypsin was ineffective.[226] Since 40 min is adequate time for circulating α_1-antitrypsin to equilibrate with the pulmonary interstitial fluid,[227] these results emphasize the importance of local inhibitory mechanisms in the lung.

The recent development of methods to depress active circulating α_1-antitrypsin levels in animals using galactosamine to impair hepatic protein synthesis[228,229] or chloramine T to inactivate the protein by oxidation[230] offer interesting new tools for analyzing the role of protease inhibitors. Neither method is as free of side effects on other metabolic systems as the genetic "model" in man, but the availability of different models, presumably with different side effects, should permit rapid progress in this area.

IV. ELASTASES

A. General Remarks Concerning the Measurement of Elastases

The attention given elastases lately as a factor in the pathogenesis of emphysema and other diseases has stimulated interest in methods to measure elastolytic activity accurately in trace amounts. Difficulties in establishing whether human alveolar macrophages have elastase activity have drawn particular attention to pitfalls in elastase assays.[231] In brief, the important lesson learned has been that elastin, in some form, is the only appropriate substrate.[232] The necessity of using elastin instead of synthetic substrates stems from findings that the use of synthetic substrates may be misleading for at least two reasons:

1. A given synthetic synthetic substrate may be attacked by some, but not all elastases.
2. Attack of a particular substrate by one type of elastase does not insure that elastolytic activity is present whenever that substrate is hydrolyzed.

Experience with two synthetic substrates for pancreatic elastase, N-tert-butoxycarbonyl-L-alanyl-p-nitrophenyl ester (NBA) and succinyl L-alanyl-L-alanyl-L-alanyl-p-nitroanalide (SLAPN), illustrate the need for caution in assaying elastases with substrates other than elastin. NBA and SLAPN can be hydrolyzed by pancreatic and neutrophil elastases, but these substrates cannot be used interchangeably, since the activity of neutrophil elastase against NBA exaggerates by a factor of about 20 the enzyme's activity against SLAPN or elastin, using pancreatic elastase as the reference enzyme. SLAPN seems to give an accurate measure of neutrophil elastase activity against elastin, but hydrolytic activity against SLAPN is not always matched by elastolytic activity. There is some evidence that human alveolar macrophages release activity against SLAPN that is associated with little or no elastolytic activity.[233] More impressive are data that hydrolytic activity against SLAPN has been found in rheumatoid synovial fluid[234] and in human bile,[235] but in neither instance is the activity matched by elastase activity.

While the use of an elastin substrate for assay of elastases is much more reliable than synthetic substrates, it may not entirely reproduce the effect of elastases in vivo. The activity of elastases against elastin may vary according to the source of the elastin substrate and even its manner of extraction. Moreover, in vivo the susceptibility of elastin to elastases may be influenced by interactions with neighboring constituents such as glycoproteins and phospholipids.

B. Elastases and Their Role in the Development of Pulmonary Emphysema

While papain and other plant proteases with elastolytic activity cause emphysema in animals, there is no evidence that such enzymes have a role in human emphysema. Indeed, it is doubtful that any exogenous elastolytic enzyme can be implicated in the human disease.

The pancreas appeared to be the only source of animal elastase until 1968 when Janoff and Scherer reported elastolytic activity in human neutrophils.[236] Subsequently,

Table 2
SOME PROPERTIES OF ELASTASES

	Porcine pancreatic elastase	Human neutrophil elastase	Human platelet elastase
Mol wt	25,000	29,000—31,000	26,000
$(E_{280}^{1\%})$	18.5	9.85	—
Carbohydrate (%)	0	21.2	0
Amino terminus	Valine	Isoleucine	Valine

elastases have been reported associated with macrophages,[237-240] monocytes,[241,242] platelets,[243] vascular tissues, and tumors.[244] Although elastases share the capacity to hydrolyze elastin, it is evident that the enzymes from different tissues are not identical and ought not be considered interchangable (see Table 2). Clear-cut differences exist in molecular weight, amino acid sequence, and carbohydrate between the pancreatic, neutrophil, platelet, and macrophage elastases. The differences between the elastolytic enzymes may be of more than biochemical interest; the physiological functions of the enzymes may also differ.

C. Endogenous Elastases with Access to the Lungs
1. Elastolytic Activity in Serum

Using a radiolabeled elastin substrate capable of detecting a few nanograms or less of elastolytic activity, we could not find elastolytic activity in serum from normal individuals.[245] This observation seems plausible in view of the high concentration of serum inhibitors of elastases. On the other hand, with a different elastin substrate, a solubilized component of elastin referred to as kappa-elastin,[246] elastase-like activity has been reported in normal serum with elevated levels in serum of patients with severe burns.[247] The same sera do not, however, solubilize intact elastin. The levels of activity against kappa-elastin are impressively high, equivalent to 50 μg of pancreatic elastase per mililiter of serum, but the significance as related to elastin metabolism is unclear. The source of the activity against Kappa-elastin is not known, but either pancreatic or leukocytic elastases or both are possible since both enzymes can be found in serum by immunological methods.[248,249] Levels of proteolytic activity in serum using elastin or kappa elastin substrates have not been reported in patients with chronic airflow obstruction.

2. Pancreatic Elastase

Pancreatic elastase, the first elastase identified in mammals, attacks a variety of proteins.[250] The possibility that pancreatic elastase is involved in human emphysema seems small, but cannot be excluded. By radioimmunoassay, a pancreatic protease can be detected in the circulation of normal adults at a concentration of approximately 70 ng/mℓ.[248] Radioimmunoassay identifies enzyme that is bound to α_1-antitrypsin, but does not recognize enzyme bound to α_2-macroglobulin. Elastase α_2-macroglobulin complexes may be important in the pathogenesis of tissue injury, since association of the ezyme with α_2-macroglobulin could provide the enzyme with protection from circulating inhibitors without blocking the activity of the enzyme against many substrates, some of large molecular weight.[225]

3. Neutrophil Elastase

The proteases of neutrophils have been discussed in detail in a recent monograph.[251] Mature, circulating neutrophils contain an abundance of elastase activity. The enzyme protein comprises 10% or more of the neutrophil granule protein.[252] Neutrophil elastase is located within the azurophil granules along with numerous other substances, including another highly cationic enzyme, cathepsin G.[253,254] Immature neutrophils contain less elastase than mature cells, but neutrophils from patients with chronic myelogenous leukemia are a plentiful source.[255]

Elastase activity has been found in neutrophils from rabbit,[253] dog,[255] mouse,[256] and man. It is likely, but still unproven that all mammals have elastase in their neutrophils. Humans with the Chediak-Higashi syndrome and its murine counterpart, the beige mouse, appear to be markedly deficient in elastase activity,[257] however, the human cells do have material that reacts with antibody directed against purified human leukocyte elastase.[258]

The large quantity of elastase in neutrophils has facilitated its purification. A number of procedures have been used with comparable success.[251,259-261] Several milligrams of the pure enzyme can be recovered from 500 mℓ of blood. Sputum from individuals with bronchitis has proven a particularly rich source, providing many milligrams.[261,262]

By acrylamide gel electrophoresis at acid pH, neutrophil elastase appears as several close bands of which the heaviest is the most cationic. The differences in charge between the forms appear to relate to carbohydrate since their amino acid composition, elastolytic activity, and immunoreactivity are similar.[260]

The first report of neutrophil elastase showed that it differed from pancreatic elastase.[236] Unlike the pancreatic enzyme, high concentrations of sodium chloride enhanced the activity and soybean trypsin inhibitor was inhibitory.

In recent years, the differences between neutrophil elastase and pancreatic elastase have been extended to include amino acid composition, peptide bond specificity, and immunological properties.[260,263] Clearly, even within the same species, pancreatic and neutrophil elastases are not the same. Purified protein with elastolytic activity obtained from human pancreas does not cross react with antiserum prepared against human neutrophil elastase.[260,264]

Apart from biochemical differences, human neutrophil elastase and porcine pancreatic elastase also differ in their effects upon tissues and isolated cells. When the enzymes were given intratracheally to hamsters, the consequences were not the same.[195] Neutrophil elastase produced severe hemorrhage with a high mortality, but only mild emphysema in the survivors. Pancreatic elastase, however, caused a low level of early mortality, but led to severe emphysema. A recent study of interactions between elastases and macrophages describes another difference. Alveolar macrophages appear to have specific receptors for neutrophil elastase, but not for pancreatic elastase (see Figure 13).[265]

Neutrophil elastase has the capacity to hydrolyze many substances (see Table 3). Some of the substrates such as fibronectin are extraordinarily sensitive to the enzyme.[266] Indeed, since the enzyme has such a wide range of potential activities, the label "elastase" may be misleading as to its important function. Neutrophil elastase also facilitates bactericidal action of the neutrophil,[267,268] stimulates lymphocytes,[269] and both generates and degrades biologically active fragments from complement components.[270-272] Accordingly, the release of neutrophil elastase may cause tissue injury not only by direct enzymatic action, but also by initiating inflammatory reactions.

4. The Relationship of Neutrophil Elastase to Chronic Obstructive Pulmonary Disease (COPD)

Galdston and associates were the first to point out that the balance between neutrophil elastase activity and α_1-antitrypsin concentration might be important in determining the development of emphysema.[273] From data in a small number of carefully selected subjects, they concluded that normal neutrophil elastase levels in the presence of reduced antitrypsin tipped the balance in favor of proteolysis and consequent em-

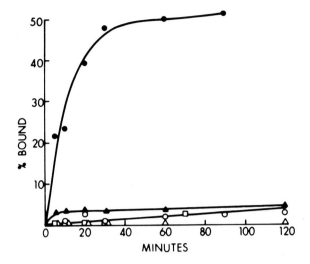

FIGURE 13. Data showing specific binding of ^{125}I-labeled human leukocyte elastase (●) to alveolar macrophages. Several other labeled proteins at comparable molar concentrations did not show specific binding: porcine pancreatic elastase, ▲; human pancreatic elastase, ○; porcine trypsin, □; and bovine serum albumin, △. (Reproduced from Campbell, E. J., White, R. R., Senior, R. M., Rodriquez, R. J., and Kuhn, C., *J. Clin. Invest.*, 64, 824, 1979. With permission.)

Table 3
BIOLOGICAL SUBSTRATES OF HUMAN NEUTROPHIL ELASTASE

Substrate	Ref.
Elastin	236
Collagen	364
Proteoglycans	364
	365
Fibronectin	266
Basal lamina	366
Fibrinogen	367
Complement components, C_3 and	270
C_5	271
	269
Complement-derived chemotactic factors	272
Immunoglobulins	368
Bacterial proteins	267
	268

physema, whereas low levels of neutrophil elastase activity offset the effects of decreased α_1-antitrypsin. This attractive concept has been tested lately in studies involving groups with various combinations of normal lung function or of chronic air flow obstruction and α_1-antitrypsin phenotypes MM, or MZ, and ZZ.[274-278] These studies are in agreement that wide differences in neutrophil elastase levels occur between individuals. Several of these studies found that among individuals with partial or severe antitrypsin deficiencies neutrophil elastase levels are higher in those with chronic air flow obstruction.[276-278] Still unsettled is whether the levels are higher in the typical patient with chronic air flow obstruction whose antitrypsin concentration is normal.

The possible association of neutrophil elastase activity with COPD strengthens the general view that elastolytic activity has a role in the pathogenesis of emphysema and incriminates neutrophil elastase as an important pathogenetic form of elastase. In addition, it provides one explanation for the variability in occurrence of chronic obstructive lung disease among individuals with partial (MZ) or severe (ZZ) antitrypsin deficiency.

5. Macrophage Elastase

Definitive proof of a macrophage elastase was reported first in 1975 in studies of mouse peritoneal macrophages in culture.[238] These cells were found to release small amounts of activity capable of digesting insoluble elastin. Only trace quantities of the activity could be recovered from cell homogenates. Besides mouse peritoneal macrophages, elastase has now been found in the culture media of alveolar and peritoneal macrophages from a number of animals, including mice, guinea pigs, hamsters, and rabbits.[238,239,279,280]

Animal macrophage elastase activity has several characteristics that distinguish it from either neutrophil or pancreatic elastases. At least some forms are barely affected by either α_1-antitrypsin or chloromethylketones, do not hydrolyze SLAPN, and require calcium for activity.[238-240]

Although observations with animal macrophages seem to offer clear-cut proof that macrophages can make elastase activity, such definite results have not been obtained in studies of human alveolar macrophages.[232,240,281,282] Indeed there is disagreement about whether the human cells contain elastase activity, whether they release elastase activity, and whether the elastase activity associated with them in some studies is a product of macrophage synthesis or is instead elastase that has been internalized as might result from binding of neutrophil elastase to cell surface receptors. Table 4 summarizes experiences with measurements of elastase activity upon human alveolar macrophages and monocytes.

From the various results with human alveolar macrophages, several conclusions can be drawn.

1. Human alveolar macrophages seem clearly different from mouse and some other animal alveolar macrophages by secreting much less elastolytic activity per cell. Whether the differences relates to using an inappropriate elastin substrate, failure to develop proper culture conditions, or lack of activation of a proenzyme remains to be determined. It is possible that under some conditions elastolytic activity might be readily apparent.
2. Because human alveolar macrophages bind and internalize neutrophil elastase,[266] macrophage extracts and conditioned media containing dead or dying alveolar macrophages may include leukocyte elastase with the quantity depending on the amount of enzyme in the macrophage's environment prior to cell collection and the rate of neutrophil elastase degradation once it is inside the cell.
3. If human alveolar macrophages have intrinsic elastase activity, it may be associated with more than one enzyme, one resembling neutrophil elastase and one or more with metalloproteinase characteristics similar to mouse macrophage elastase.[283]

6. Effects of Smoking on Elastase Production by Alveolar Macrophages

A number of indirect observations suggest the involvement of macrophages in the pathogenesis of emphysema. Macrophages are the characteristic inflammatory cell of

Table 4

EVIDENCE FOR ELASTOLYTIC ACTIVITY ASSOCIATED WITH HUMAN MONONUCLEAR PHAGOCYTIC CELLS

Cell type	Material assayed	Test substrate	Comment	Ref.
Alveolar macrophage (postmortem lungs)	Cell homogenate and granule extract	Elastin-orcein		237
Alveolar macrophage	Culture media	Elastin in agar	Activity only with smokers' cells	282
Alveolar macrophage	Cell homogenate	^{3}H-labeled elastin	No relationship of activity to degree of obstructive lung disease	289
Alveolar macrophage	Culture media	Elastin in agarose	Increased release of activity in the presence of phagocytosis of latex particles	240
Alveolar macrophage	Lysosomal extracts and culture media	Oxalic acid solubilized elastin	No relationship of activity to smoking; continuous release of activity over 6 weeks; activity inhibited by elastase specific chloromethyl ketones	281
Alveolar macrophage	Cell homogenate	^{3}H-labeled elastin	Low-level activity resembling neutrophil elastase; its presence not influenced by inhibition of protein synthesis	234
Monocytes	Intact cells	Fluorescein conjugated monospecific antiserum against human neutrophil elastase	Immunoreactive material in 30% of glass attached cells, but not in freshly harvested cells	241
Monocytes	Culture media of cells exposed to immune complexes	^{125}I-labeled fibrin	Elastase activity detected indirectly by using elastase specific chloromethyl ketones to decrease fibrinolysis; the elastase activity resembled neutrophil elastase	242

the early lesions of emphysema.[284] In cigarette smokers, the number of macrophages which can be recovered from the lung is increased severalfold.[285] In a study of the lungs of young cigarette smokers at autopsy, accumulations of macrophages loaded with brown pigment in respiratory bronchioles was the only consistent morphologic feature which distinguished the smokers from nonsmokers.[286]

Although smoking clearly produces a number of alterations in the properties of alveolar macrophages, (see Chapter 1) the relationship of smoking to elastase release by human macrophages remains unsettled. Rodriguez et al. observed elastolytic activity in culture media containing smokers' cells, but not in media with cells from nonsmokers.[282] Others, however, have found no difference in the amounts of elastase activity released by human alveolar macrophages, irrespective of whether the cells come from smokers or nonsmokers.[281] As noted earlier, some workers find no elastase release by human alveolar macrophages whether the cells are from smokers or nonsmokers.[234]

Where experimental animals have been examined, the results favor the conclusion that smoking does enhance the release of elastase activity from macrophages. In mice and baboons, smoking leads to increases in the elastase activity released per cell.[287,288] The enhanced macrophage elastase associated with smoking in mice does not, however, appear to involve direct action upon the cells since the effects of cigarette smoking in vivo cannot be duplicated in vitro simply by exposing cells to smoke. White et al.

suggest that cigarette smoke may produce its effect upon elastase production indirectly either by recruiting activated cells into the alveolar spaces or by stimulating other cells, probably lymphocytes, to release factors that stimulate the resident macrophages.[287]

With the data at hand, it appears that a relationship between emphysema and macrophage elastase will be difficult to establish. The only report thus far that looked specifically at macrophage elastase levels in patients with chronic air flow obstruction came to a negative conclusion. In this study, macrophage elastase was found in the cells and varied nearly 20-fold between individuals, yet the elastase levels showed no relation to a battery of pulmonary function abnormalities.[289]

7. Platelet Elastase

Human platelets contain an elastase that is associated in part with the α-granule and in part with the membrane, a distribution similar to the platelet collagenase.[243,290] An interesting feature that distinguishes platelet elastase from neutrophil elastase is that it can be found in a precursor form.[291] The active form may be generated by exposing the precursor to trypsin. There is no evidence implicating platelet elastase in the pathogenesis of emphysema, but it seems reasonable to suspect at the least that the enzyme may be involved in some forms of lung injury such as caused by disseminated intravascular coagulation.

8. Release of Elastases from Neutrophils and Macrophages

For many years, neutrophils and macrophages were regarded exclusively as phagocytic cells having as functions only ingestion and digestion. This concept has had to be revised extensively to incorporate the discovery that viable phagocytic cells release many biologically active substances.[292,293] The variety of substances released, the mechanisms of release, and factors that modulate release are currently topics of considerable interest and a large mass of experimental data is accumulating quickly.

It is already clear that many factors influence the release of substances from neutrophils and macrophages and that the release processes are complex. Potentially releasable substances are not necessarily affected in a uniform way from the same cell. Thus, an agent acting on neutrophils may selectively favor release of primary granule contents over the constituents of azurophil granules.[293a] Likewise, some agents have divergent effects upon the secretion of different enzymes from macrophages.[294]

Important differences exist between neutrophils and macrophages relating to the storage, speed of release, and the factors that influence the release of elastase and other substances. Neutrophils contain large quantities of elastase and can release within minutes as much as 35% of the total enzyme content. In contrast, macrophages do not have bursts of enzyme release even when stimulated. Macrophages, at least those from animals, are capable of secreting elastase steadily for long periods when held in culture, unless protein synthesis is blocked.[238,239]

a. Neutrophils

Four principal mechanisms have been described for the release of neutrophil lysosomal contents.[295]

1. Cell death
2. Cell perforation from within, a phenomenon occurring after the cell internalizes certain materials such as crystalline silica
3. So called "regurgitation during feeding" a designation of the discharge of lysosomal contents into an incompletely formed phagocytic vacuole
4. Reverse endocytosis, or the release of lysosomal contents directly into the exterior of the cell coincident with the cell's efforts to internalize a large, nonphagocytosable surface

Neutrophils also discharge lysosomal enzymes when the cell surface makes contact with appropriately altered IgG or C3 fragments and when chemotactic agents react with the cell in the presence of cytochalasin B.[292,295]

A variety of pharmacologic agents affect the quantities of lysosomal contents released during endocytic events. Among the agents that are inhibitory are glucocorticoids, theophylline, β-adrenergic agonists, and cyclic AMP. Substances that augment lysosomal release include cyclic GMP and cholinergic agonists.

With specific reference to the pathogenesis of emphysema, relatively little is known about factors in the lungs that might promote neutrophil lysosomal enzyme release. Among the few relevant facts are that ingredients in cigarette smoke cause rapid release of active elastase from neutrophils and that alveolar macrophages upon stimulation produce chemotactants for neutrophils.[297-299] The interplay between neutrophils, other inflammatory cells, and toxic inhaled substances is an area that needs much investigation.

b. Macrophages

The mechanism for release of elastase and other substances from macrophages can only be described in general terms. As outlined by Cohn, the release of macrophage products would appear to involve events such as fusion of either tiny Golgi vesicles or secondary lysosomes with incompletely formed endocytic vacuoles and with the plasma membrane itself.[300] Whether the different products utilize different pathways and whether a substance follows the same routes at all times are not known.

Substances released by mouse macrophages appear to be under various controls. Lysozyme is released irrespective of the state of activation of the cells, while other products, including collagenase, elastase, and plasminogen activator, are released differently according to the state of macrophage stimulation.[301] The release of macrophage products can be influenced by agents such as colchicine, prostaglandins, glucocorticoids, and factors derived from lymphocytes.

The control of releaseable substances from the cells is complex and cannot even be generalized for elastase and the other neutral proteases. An agent does not necessarily affect the release of the various neutral proteases in a uniform manner. Colchicine, for example, inhibits release of plasminogen activator, but enhances release of elastase and collagenase.[294] Tumor lines derived from murine macrophages highlight the variability of neutral protease release that can occur. These neoplastic cells distinguish themselves by producing different patterns of neutral proteases depending upon the cell line.[302,303] It would appear that each macrophage product may need to be examined separately to understand production, release, and controlling factors.

With reference to macrophage elastase, studies have been done primarily using murine cells. Resident mouse peritoneal macrophages release low levels of elastase that can be boosted by giving the cells phagocytosable material.[238] Even then the cells do not release as much elastase activity as peritoneal exudative cells which are elicited by instilling thioglycollate medium into the peritoneal cavity a few days before harvesting cells. Mouse alveolar macrophages secrete still more elastase activity, suggesting that they have been stimulated spontaneously.[239] Although phagocytosis will not increase the output of elastase activity by alveolar cells, their release of elastase can be increased with chemical agents including cytochalasin B and colchicine. Glucocorticoids inhibit the release of elastase activity by peritoneal exudate cells, an effect also seen upon rabbit and guinea pig alveolar macrophages.[279]

Since macrophages are known to release elastase and elastases have been implicated in emphysema, macrophages have been thought important in the pathogenesis of emphysema. Unfortunately, there is only limited support from a study of human alveolar macrophages. As noted above, it remains uncertain whether human alveolar cells pro-

Table 5
SERUM PROTEASE INHIBITORS[a]

Inhibitor	Mol wt	Carbohydrate content (%)	Active on elastase
α_1-Antitrypsin	56,000	12	Yes
α_1-Antichymotrypsin	69,000	25	No
Inter α-trypsin inhibitor	160,000	8	No
Antithrombin III	65,000	13	No
Cl-inactivator	104,000	35	No
α_2 Macroglobulin	780,000	7.7	Yes
α_1-Anticollagenase	40,000	—[b]	No

[a] Based largely on Heimberger et al.[311] and Wooley et al.[312]
[b] Not reported.

duce elastase. At this writing, caution must be expressed that the attractiveness of assigning a role to macrophage elastase in the development of emphysematous lesions should not be mistaken for evidence that it is actually involved.

c. Evidence that Elastases are Released from Phagocytic Cells In Vivo

Using immunoassay, human neutrophil elastase has been detected in blood and other materials from diseased sites, such as inflamed gingivae, rheumatoid joints, bronchitic airways, and inflamed peritoneal cavities.[304-307] The enzyme has been found free and in association with inhibitor. Even plasma from healthy persons contains immunoreactive enzyme bound to α_1-antitrypsin. The mechanism for entry of the enzyme into the plasma is not known.

Whether neutrophil elastase has a role in the pathogenesis of pulmonary emphysema is still unproved, but it appears likely from indirect evidence and from the fact that the enzyme with inhibitor probably enters lung tissue regularly along with other plasma constituents that diffuse out of plasma into the interstitial spaces. The enzyme may also gain access to lung tissues as a result of neutrophil decay in the lung,[308,309] a phenomenon believed to be normal in the turnover of neutrophils. However, there are as yet no data showing a positive balance across the pulmonary circulation for neutrophil elastase or other neutrophil constituents. Only small numbers of neutrophils can be found in alveoli normally.[310] Bronchopulmonary lavage from smokers yields a low percentage of neutrophils among the cells, and their source, whether alveolar or small airway, is not clear.

Macrophage elastase has not been identified in vivo either in normal or diseased tissues and fluids. As occurred with neutrophil elastase, identification of macrophage elastase in tissue awaits developments of radioimmunoassays and other immunological techniques.

V. PROTEASE INHIBITORS

A major line of defense against damage due to proteases released in the tissues is provided by macromolecular inhibitors, proteins which bind with proteases and inactivate them. Both serum proteins and nonserum inhibitors produced locally are available to control extracellular proteolysis in the lung. Table 5 lists the serum protease inhibitors. At least two, α_1-antitrypsin and α_2-macroglobulin, complex with pancreatic and granulocyte elastase. It appears that mouse macrophage elastase is not inhibited by α_1-antitrypsin. Two nonserum elastase inhibitors also have been identified in the lung.[313,314]

Weinbaum et al. studied a heat stable inhibitor present in dog lung lavage which was distinguishable from α_1-antitrypsin and α_2-macroglobulin and was effective against chymotrypsin, pancreatic elastase, and granulocyte elastase, but not trypsin.[313] Of the enzymes tested, granulocyte elastase was the most sensitive to inhibition. This inhibitor may also be effective against macrophage elastase, since unfractionated lavage fluid inhibits macrophage elastase, despite the resistance of this enzyme to α_1-antitrypsin.[239]

Hochstrasser and colleagues originally isolated a low molecular weight protease inhibitor from sputum which is an effective inhibitor of bovine trypsin, human or dog leukocyte elastase, and cathepsin G.[314,315] It does not inhibit pancreatic elastases or leukocyte collagenase. The inhibitor is acid stable, has a mol wt of approximately 11,000 daltons, and shares antigenic determinants with the interalpha trypsin inhibitor in serum.[316] It appears to be identical with an inhibitor found in other mucous secretions, notably cervical mucus and seminal plasma.[317] It has been localized to the cytoplasm of bronchial and paranasal sinus epithelial cells by immunocytochemistry. This suggests that it is synthesized in large airways where it is thought to help to protect mucous epithelia from damage by leukocyte proteases.[318] Since it has not been demonstrated at the alveolar level, it may not be directly relevant to emphysema.

α_1-Antitrypsin not only circulates in the plasma, it is distributed in the extracellular fluid[319] and has been identified in a wide variety of body fluids.[103] It is consistently found in bronchoalveolar lavage fluid[320-324] and has been localized to the alveolar lining by immunofluorescence.[325] Hence it is available to inactivate leukoproteinases released in the alveoli under normal conditions. Under conditions of overt inflammation in which there is a large influx and accelerated degranulation of neutrophils, the accompanying edema would be expected to provide a large increment of α_1-antitrypsin from the serum. In fact, during acute inflammation arteriovenous differences in α_1-antitrypsin can be measured across the lung indicating sequestration of this protein in the inflamed tissue.[326]

α_1-Antitrypsin is mainly effective against serine proteases. It inhibits through the formation of an equimolar complex with the target protease. The protease cleaves the antitrypsin molecule during the process, with the generation of a new amino terminal amino acid.[327,328] There is evidence that there are in fact two bonds susceptible to cleavage by pancreatic elastase. If one specific bond near the carboxyterminal end of the α_1-antitrypsin molecule is cleaved, the α_1-antitrypsin is inactivated as an inhibitor without forming a stable complex with the enzyme.[327] If the other bond, a methionyl-serine or methionyl-threonine bond near the amino terminal end of the α_1-antitrypsin molecule is cleaved, the protease forms a stable complex and is thereby inhibited.[327,329] The same bond appears to be involved in the inhibition of trypsin, chymotrypsin, and elastase.

If inadequate amounts of α_1-antitrypsin due to an abnormal gene can lead to emphysema, it is possible that interference with its function could also lead to unchecked proteolysis. This possibility was suggested by Chowdhury and Louria, who compared the effects of Cd and other trace metals on the α_1-antitrypsin content and trypsin-inhibitory capacity (TIC) of serum.[330] Cd over the range 10 to 50 $\mu g/m\ell$ produced a dose related fall in α_1-AT and TIC in serum. The authors noted that similar concentrations of Cd occur in industrial workers heavily exposed to Cd and suggested that interference with α_1-AT could explain the emphysema in Cd workers. Their experiments were not well controlled for the fall in pH which accompanied the addition of the particular Cd preparation which they used and which may have contributed to the loss of α_1-AT.[332]

Cigarette smoke, in addition to its other pertinent effects, can interfere with the function of α_1AT.[332] Janoff and Carp found that crude cigarette smoke condensate prevented the inhibition of elastase by α_1AT, serum, or lung lavage fluid. The inactivation of α_1AT could be prevented by the use of phenolic antioxidants.[333] This suggested that oxication of critical groups in α_2AT by cigarette smoke might impair its function and contribute to the pathogenesis of emphysema.

Oxidation under controlled conditions in vitro can inactivate α_1AT.[230,329,334] Oxidation of the single cysteine residue does not affect its effectiveness as an inhibitor, but oxidation of two of the eight methionyl residues to methionyl sulfoxide will inactivate α_1AT.[329] Presumably the methionyl residue at the active site is one of the critical methionines. In vivo, injection of a strong oxidant, chloramine T, in monkeys, depresses serum α_1AT.[230]

The oxidation of α_1AT by oxidant air pollutants might in principle help to upset the protease-inhibitor balance. Leh et al. observed that 88 mol of ozone were required to inactivate 1 mol of α_1AT. Breathing an ambient ozone concentration of 0.33 ppm, an individual would inactivate 0.5 mg of α_1AT in 3 hr. With a serum concentration of 1.8 mg/mℓ, the biological effect of this concentration of ozone on serum α_1AT would be negligible.[334]

Powerful oxidants are produced in the body as well as introduced by inhalation. In an ingenious series of experiments, Carp and Janoff showed that oxidants produced by stimulated granulocytes could inactivate α_1AT.[335] Inhibitor studies indicated that superoxide anion and hydroxyl radicals were among the reactive species. The coincident production of oxidant radicals at local sites of granulocyte enzyme release might protect the proteases from inactivation and promote local degradation of elastic tissue.

The idea that the α_1-antitrypsin molecule itself may be a target for toxic inhalants is of recent origin, but seems solidly based in terms of the chemistry of the α_1-antitrypsin molecule. It is doubtful that the levels of oxidants in cigarette smoke or ambient air pollution could produce significant depression of circulating α_1-antitrypsin levels, especially in view of the capacity of the liver to replace consumed inhibitor.[336] Nevertheless, transient effects on the much smaller extravascular local pool of α_1-antitrypsin in the lung could be of significance in initiating elastolytic damage.

α_2-Macroglobulin is the second major serum elastase inhibitor. It is a glycoprotein of mol wt 780,000 composed of 4 similar peptide chains of approximately 185,000 daltons each.[337,338] α_2-Macroglobulin (α_2M) has a much broader specificity than α_1AT. It inhibits proteases of all the major classes, i.e., serine proteases, carboxyl proteases, thiol proteases, and metalloproteases.[339] Although some studies have suggested a 1:1 molar ratio between α_2M and proteases,[339,340] the majority of investigators have found that 1 mol of α_2M complexes with 2 mol of enzyme. The enzyme-inhibitor complexes are stable and retain enzymatic activity against low molecular weight substrates such as synthetic esters, although inactive against many, but not all, large molecular weight proteins.[341] Complex formation has been postulated to involve cleavage of a susceptible region of the α_2M molecule. End group analysis indicates that two of the 185,000-dalton peptide chains are cleaved for each mole of protease bound.[338] This results in a conformational change in the α_2M molecule which "entraps" the protease. Large protein substrates are generally sterically prevented from reaching the protease, whereas many small substrates are hydrolyzed, but at a reduced rate.[339] In the case of complexes with granulocyte elastase, as well as a few other enzymes, the activity toward low molecular weight substrates is paradoxically enhanced.[342] Activity is retained toward tropoelastin, an uncross-linked elastin monomer which may be the precursor of mature elastin, although the level of activity for this substrate is much reduced.[225]

Some α_2M is probably available in lung tissue. Because of its large size, little circulating α_2M would be expected to leave the vascular compartment. Ganrot et al. compared the concentrations of α_1AT and α_2M in lymph from various organs.[319] As expected, α_2M was present in lower concentrations than α_1AT. Nevertheless, the concentration of α_2M was higher in lymph from lung and liver than from other tissues.

Since α_2M can be synthesized by cultured fetal lung fibroblasts,[343,344] local synthesis seems a more likely explanation for the relatively high concentration in pulmonary lymph than unusual permeability of the pulmonary endothelium. Local synthesis of α_2M in the lung interstitium could provide high concentrations of α_2M in the same tissue compartment with the connective tissue fibers. Despite the observation that α_2M can also be synthesized by cells of the mononuclear phagocyte system,[346] α_2M is absent from bronchopulmonary lavage fluid[320,323] or is only detectable in tiny amounts.[322,324]

The interactions of pancreatic and granulocyte elastases with the two major serum protease inhibitors are similar. If small amounts of enzyme are administered i.v. or mixed with human or dog serum, 90% of the enzyme complexes with α_1AT; most of the remainder complexes with α_2M.[346,347] This reflects the 10:1 molar excess of α_1AT over α_2M in serum; the affinity of the elastase is of a similar order for both inhibitors. Granulocyte collagenase, in contrast, has a much greater affinity for α_2M than for α_1AT. In the circulation, the clearance of complexes with the two inhibitor molecules is quite different. Complexes of proteases with α_2M are rapidly cleared from the circulation with half times of 6 to 9 min,[348,350] and accumulate in the reticuloendothelial organs, especially the Von Kuppfer cells of the liver.[348,351] The complexes are taken into lysosomes where they can be degraded, possibly by cathepsin B-1 and D.[351,352]

Complexes of elastase with αAT disappear from the circulation more slowly; half times of 45 min[350] to 3 hr[347] have been reported. Using complexes in which both the elastase and α_1AT were labeled, Ohlsson and Delshammar found that the clearance of the elastase was more rapid than that of the α_1AT portion of the complex and that elastase was gradually released from complexes with α_1AT and could then be bound by α_2M for rapid clearance.[347]

If elastases are released in the lung, their fate is less certain. Like the mononuclear phagocytes of the liver, the alveolar macrophages can rapidly bind and sequester complexes of proteases with α_2M.[353-355] As noted above, however, there is considerable uncertainty about the quantity of α_2M in the interstitium or alveoli of the lung in the absence of overt edema. α_1-Antitrypsin certainly is available, and when large doses of elastase are injected into the lungs of animals, complexes with α_1AT have been identified.[221] Such complexes are probably cleared mainly via the lymph and circulation. Although the uptake of protease complexes with α_1AT by macrophages is slow and probably nonselective,[353] α_1AT has been found in the cytoplasm of alveolar macrophages from smokers[321,356,357] suggesting that cellular uptake of complexes with α_1AT may indeed occur.

If α_1AT is genetically diminished or inactivated by environmental insults, more of the burden falls on other defenses, α_2M in the serum and lung as well as local nonserum inhibitors. Since the complexes with α_2M retain activity toward soluble elastin precursors,[225] they might interfere with the reparative synthesis of new elastin, unless removed by macrophages.

The consequences of the uptake of elastase complexes with α_2M, as well as of free granulocyte elastase, are unknown. The elastase and complexes are probably degraded within lysosomes and rendered harmless.[349,352,355] However, they may be concentrated by the macrophages which in turn collect in the respiratory bronchioles of smokers.[286] Here, eventually, the enzyme or enzymatically active complexes could be released to produce additional injury. Clearly more information is needed about the fate of internalized elastase and elastase-inhibitor complexes.

VI. CONCLUSIONS

The available evidence suggests that the pathogenesis of emphysema involves injury to pulmonary connective tissue, specifically to elastic tissue. This conclusion is supported by the occurrence of emphysema in disease states in which the connective tissue is abnormal, such as the Marfan syndrome and cutis laxa in man and the blotchy mouse and congenital copper deficiency in animals; by the experimental production of emphysema in animals using enzymes with elastolytic activity and only with such enzymes; by the association of emphysema with deficient serum elastase inhibitory capacity in α_1-antitrypsin deficiency; and by morphological evidence of elastic fiber damage in emphysematous lungs.

Transient reductions in lung elastin occur in enzyme-induced experimental emphysema. Whether there is depletion of elastin in emphysematous human lung remains controversial. The results of such measurements may depend on sampling and also upon whether emphysema formation continued up until the time the tissue was obtained for analysis. If the putative elastolytic process has been persistent, elastin may be depleted, but if it was operative only in the past, the elastin content of the lung may have been restored to normal by reparative processes.

The increased compliance and decreased elastic recoil of emphysematous lung are consistent with the hypothesis that elastin is damaged. The observation that simple treatment of lung tissue in vitro with elastase[43] does not reproduce all the length-tension properties of emphysematous lung is not surprising. Lung tissue treated with elastase in vitro is simply depleted of elastin. In emphysema the elastic tissue is disorganized and remodeled.

The importance of changes in other connective tissue components in emphysema is less clear. The detection of antibodies to collagen in patients with emphysema[358] indicates that immunogenic collagen peptides have been exposed to the immune system and suggests pathologic destruction of collagen. Small changes in the collagen content of the lung occur in experimental enzyme-induced emphysema[214] and reorganization of collagen is evident by electron microscopy in man as well.[51] Changes in glycosaminoglycans[359] may also be important by influencing the accessability of elastic fibers to degradative enzymes or the physical interaction of elastic fibers with other tissue components.[360]

Despite a considerable amount of circumstantial evidence, there is no conclusive evidence of accelerated pulmonary connective tissue breakdown in emphysema in man. A pressing research need is to develop methods for the measurement of elastin turnover suitable to human studies. Desmosine-containing peptides derived from elastin can be recognized in urine after experimental administration of elastase to hamsters.[215] The development of a sensitive radioimmunoassay for elastin cross-links in human urine[361] opens the possibility of measuring elastin turnover in man in the near future.

The net quantity of pulmonary connective tissue is a balance between synthesis and turnover. The lung responds to enzymatic destruction of connective tissue with the synthesis of new connective tissue. It is likely that this response plays a role in limiting the severity of the resultant lesions. Nothing is known currently of the mechanisms regulating this response or whether it is a target of emphysemaproducing agents. Some insights have been gained recently into factors involved in turnover, however.

Under normal circumstances, the turnover of connective tissue is slow, despite the capacity of phagocytes to release enzymes capable of destroying connective tissue. This is partly because the lung contains protease inhibitors both of the serum type, exemplified by α_1AT, and locally produced nonserum inhibitors. Emphysema-producing agents may increase turnover by disturbing the balance between proteases and their inhibitors. Stimuli such as tobacco smoke may raise levels of extracellular proteases by stimulating release of the enzymes from intracellular stores, by activating phagocytes to produce more enzyme, or by stimulating the recruitment of new phagocytes into the lung. In vitro, oxidants including ozone and cigarette smoke can inactivate α_1AT. In vivo, inhibitor oxidation resulting from either exogenous or endogenous oxidizing agents might permit normal levels of proteases to produce tissue damage.

The roles of specific cells in the production of emphysema have not been defined. Granulocytes contain an elastase which is capable of producing emphysema and which is inhibitable by α_1AT. There is evidence that levels of granulocyte elastase may influence susceptibility to emphysema especially in those with borderline α_1AT levels. When stimulated to phagocytosis, granulocytes not only release granule-associated enzymes, but strong oxidants such as hydroxyl radicals and superoxide anion capable of oxidizing and inactivating α_1AT. It is interesting to contrast this scheme with the many diseases, exemplified by pneumococcal lobar pneumonia, where the lung is flooded with phagocytosing granulocytes and yet emphysema does not result. The explanation for failure to get emphysema in these acute processes may lie in the marked changes in capillary permeability early in the diseases such that edema fluid containing circulating protease inhibitors preceeds the major influx of granulocytes into the tissue. Even elastases given experimentally may not express their full emphysema-producing potential because they produce capillary damage allowing serum inhibitors to enter the airspaces. An abundance of particle-laden macrophages is characteristic of the smoker's lung[286] and of early emphysema.[284] Macrophages have a number of activities which may influence the pathogenesis of emphysema. Animal macrophages produce elastolytic enzymes and can be activated to produce greater levels by cigarette smoke, as well as other stimuli.[287] A comparable elastase has yet to be conclusively identified from human alveolar macrophages. Macrophages produce chemotactic factors[297-299] and leukocyte mitogens (colony stimulating factors)[362] which influence the numbers and activity of other cells which are potential sources of proteases. However, the ability of macrophages to bind and sequester both uncomplexed leukocyte elastase[265] and complexes of proteases and α_2-M[353,354] (which retain some enzymatic activities) may give macrophages a protective function in the context of the pathogenesis of emphysema. Clearly, much more detailed knowledge of the interaction of toxic agents with the phagocyte system is required for a complete understanding of the pathogenesis of emphysema.

The continuous mechanical traction applied to the alveolar walls by transpulmonary pressure may play a role in producing the anatomic lesions of emphysema. Although not proven experimentally, it seems likely *a priori* that the stresses which produce air space enlargement derive ultimately from those which maintain lung expansion. One may speculate that destruction of elastin removes the main connective tissue component responsible for returning the tissue elements to their normal resting configuration after each inspiration, and progressive tissue deformation results. Resynthesis of the elastin helps to restabilize the tissue, but cannot restore the disordered architecture. If this concept is correct, then the tissue injury which causes centriacinar emphysema need not be selective regionally within the lung; the greater stress in the alveolar walls of the upper portions of the lung due to the gradient of transpulmonary pressure in the erect posture[363] offers an explanation for the upper-lobe distribution so characteristic of that form of emphysema.

By the same logic, the lower lobe distribution of emphysema in α_1-antitrypsin deficiency implies a predominance of injury in the lower lobes. Since both ventilation and perfusion are greater to the lower lobes, the explanation for that injury could be either greater exposure of the tissue to inhaled toxic materials or greater delivery of leukocytes, enzymatically active enzyme-inhibitor complexes or, less likely, free enzymes through the circulation.

REFERENCES

1. Kilburne, K. H., New clues for the emphysemas, *Am. J. Med.*, 58, 591, 1975.
2. Sweet, H. C., Wyatt, J. P., Fritsch, A. J., and Kinsella, P. W., Panlobular and centrilobular emphysema. Correlation of clinical findings with pathologic patterns, *Ann. Intern. Med.*, 55, 565, 1961.
3. Anderson, J. A., Dunnill, M. S., and Ryder, R. C., Dependence of the incidence of emphysema on smoking history, age and sex, *Thorax*, 27, 547, 1972.
4. Scott, K. W. M., A pathological study of the lungs and heart in fatal and non-fatal chronic airways obstruction, *Thorax*, 31, 70, 1976.
5. Pulmonary Terms and Symbols. A report of the ACCP-ATS Joint Committee on Pulmonary Nomenclature, *Chest*, 67, 583, 1975.
6. Heppleston, A. G., The pathology of honeycomb lung, *Thorax*, 11, 77, 1956.
7. Reid, L., *The Pathology of Emphysema*, Yearbook Medical Publishers, Chicago, 1967.
8. Heard, B. E., *Pathology of Chronic Bronchitis and Emphysema*, J. and A. Churchill, London, 1969.
9. Thurlbeck, W. M., *Chronic Airflow Obstruction in Lung Disease*, W. B. Saunders, Philadelphia, 1976.
10. Heppleston, A. G. and Leopold, J. G., Chronic pulmonary emphysema. Anatomy and pathogenesis, *Am. J. Med.*, 31, 279, 1961.
11. Gough, J., The pathogenesis of emphysema, in *The Lung*, Liebow, A. A. and Smith, D. E., Eds., Williams & Wilkins, Baltimore, 1968, 109.
12. Pump, K. K., Morphology of the acinus of the human lung, *Chest*, 56, 126, 1969.
13. Boyden, E. A., The structure of the pulmonary acinus in a child of six years and eight months, *Am. J. Anat.*, 132, 275, 1971.
14. Pratt, P. C. and Kilburn, K. H., A modern concept of the emphysemas based on correlation of structure and function, *Hum. Pathol.*, 1, 443, 1970.
15. Bignon, J., Andre-Bougaran, J., and Brouet, G., Parenchymal, bronchiolar and bronchial measurements in centrilobular emphysema. Relation to weight of right ventricle, *Thorax*, 25, 556, 1970.
16. Despierre, A., Bignon, J., Lebeau, A., and Brouet, G., Quantitative study of parenchyma and small conductive airways in chronic non-specific lung disease, *Chest*, 62, 699, 1972.
17. Linhartova, A., Anderson, A. E., and Foraker, A. G., Further observations on luminal deformity and stenosis of non-respiratory bronchioles in pulmonary emphysema, *Thorax*, 32, 53, 1977.
18. Laurell, C. B. and Eriksson, S., The electrophoretic alpha$_1$ globulin pattern of serum in alpha-1-antitrypsin deficiency, *Scand. J. Lab. Clin. Invest.*, 15, 132, 1963.
19. Eriksson, S., Studies in alpha-1-antitrypsin deficiency, *Acta Med. Scand.*, 177 (Suppl. 432), 1, 1965.
20. Martelli, N. A., Lower-zone emphysema in young patients without α_1-antitrypsin deficiency, *Thorax*, 29, 237, 1974.
21. Gough, J., Pneumoconiosis in coal trimmers, *J. Pathol. Bacteriol.*, 51, 277, 1940.
22. Heppleston, A. G., The pathogenesis of simple pneumokoniosis in coal workers, *J. Pathol. Bacteriol.*, 67, 51, 1954.
23. Heppleston, A. G., The pathological recognition and pathogenesis of emphysema and fibrocytic disease of the lung with special reference to coal workers, *Ann. N.Y. Acad. Sci.*, 200, 347, 1972.
24. Wyatt, J. P., Morphogenesis of penumoconiosis occurring in Southern Illinois bituminous workers, *Arch. Ind. Health*, 21, 445, 1961.
25. Naeye, R. L., Black lung disease, the anthracotic pneumoconioses, *Pathol. Annu.*, 8, 349, 1973.
26. Mitchell, R. S., Silvers, G. W., Goodman, N., Dart, G., and Maisel, J. C., Are centrilobular emphysema and panlobular emphysema two different diseases?, *Hum. Pathol.*, 1, 433, 1970.
27. Anderson, A. E. and Foraker, A. G., Centrilobular emphysema and panlobular emphysema: two different diseases, *Thorax*, 28, 547, 1973.
28. Thurlbeck, W. M. and Simon, G., Radiologic appearance of the chest in emphysema, *Am. J. Roentgenol.*, 130, 429, 1978.
29. Thurlbeck, W. M., Internal surface area and other measurements in emphysema, *Thorax*, 22, 483, 1967.
30. Park, S. S., Janis, M., Shim, C. S., and Williams, M. H., Relationship of bronchitis and emphysema to altered pulmonary function, *Am. Rev. Respir. Dis.*, 102, 927, 1970.
31. Boushy, S. F., Aboumrad, M. H., North, L. B., and Helgason, A. H., Lung recoil pressure, airway resistance and forced flows related to morphologic emphysema, *Am. Rev. Respir. Dis.*, 104, 551, 1971.
32. Berend, N., Woolcock, A. J., and Marlin, G. E., Correlation between the function and structure of the lung in smokers, *Am. Rev. Respir. Dis.*, 119, 695, 1979.
33. Christie, R. V., The elastic properties of the emphysematous lung and their clinical significance, *J. Clin. Invest.*, 13, 295, 1934.
34. Stead, W. W., Fry, D. L., and Ebert, R. V., The elastic properties of the lung in normal men and in patients with chronic pulmonary emphysema, *J. Lab. Clin. Med.*, 40, 674, 1952.

35. Turner, J. M., Mead, J., and Wohl, M. E., Elasticity of human lungs in relation to age, *J. Appl. Physiol.*, 25, 664, 1968.

36. Niewoehner, D. E., Kleinerman, J. E., and Liolta, L., Elastic behavior of postmortem human lung: effects of aging and mild emphysema, *J. Appl. Physiol.*, 39, 943, 1975.

37. Fry, D. L., Ebert, R. V., Stead, W. W., and Brown, C. C., The mechanics of pulmonary ventilation in normal subjects and in patients with emphysema, *Am. J. Med.*, 16, 80, 1954.

38. Mead, J., Lindgren, I., and Gaensler, E. A., The mechanical properties of the lungs in emphysema, *J. Clin. Invest.*, 34, 1005, 1956.

39. Leaver, D. G., Tattersfield, A. E., and Pride, N. B., Bronchial and extrabronchial factors in chronic airflow obstruction, *Thorax*, 29, 394, 1974.

40. Colebatch, H. J. H., Finucane, K. E., and Smith, M. M., Pulmonary conductance and elastic recoil relationships in asthma and emphysema, *J. Appl. Physiol.*, 34, 143, 1973.

41. Johanson, W. G. and Pierce, A. K., Effects of elastase, collagenase, and papain on structure and function of rat lungs *in vitro*, *J. Clin. Invest.*, 51, 288, 1972.

42. Karlinsky, J. B., Snider, G. L., Franzblau, C., Stone, P. J., and Hoppin, F. G., In vitro effects of elastase and collagenase on mechanical properties of hamster lungs, *Am. Rev. Respir. Dis.*, 113, 769, 1976.

43. Martin, C. J. and Sugihara, T., Simulation of tissue properties in irreversible diffuse obstructive pulmonary syndromes. Enzyme digestion, *J. Clin. Invest.*, 52, 1918, 1973.

44. Senior, R. M., Bielefeld, D. R., and Abensohn, M. K., The effects of proteolytic enzymes on the tensile strength of the human lung, *Am. Rev. Respir. Dis.*, 111, 184, 1975.

45. Sugihara, T., Martin, C. J., and Hildebrandt, J., Length-tension properties of alveolar wall in man, *J. Appl. Physiol.*, 30, 874, 1971.

46. Eppinger, H., Das Emphysem der Lungen, *Vierteljahresschr. Prakt. Heilk.*, 4, 1, 1876.

47. Orsos, F., Uber das elastische Gerust der normalen und der emphysematosen Lunge, *Beitr. Pathol. Anat.*, 41, 95, 1907.

48. Wright, R. R., Elastic tissue of normal and emphysematous lungs. A tridimensional histologic study, *Am. J. Pathol.*, 39, 355, 1961.

49. Pump, K. K., Fenestrae in the alveolar membrane of the human lung, *Chest*, 65, 431, 1974.

50. Reynolds, R. C., Electron microscopy of obstructive pulmonary emphysema, *Med. Thorac.*, 22, 161, 1965.

51. Belton, J. C., Crise, N., McLaughlin, R. F., and Tueller, E. E., Ultrastructural alterations in collagen associated with microscopic foci of human emphysema, *Hum. Pathol.*, 8, 669, 1977.

52. Mead, J., Mechanical properties of lungs, *Physiol. Rev.*, 41, 281, 1961.

53. Snider, G. L. and Karlinsky, J. B., Relation between the elastic behavior and the connective tissues of the lungs, *Pathobiol. Annu.*, 7, 115, 1977.

54. Briscoe, A. M. and Loring, W. E., Elastin content of the human lung, *Proc. Soc. Exp. Biol. Med.*, 99, 162, 1958.

55. Pierce, J. A., Hocott, J. B., and Ebert, R. V., Studies of lung collagen and elastin, *Am. Rev. Respir. Dis.*, 80, 45, 1959.

56. Pierce, J. A. and Hocott, J. B., Studies on the collagen and elastin content of the human lung, *J. Clin. Invest.*, 39, 8, 1960.

57. Johnson, J. R. and Andrews, F. A., Lung scleroproteins in age and emphysema, *Chest*, 57, 239, 1970.

58. John, R. and Thomas, J., Chemical compositions of elastins isolated from aortas and pulmonary tissues of humans of different ages, *Biochem. J.*, 127, 261, 1972.

59. Pierce, J. A. and Ebert, R. V., Fibrous network of the lung and its change with age, *Thorax*, 20, 469, 1965.

60. Pierce, J. A., Hocott, J. B., and Ebert, R. V., The collagen and elastin content of the lung in emphysema, *Ann. Intern. Med.*, 55, 210, 1961.

61. Wright, G. W., Kleinerman, J., and Zorn, E. M., The elastin and collagen content of normal and emphysematous human lungs, *Am. Rev. Respir. Dis.*, 81, 938, 1960.

62. Fitzpatrick, M., Studies of human pulmonary connective tissue. Chemical changes in structural proteins with emphysema, *Am. Rev. Respir. Dis.*, 96, 254, 1967.

63. Keller, S. and Mandl, I., Qualitative differences between normal and emphysematous human lung elastin, in *Pulmonary Emphysema and Proteolysis*, Mittman, C., Ed., Academic Press, New York, 1972, 251.

64. Chrzanowski, P., Keller, S., Cerreta, J., Mandl, I., and Turino, G. M., Elastin Content of Normal and emphysematous lung, *Am. J. Med.*, 69, 351, 1980.

65. Smoking and Health, report of the Advisory Committee to the Surgeon General of the Public Health Service, U.S. Department of Health, Education, and Welfare, Washington, D.C., 1964.

66. Anderson, J. A., Dunnill, M. S., and Ryder, R. C., Dependence of the incidence of emphysema on smoking history, age and sex, *Thorax*, 27, 547, 1972.

67. Sutinen, S., Vaajulahti, P., and Prakko, P., Prevalence, severity and types of pulmonary emphysema in a population of deaths in a Finnish city. Correlation with age, sex and smoking, *Scand. J. Respir. Dis.*, 59, 101, 1978.

68. Thurlbeck, W. M., A clinicopathological study of emphysema in an American hospital, *Thorax*, 18, 59, 1963.

69. Mitchell, R. S., Vincent, T. N., and Filley, G. F., Cigarette smoking, chronic bronchitis and emphysema, *JAMA*, 188, 12, 1964.

70. Auerbach, O., Hammond, E. C., Garfinkel, L., and Benante, C., Relation of smoking and age to emphysema. Whole-lung section study, *N. Engl. J. Med.*, 286, 853, 1972.

71. Spain, D. M., Siegel, H., and Brodess, V. A., Emphysema in apparently healthy adults. Smoking, age and sex. *JAMA*, 224, 322, 1973.

72. Ryder, R. C., Dunnill, M. S., and Anderson, J. A., A quantitative study of bronchial mucous gland volume, emphysema, and smoking in a necropsy population, *J. Pathol.*, 104, 59, 1971.

73. Doll, R. and Peto, R., Mortality in relation to smoking: 20 years' observations on male British doctors, *Br. Med. Jr.*, 2, 1525, 1976.

74. Shy, C. M., Goldsmith, J. R., Hackney, J. D., Lebowitz, M. D., and Menzel, D. B., Health effects of air pollution, *Am. Thorac. Soc. News*, 4, 22, 1978.

75. Ishikawa, S., Bowden, D. H., Fisher, V., and Wyatt, J. P., The emphysema profile in two midwestern cities in North America, *Arch. Environ. Health*, 18, 660, 1969.

76. Lane, R. E. and Campbell, A. C. P., Fatal emphysema in two men making a copper cadmium alloy, *Br. J. Ind. Med.*, 11, 118, 1954.

77. Bonnell, J. A., Kazantzis, G., and King, E., A follow-up study of men exposed to cadmium oxide fume, *Br. J. Ind. Med.*, 16, 135, 1959.

78. Smith, T. S., Petty, T. L., Reading, J. C., and Lakshminarayan, S., Pulmonary effects of chronic exposure to airborn cadmium, *Am. Rev. Respir. Dis.*, 114, 161, 1976.

79. Hirst, R. N., Perry, H. M., Cruz, M. G., and Pierce, J. A., Elevated cadmium concentration in emphysematous lungs, *Am. Rev. Respir. Dis.*, 108, 30, 1973.

80. Lewis, G. P., Lyle, H., and Miller, S., Association between elevated hepatic water soluble protein-bound cadmium levels and chronic bronchitis and/or emphysema, *Lancet*, 2, 1330, 1969.

81. Morgan, J. M., Burch, H. B., and Watkins, J. B., Tissue cadmium and zinc content in emphysema and bronchogenic carcinoma, *J. Chronic Dis.*, 24, 107, 1971.

82. Nandi, M., Jick, H., Slone, D., Shapiro, S., and Lewis, G. P., Cadmium content of cigarettes, *Lancet*, 2, 1329, 1969.

83. Larson, R. K. and Barman, M. L., Familial occurence of chronic obstructive pulmonary disease, *Ann. Intern. Med.*, 63, 1001, 1965.

84. Larson, R. K., Barman, M. L., Kueppers, F., and Fudenberg, H. H., Genetic and environmental determinants of chronic obstructive pulmonary disease, *Ann. Intern. Med.*, 72, 627, 1970.

85. McKusick, V. A., *Heritable Disorders of Connective Tissue*, 4th ed., C. V. Mosby, St. Louis, 1972.

86. Uitto, J., Biochemistry of the elastic fiber in normal connective tissues and its alterations in diseases, *J. Invest. Dermatol.*, 72, 1, 1979.

87. Fuleihan, F. J. D., Suh, S. K., and Shepard, R. H., Some aspects of pulmonary function in the Marfan syndrome, *Bull. Johns Hopkins Hosp.*, 113, 320, 1963.

88. Chisholm, J. C., Chernick, N. S., and Carton, R. W., Results of pulmonary function testing in 5 persons with the Marfan syndrome, *J. Lab. Clin. Med.*, 71, 25, 1968.

89. Bolande, R. P. and Tucker, A. S., Pulmonary emphysema and other cardiorespiratory lesions as part of the Marfan abiotrophy, *Pediatrics*, 33, 356, 1964.

90. Reye, R. D. V. and Bale, P. M., Elastic tissue in pulmonary emphysema in Marfan syndrome, *Arch. Pathol.*, 96, 427, 1973.

91. Sayers, C. P., Golz, R. W., and Mottaz, J., Pulmonary elastic tissue in generalized elastolysis (cutis laxa) and Marfan's syndrome. A light and electron microscopic study, *J. Invest. Dermatol.*, 65, 451, 1975.

92. Turner, J. A. McM. and Stanley, N. N., Fragile lung in the Marfan syndrome, *Thorax*, 31, 771, 1976.

93. Harris, R. B., Heaphy, M. R., and Perry, H. O., Generalized elastolysis (cutis laxa), *Am. J. Med.*, 65, 815, 1978.

94. Byers, P. H., Narayanan, A. S., Bornstein, P., and Hall, J. G., An X-linked form of cutis laxa due to deficiency of lysyl oxidase, *Birth Defects*, 12, 293, 1976.

95. Turino, G. M., Senior, R. M., Garg, B. D., Keller, S., Levi, M. M., and Mandl, I., Serum elastase inhibitor deficiency and α_1-antitrypsin deficiency in patients with obstructive emphysema, *Science*, 165, 709, 1969.

96. Talamo, R. C., Blennerhassett, J. B., and Austen, K. F., Familial emphysema and alpha$_1$-antitrypsin, *N. Engl. J. Med.*, 275, 1301, 1966.

97. Mazodier, P., Orell, S. R., Siken, L., and Svanborg, N., Déficit constitutionnel en alpha₁-antitrypsine et emphyseme panlobulaire, *J. Fr. Med. Chir. Thorac.*, 25, 5, 1971.
98. Greenberg, S. D., Jenkins, D. E., Stevens, P. M., and Schweppe, H. I., The lungs in homozygous alpha-1-antitrypsin deficiency, *Am. J. Clin. Pathol.*, 60, 581, 1973.
99. Guenter, C. A., Welch, M. H., Russell, T. R., Hyde, R. M., and Hammarsten, J. F., The pattern of lung disease associated with alpha₁ antitrypsin deficiency, *Arch. Intern. Med.*, 122, 254, 1968.
100. Larsson, C., Natural history and life expectancy in severe alpha₁-antitrypsin deficiency, Pi Z, *Acta Med. Scand.*, 204, 345, 1978.
101. Sharp, H. L., Bridges, R. A., Krivit, W., and Freier, E. F., Cirrhosis associated with alpha-1-antitrypsin deficiency: a previously unrecognized inherited disorder, *J. Lab. Clin. Med.*, 73, 934, 1969.
102. Sharp, H. L., Alpha-1-antitrypsin deficiency, *Hosp. Pract.*, 6, 83, 1971.
103. Morse, J. O., Alpha₁-antitrypsin deficiency, *N. Engl. J. Med.*, 299, 1045 and 1099, 1978.
104. Berg, N. O. and Eriksson, S., Liver disease in adults with alpha-₁-antitrypsin deficiency, *N. Engl. J. Med.*, 287, 1264, 1972.
105. Eriksson, S. and Hogerstrand, I., Cirrhosis and malignant hepatoma in α_1 antitrypsin deficiency, *Acta Med. Scand.*, 195, 451, 1974.
106. Greenwald, A. J., Johnson, D. S., Oskvig, R. M., Aschenbrener, C. A., and Randa, D. C., α_1-antitrypsin deficiency, emphysema, cirrhosis and intestinal mucosal atrophy, *JAMA*, 231, 273, 1975.
107. Laurell, C.-B., Pierce, J. A., Persson, U., and Thulin, E., Purification of α_1-antitrypsin from plasma through thiol-disulfide interchange, *Eur. J. Biochem.*, 57, 107, 1975.
108. Jeppsson, J. O., Laurell, C.-B., and Fagerhol, M., Properties of isolated human α_1-antitrypsins of Pi types M, S and Z, *Eur. J. Biochem.*, 83, 143, 1978.
109. Fagerhol, M. K. and Braend, M., Serum prealbumins: polymorphism in man, *Science*, 149, 986, 1965.
110. Fagerhol, M. K. and Laurell, C. B., The polymorphism of "prealbumin" and alpha₁-antitrypsin in human sera, *Clin. Chim. Acta*, 16, 199, 1967.
111. Fagerhol, M. K., The incidence of α_1-antitrypsin variants in chronic obstructive pulmonary disease, in *Pulmonary Emphysema and Proteolysis*, Mittman, C., Ed., Academic Press, New York, 1972, 51.
112. Larsson, C., Dirksen, H., and Sundström, G., Lung function studies in assymptomatic individuals with moderately (PiSZ) and severely (PiZ) reduced levels of α_1 antitrypsin, *Scand. J. Respir. Dis.*, 57, 267, 1976.
113. Talamo, R. C., Langley, C. E., Reed, C. E., and Makino, S., α_1-antitrypsin deficiency. A variant with no detectable α_1-antitrypsin, *Science*, 181, 70, 1973.
114. Mittman, C., The PiMZ phenotype: is it a significant risk factor for the development of chronic obstructive lung disease?, *Am. Rev. Respir. Dis.*, 118, 649, 1978.
115. Eriksson, S., Moestrup, T., and Hagerstrand, I., Liver, lung and malignant disease in heterozygous (PiMZ) alpha₁ antitrypsin deficiency, *Acta Med. Scand.*, 198, 243, 1975.
116. Larsson, C., Eriksson, S., and Dirksen, H., Smoking and intermediate alpha₁-antitrypsin deficiency and lung function in middle aged men, *Br. Med. J.*, 2, 922, 1977.
117. Owen, M. C. and Carrell, R. W., Alpha₁-antitrypsin: molecular abnormality of the S variant, *Br. Med. J.*, 1, 130, 1976.
118. Jeppsson, J. O., Amino acid substitution glu-lys in alpha₁-antitrypsin Pi Z, *FEBS Lett.*, 65, 195, 1976.
119. Yoshida, A., Lieberman, J., Gaidulis, L., and Ewing, C., Molecular abnormality of human alpha₁-antitrypsin variant (Pi ZZ) associated with plasma activity deficiency, *Proc. Natl. Acad. Sci. U.S.A.*, 73, 1324, 1976.
120. Eriksson, S. and Larssen, C., Purification and partial characterization of PAS-positive inclusion bodies from the liver in alpha₁-antitrypsin deficiency, *N. Engl. J. Med.*, 292, 176, 1975.
121. Jeppsson, J. O., Larssen, C., and Eriksson, S., Characterization of alpha₁-antitrypsin deficiency, *N. Engl. J. Med.*, 293, 576, 1975.
122. Bell, O. F. and Carell, R. W., Basis of the defect in α_1-antitrypsin deficiency, *Nature (London)*, 243, 410, 1973.
123. Cox, D. W., Defect in alpha₁-antitrypsin deficiency, *Lancet*, 2, 844, 1973.
124. Thurlbeck, W. M., The diagnosis of emphysema, *Thorax*, 19, 571, 1964.
125. Kuhn, C. and Tavassoli, F., The scanning electron microscopy of elastase-induced emphysema: a comparison with emphysema in man, *Lab. Invest.*, 34, 2, 1976.
126. Weibel, E. R. and Vidone, R. A., Fixation of the lung by formalin steam in a controlled state of air inflation, *Am. Rev. Respir. Dis.*, 84, 856, 1961.
127. Heard, B. E., Pathology of pulmonary emphysema. Methods of study, *Am. Rev. Respir. Dis.*, 82, 792, 1960.
128. Gough, J. and Wentworth, J. E., Thin sections of entire organs mounted on paper, in *Recent Advances in Pathology*, 7th ed., Harrison, C. V., Ed., Churchill, London, 1969, 80.

129. Dunnill, M. S., Quantitative methods in the study of pulmonary pathology, *Thorax*, 17, 320, 1962.

130. Thurlbeck, W. M., The internal surface area of nonemphysematous lungs, *Am. Rev. Respir. Dis.*, 95, 765, 1967.

131. Snider, G. L. and Korthy, A., Internal surface area and numbers of respiratory air spaces in elastase-induced emphysema in hamsters, *Am. Rev. Respir. Dis.*, 117, 685, 1978.

132. Hernandez, J. A., Anderson, A. E., Holmes, W. L., and Foraker, A. G., Pulmonary parenchymal defects in dogs following prolonged cigarette smoke exposure, *Am. Rev. Respir. Dis.*, 93, 78, 1966.

133. Thurlbeck, W. M., Dunnill, M. S., Hartung, W., Heard, B. E., Heppleston, A. G., and Ryder, R. C., A comparison of three methods of measuring emphysema, *Hum. Pathol.*, 1, 215, 1970.

134. Auerbach, O., Hammond, E. C., Kirman, D., and Garfinkel, L., Emphysema produced in dogs by cigarette smoking, *JAMA*, 199, 241, 1967.

135. Frasca, J. M., Auerbach, O., Parks, V. R., and Jamieson, J. D., Electron microscopic observations on pulmonary fibrosis and emphysema in smoking dogs, *Exp. Mol. Pathol.*, 15, 108, 1971.

136. Holland, R. H., Kozlowski, E. J., and Booker, L., The effect of cigarette smoke on the respiratory system of the rabbit. A final report, *Cancer*, 16, 612, 1963.

137. Strawbridge, H. T. G., Chronic pulmonary emphysema (an experimental study). II Spontaneous pulmonary emphysema in rabbits, *Am. J. Pathol.*, 37, 309, 1960.

138. Park, S. S., Kikkawa, Y., Goldring, I. P., Daly, M. M., Zelefsky, M., Shim, C., Spierer, M., and Morita, T., An animal model of cigarette smoking in beagle dogs. Correlative evaluation of effects on pulmonary function, defense and morphology, *Am. Rev. Respir. Dis.*, 115, 971, 1977.

139. Health effects of nitrogen oxides, in *Medical and Biologic Effects of Environmental Pollutants*, National Academy of Sciences, Washington, D.C., 1977, 215.

140. Goldstein, E., Evaluation of the role of nitrogen dioxide in the development of respiratory diseases in man, *Calif. Med.*, 115, 21, 1971.

141. Kleinerman, J., Some effects of nitrogen dioxide on the lung, *Fed. Proc. Fed. Am. Soc. Exp. Biol.*, 36, 1714, 1977.

142. Blair, W. H., Henry, M. C., and Ehrlich, R., Chronic toxicity of nitrogen dioxide. II. Effect on histopathology of lung tissue, *Arch. Environ. Health*, 18, 186, 1969.

143. Freeman, G., Crane, S. C., Furiosi, N. J., Stephens, R. J., Evans, M. J., and Moore, W. D., Covert reduction in ventilatory surface in rats during prolonged exposure to subacute nitrogen dioxide, *Am. Rev. Respir. Dis.*, 106, 563, 1972.

144. Freeman, G., Crane, S. C., Stephens, R. J., and Furiosi, N. J., Pathogenesis of the nitrogen dioxide-induced lesion in the rat lung: a review and presentation of new observations, *Am. Rev. Respir. Dis.*, 98, 429, 1968.

145. Azoulay, E., Soler, P., and Blayo, M. C., The absence of lung damage in rats after chronic exposure to 2 ppm nitrogen dioxide, *Bull. Eur. Physiopathol. Respir.*, 14, 311, 1978.

146. Hayden, G. B., Davidson, J. T., Lillington, G. A., and Wasserman, K., Nitrogen dioxide-induced emphysema in rabbits, *Am. Rev. Respir. Dis.*, 95, 797, 1967.

147. Kleinerman, J. and Rynbrandt, D., Lung proteolytic activity and serum protease inhibition after NO_2 exposure, *Arch. Environ. Health*, 31, 33, 1976.

148. Rynbrandt, D. and Kleinerman, J., Nitrogen dioxide and pulmonary proteolytic enzymes. Effect on lung tissue and macrophages, *Arch. Environ. Health*, 32, 165, 1977.

149. Boren, H. G., Carbon as a carrier mechanism for irritant gases, *Arch. Environ. Health*, 8, 119, 1964.

150. Furiosi, N. J., Crane, S. C., and Freeman, G., Mixed sodium chloride aerosol and nitrogen dioxide in air. Biological effects on monkeys and rats, *Arch. Environ. Health*, 27, 405, 1973.

151. Clay, J. R. and Rossing, R. G., Histopathology of exposure to phosgene. An attempt to produce pulmonary emphysema experimentally, *Arch. Pathol.*, 78, 544, 1964.

152. Thurlbeck, W. M. and Foley, F. D., Experimental pulmonary emphysema. The effect of intratracheal injection of cadmium chloride solution in the guinea pig, *Am. J. Pathol.*, 42, 431, 1963.

153. Harrison, H. E., Bunting, H., Ordway, N. K., and Albrink, W. S., The effects and treatment of inhalation of cadmium chloride aerosols in the dog, *J. Ind. Hyg. Toxicol.*, 29, 302, 1947.

154. Snider, G. L., Hayes, J. A., Korthy, A. L., and Lewis, G. P., Centrilobular emphysema experimentally induced by cadmium chloride aerosols, *Am. Rev. Respir. Dis.*, 108, 40, 1973.

155. Karlinsky, J. B. and Snider, G. L., Animal models of emphysema, *Am. Rev. Respir. Dis.*, 117, 1109, 1978.

156. Eiseman, B., Petty, T., and Silen, W., Experimental emphysema, *Am. Rev. Respir. Dis.*, 80 (Suppl.), 147, 1959.

157. Strawbridge, H. T. G., Chronic pulmonary emphysema (an experimental study). I. Historical review, *Am. J. Pathol.*, 37, 161, 1960.

158. Rackemann, F. M. and Edwards, M. C., Asthma in children: a follow-up study of 688 patients after an interval of 20 years, *N. Engl. J. Med.*, 246, 815, 1952.

159. Anderson, A. E., Azcuy, A., Batchelder, T. L., and Foraker, A. G., Experimental analysis in dogs of the relationship between pulmonary emphysema, alveolitis and hyperinflation, *Thorax*, 420, 1964.

160. Tura, S., Pulmonary emphysema and polycythemia induced in rats by forced swimming, *Proc. Soc. Exp. Biol. Med.,* 103, 713, 1960.
161. Cowdrey, C. R., Wright, G. W., and Kleinerman, J., The attempted experimental production of pulmonary emphysema in rats by forced swimming, *Am. Rev. Respir. Dis.,* 87, 444, 1963.
162. Kuhn, C., unpublished.
163. Strawbridge, H. T. G., Chronic pulmonary emphysema (an experimental study). III. Experimental pulmonary emphysema, *Am. J. Pathol.,* 37, 391, 1960.
164. Wright, G. W. and Kleinerman, J., A consideration of the etiology of emphysema in terms of contemporary knowledge, *Am. Rev. Respir. Dis.,* 88, 605, 1963.
165. Boatman, E. S. and Martin, H. B., Electron microscopy in pulmonary emphysema of rabbits, *Am. Rev. Respir. Dis.,* 91, 197, 1965.
166. McLaughlin, R. F., Tyler, W. S., Edwards, D. W., Crenshaw, G. L., Canada, R. O., Fowler, M. A., Parker, E. A., and Reifenstein, G. H., Chlorpromazine induced emphysema. Results of an initial study in the horse, *Am. Rev. Respir. Dis.,* 92, 597, 1964.
167. Hance, A. J. and Crystal, R. G., The connective tissue of lung, *Am. Rev. Respir. Dis.,* 112, 657, 1975.
168. Tanzer, M. L., Cross-linking of collagen. Endogenous aldehydes in collagen react in several ways to form a variety of unique covalent cross-links, *Science,* 180, 561, 1973.
169. Barrow, M. V., Simpson, C. F., and Miller, E. J., Lathyrism: a review, *Q. Rev. Biol.,* 49, 101, 1974.
170. Stanley, N. M., Cherniak, N. S., Altose, M. D., Saldana, M., and Fishman, A. P., Effects of beta-aminoproprionitrile on the mechanical properties of rat lung, (abstract), *Am. Rev. Respir. Dis.,* 105, 999, 1972.
171. Hoffman, L., Mondshine, R. B., and Park, S. S., Effect of DL-penicillamine on elastic properties of rat lung, *J. Appl. Physiol.,* 30, 508, 1971.
172. Hoffman, L., Blumenfeld, O. O., Mondshine, R. B., and Park, S. S., Effect of DL-penicillamine on fibrous proteins of rat lung, *J. Appl. Physiol.,* 33, 42, 1972.
173. Stanley, N. N., Alper, R., Cunningham, E. L., Cherniack, N. S., and Kefalides, N. A., Effects of a molecular change in collagen on lung structure and mechanical function, *J. Clin. Invest.,* 55, 1195, 1975.
174. Slack, H. G. B., Metabolism of elastin in the adult rat, *Nature (London),* 174, 512, 1954.
175. Walford, R. L., Carter, P. K., and Schneider, R. B., Stability of labeled aortic elastic tissue with age and pregnancy in the rat, *Arch. Pathol.,* 78, 43, 1964.
176. Dubreuil, G., LaCoste, A., and Raymond, R., Observations sur le développement du poumon humain, *Bull. Histol. Appl. Physiol. Pathol.,* 13, 236, 1936.
177. Loosli, C., and Potter, E. L., Pre- and postnatal development of the respiratory portion of the human lung, *Am. Rev. Respir. Dis.,* 80, 5, 1959.
178. Burri, P. H., The postnatal growth of the rat lung. III. Morphology, *Anat. Rec.,* 180, 77, 1974.
179. Rowe, D. W., McGoodwin, E. B., Martin, G. R., and Grahn, D., Decreased lysyl oxidase activity in the aneurysmprone mottled mouse, *J. Biol. Chem.,* 252, 939, 1977.
180. Starcher, B. C., Madaras, J. A., and Tepper, A. S., Lysyl oxidase deficiency in lung and fibroblasts from mice with hereditary emphysema, *Biochem. Biophys. Res. Commun.,* 78, 706, 1977.
181. Fisk, D. E. and Kuhn, C., Emphysema-like changes in the lungs of the Blotchy mouse, *Am. Rev. Respir. Dis.,* 113, 787, 1976.
182. O'Dell, B. L., Kilburn, K. H., McKenzie, W. N., and Thurston, R. J., The lung of the copper-deficient rat, *Am. J. Pathol.,* 91, 413, 1978.
183. Gross, P. M., Babjak, M. A., Tolker, E., and Kaschak, M., Enzymatically induced pulmonary emphysema. A preliminary report, *J. Occup. Med.,* 6, 481, 1964.
184. Gross, P., Pfitzer, E. A., Tolker, E., Babjak, M. A., and Kaschak, M., Experimental emphysema. Its production with papain in normal and silicotic rats, *Arch. Environ. Health,* 11, 50, 1965.
185. Goldring, I. P., Greenburg, L., and Ratner, I. M., On the production of emphysema in Syrian hamsters by aerosol inhalation of papain, *Arch. Environ. Health,* 16, 59, 1968.
186. Giles, R. E., Finkel, M. P., and Leeds, R., The production of an emphysema-like condition in rats by the administration of papain aerosol, *Proc. Soc. Exp. Biol. Med.,* 134, 157, 1970.
187. Pushpackom, R., Hogg, J. C., Woocock, A. J., Angus, A. E., Macklem, P. T., and Thurlbeck, W. M., Experimental papain induced emphysema in dogs, *Am. Rev. Respir. Dis.,* 102, 778, 1970.
188. Caldwell, E. J., Physiologic and anatomic effects of papain on the rabbit lung, *J. Appl. Physiol.,* 31, 458, 1972.
189. Johanson, W. G., Jr. and Pierce, A. K., Lung structure and function with age in normal rats and rats with papain emphysema, *J. Clin. Invest.,* 52, 2921, 1973.
190. Blackwood, C. E., Hosannah, Y., Perman, E., Keller, S., and Mandl, I., Experimental emphysema in rats: elastolytic titer of inducing enzyme as determinant of response, *Proc. Soc. Exp. Biol. Med.,* 144, 450, 1973.

191. Mass, B., Ikeda, T., Meranze, D. R., Weinbaum, G., and Kimbel, P., Induction of experimental emphysema: cellular and species specificity, *Am. Rev. Respir. Dis.*, 106, 384, 1972.

192. Kaplan, P. D., Kuhn, C., and Pierce, J. A., The induction of emphysema with elastase. I. The evolution of the lesion and influence of serum, *J. Lab. Clin. Med.*, 82, 349, 1973.

193. Hayes, J. A., Korthy, A. L., and Snider, G. L., Pathology of elastase induced panacinar emphysema, *J. Pathol. (London)*, 117, 1, 1975.

194. Janoff, A., Sloan, B., Weinbaum, G., Damiano, V., Sandhaus, R. A., Elias, J., and Kimbel, P., Experimental emphysema induced with purified human neutrophil elastase: tissue localization of the instilled protease, *Am. Rev. Respir. Dis.*, 115, 461, 1977.

195. Senior, R. M., Tegner, H., Kuhn, C., Ohlsson, K., Starcher, B. C., and Pierce, J. A., The induction of pulmonary emphysema with human leukocyte elastase, *Am. Rev. Respir. Dis.*, 116, 469, 1977.

196. Snider, G. L., Hayes, J. A., Franzblau, C., Kagan, H. M., Stone, P. S., and Korthy, A. L., Relationship between elastolytic activity and experimental emphysema-inducing properties of papain preparations, *Am. Rev. Respir. Dis.*, 110, 254, 1974.

197. Senior, R. M., Kaplan, P. D., Kuhn, C., and Linder, H. E., Enzyme-induced emphysema, in *Fundamental Problems of Cystic Fibrosis and Related Diseases*, Mangos, J. A., and Talamo, R. C., Eds., Symposia Specialists, Miami, Fla., 1973, 183.

198. Rosenbloom, J., Christner, P., Weinbaum, G., and Damato, D., Sequential elastase-trypsin administration: a new model for emphysema in the hamster, *Am. Rev. Respir. Dis.*, 119 (Abstr.), 354, 1979.

199. Takaro, T. and White, S. M., Unilateral severe experimental pulmonary emphysema, *Am. Rev. Respir. Dis.*, 108, 334, 1973.

200. Weinbaum, G., Marco, V., Ikeda, T., Mass, B., Meranze, D. R., and Kimbel, P., Enzymatic production of experimental emphysema in the dog. Route of exposure, *Am. Rev. Respir. Dis.*, 109, 351, 1974.

201. Turino, G. M., Hornbeck, W., and Robert, B., In vivo effects of pancreatic elastase. I. Studies on the serum inhibitors, *Proc. Soc. Exp. Biol. Med.*, 146, 712, 1974.

202. Fierer, J. A., Cerreta, J. M., Turino, G. M., and Mandl, I., Ultrastructural studies of lung elastin in elastase-induced emphysema, *Am. J. Pathol.*, 82, 42a, 1976.

203. Schuyler, M. R., Rynbrandt, D. J., and Kleinerman, J., Physiologic and morphologic observations of the effects of intravenous elastase on the lung, *Am. Rev. Respir. Dis.*, 117, 97, 1978.

204. Schneeberger, E. E. and Karnovsky, M. J., The influence of intravascular fluid volume on the permeability of newborn and adult mouse lungs to ultrastructural protein tracers, *J. Cell Biol.*, 49, 319, 1971.

205. Taylor, A. E. and Gaar, K. A., Estimation of equivalent pore radii of pulmonary capillary and alveolar membranes, *Am. J. Physiol.*, 218, 1133, 1970.

206. Staub, N. C., Pulmonary edema, *Physiol. Rev.*, 54, 678, 1974.

207. Becker, C. G. and Harpel, P. C., α_2 macroglobulin on human vascular endothelium, *J. Exp. Med.*, 144, 1, 1976.

208. Snider, G. L. and Sherter, C. B., A one-year study of the evolution of elastase-induced emphysema in hamsters, *J. Appl. Physiol. Respir. Environ. Exercise Physiol.*, 43, 721, 1977.

209. Christensen, T. G., Korthy, A. L., Snider, G. L., and Hayes, J. A., Irreversible bronchial goblet cell metaplasia in hamsters with elastase-induced panacinar emphysema, *J. Clin. Invest.*, 59, 397, 1977.

210. Cooper, B. and Kuhn, C., Cor pulmonale in elastase-induced emphysema, *Am. Rev. Respir. Dis.*, 117 (Abstr.), 324, 1978.

211. Park, S. S., Goldring, I. P., Shim, C. S., and Williams, M. H., Jr., Mechanical properties of the lung in experimental pulmonary emphysema, *J. Appl. Physiol.*, 26, 738, 1969.

212. Marco, V., Meranze, D. R., Yoshida, M., and Kimbel, P., Papain-induced experimental emphysema in the dog, *J. Appl. Physiol.*, 33, 293, 1972.

213. Snider, G. L., Sherter, C. B., Koo, K. W., Karlinsky, J. B., Hayes, J. A., and Franzblau, C., Respiratory mechanics in hamsters following treatment with endotracheal elastase or collagenase, *J. Appl. Physiol. Respir. Environ. Exercise Physiol.*, 42, 206, 1977.

214. Kuhn, C., Yu, S-Y., Chraplyvy, M., Linder, H. E., and Senior, R. M., The induction of emphysema with elastase. II. Changes in connective tissue, *Lab. Invest.*, 34, 372, 1976.

215. Goldstein, R. A. and Starcher, B. C., Urinary excretion of elastin peptides containing desmosine after intratracheal injection of elastase in hamsters, *J. Clin. Invest.*, 61, 1286, 1978.

216. Martorana, P. A., Share, N. N., and Richard, J. W., Free alveolar cells in papain-induced emphysema in the hamster, *Am. Rev. Respir. Dis.*, 116, 57, 1977.

217. Kovnat, D. M., Snider, G. L., and Brody, J. S., Pattern of injury and phagocyte function in elastase induced emphysema, *Clin. Res.*, 23, 349A, 1975.

218. Smith, T. and Kuhn, C., unpublished.

219. Sahebjami, H. and Vassallo, C. L., Exercise stress and enzyme-induced emphysema, *J. Appl. Physiol.*, 41, 332, 1976.
220. Goldring, I. P., Greenburg, L., Park, S. S., and Ratner, I. M., Pulmonary effects of sulfur dioxide exposure in the Syrian hamster. II. Combined with emphysema, *Arch. Environ. Health*, 21, 32, 1970.
221. Sandhaus, R. A. and Janoff, A., Animal models of emphysema. Distribution and fate of endotracheally instilled protease, *Fed. Proc. Fed. Am. Soc. Exp. Biol.*, 34 (Abstr.), 839, 1975.
222. Stone, P. J., Pereira, W., Biles, D., Snider, G. L., Kagan, H. M., and Franzblau, C., Studies on the fate of pancreatic elastase in the hamster lung. ^{14}C-guanidinated elastase, *Am. Rev. Respir. Dis.*, 116, 49, 1977.
223. Collins, J. F., Durnin, L. S., and Johanson, W. G., Papain-induced lung injury: alterations in connective tissue metabolism without emphysema, *Exp. Mol. Pathol.*, 29, 29, 1978.
224. Kuhn, C. and Starcher, B., The effect of lathyrogens on the evolution of elastase-induced emphysema, *Am. Rev. Resp. Dis.*, 122, 453, 1980.
225. Galdston, M., Levytska, V., Liener, I. E., and Twumasi, D. Y., Degradation of tropoelastin and elastin substrates by human neutrophil elastase free and bound to alpha$_2$-macroglobulin in serum of the M and Z (Pi) phenotypes for alpha$_1$-antitrypsin, *Am. Rev. Respir. Dis.*, 119, 435, 1979.
226. Martorana, P. A. and Share, N. N., Effect of human alpha1-antitrypsin on papain-induced emphysema in the hamster, *Am. Rev. Respir. Dis.*, 113, 607, 1976.
227. Makino, S. and Reed, C. E., Distribution and elimination of exogenous alpha$_1$-antitrypsin, *J. Lab. Clin. Med.*, 75, 742, 1970.
228. Kleinerman, J. and Rynbrandt, D. J., The depression of serum trypsin inhibition by galactosamine. A possible experimental model of α_1-antitrypsin deficiency, *Fed. Proc. Fed. Am. Soc. Exp. Biol.*, 33, 635, 1974.
229. Blackwood, R. A., Cerreta, J. M., Mandl, I., and Turino, G. M., Alpha$_1$ Antitrypsin Deficiency and Increased Susceptibility to Elastase Induced Experimental Emphysema in a Rat Model, submitted for publication.
230. Cohen, A. B., The effects in vivo and in vitro of oxidative damage to purified α_1-antitrypsin and to the enzyme-inhibiting activity of plasma, *Am. Rev. Respir. Dis.*, 119, 953, 1979.
231. Levine, E. A., Senior, R. M., and Butler, J. V., The elastase activity of alveolar macrophages: measurements using synthetic substrates and elastin, *Am. Rev. Respir. Dis.*, 113, 25, 1976.
232. Bielefeld, D. R., Senior, R. M., and Yu, S. Y., A new method for determination of elastolytic activity using [^{14}C] labeled elastin and its application to leukocytic elastase, *Biochem. Biophys. Res. Commun.*, 67, 1553, 1975.
233. Saklatula, J., Hydrolysis of the elastase substrate succinyltrialanine nitroanilide by a metal-dependent enzyme in rheumatoid synovial fluid, *J. Clin. Invest.*, 59, 794, 1977.
234. Hinman, L., Stevens, C. A., Matthay, R. A., and Gee, J. B. L., Elastase and lysozyme activities in human alveolar macrophages: effects of cigarette smoking, *Am. Rev. Resp. Dis.*, 21, 263, 1980.
235. Ogawa, M., Kosaki, G., Tanaka, S., Iwaki, K., and Nomoto, M., An activity of hydrolyzing elastase substrate succinyltrialanine *p*-nitro-anilide in human bile, *Clin. Chim. Acta*, 93, 235, 1979.
236. Janoff, A. and Scherer, J., Mediators of inflammation in leukocyte lysosomes. IX. Elastolytic activity in granules of human polymorphonuclear leukocytes, *J. Exp. Med.*, 128, 1137, 1968.
237. Janoff, A., Rosenberg, R., and Galdston, M., Elastase-like esteroprotease activity in human and rabbit alveolar macrophage granules, *Proc. Soc. Exp. Biol. Med.*, 136, 1054, 1971.
238. Werb, Z. and Gordon, S., Elastase secretion by stimulated macrophages. Characterization and regulation, *J. Exp. Med.*, 142, 361, 1975.
239. White, R., Lin, H. S., and Kuhn, C., Elastase secretion by peritoneal exudative and alveolar macrophages, *J. Exp. Med.*, 146, 802, 1977.
240. DeCremoux, H., Hornebeck, W., Jaurand, M-C., Bignon, J., and Robert, L., Partial characterization of an elastase-like enzyme secreted by human and monkey alveolar macrophages, *J. Pathol.*, 125, 170, 1978.
241. Pryzwansky, K. B., Martin, L. E., and Spitznagel, J. K., Immunocytochemical localization of myeloperoxidase, lactoferrin, lysozyme and neutral proteases in human monocytes and neutrophilic granulocytes, *J. Reticuloendothel. Soc.*, 24, 295, 1978.
242. Ragsdale, C. G. and Arend, W. P., Neutral protease secretion by human monocytes: effect of surface-bound immune complexes, *J. Exp. Med.*, 149, 954, 1979.
243. Legrand, Y., Caen, J., Booyse, F. M., Rafelson, M. E., Robert, B., and Robert, L., Studies on a human blood platelet protease with elastolytic activity, *Biochem. Biophys. Acta*, 309, 406, 1973.
244. Hornebeck, W., Adnet, J. J., and Robert, L., Age dependent variation of elastin and elastase in aorta and human breast cancers, *Exp. Gerontol.*, 13, 293, 1978.
245. Senior, R. M. and Griffin, G., unpublished.
246. Bellon, G., Hornebeck, W., Derouette, J. C., and Robert, L., Methodes simples pour quantifier l'elastase et ses inhibiteurs dans le serum humain, *Pathiol. Biol.*, 26, 515, 1978.
247. Miskulin, M., Moati, F., Robert, A. M., Robert, L., and Guilband, J., Serum elastase and its inhibitors in the blood of heavily burnt patients, *J. Clin. Pathol.*, 31, 866, 1978.

248. Geokas, M. C., Brodrick, J. W., Johnson, J. H., and Largman, C., Pancreatic elastase in human serum: determination by radioimmunoassay, *J. Biol. Chem.*, 252, 61, 1977.

249. Ohlsson, K. and Olsson, A-S., Immunoreactive granulocyte elastase in human serum, *Hoppe-Seyler's Z. Physiol. Chem.*, 359, 1531, 1978.

250. Mandl, I., Collagenases and elastases, *Adv. Enzymol.*, 2, 163, 1961.

251. Havemann, K. and Janoff, A., *Neutral Proteases of Human Polymorphonuclear Leukocytes*, Urban and Schwarzenberg, Baltimore, 1978.

252. Taylor, J. C. and Crawford, J., Purification and preliminary characterization of human leukocyte elastase, *Arch. Biochem. Biophys.*, 169, 91, 1975.

253. Dewald, B., Rindler-Ludwig, R., Bretz, U., and Baggiolini, M., Subcellular localization and heterogeneity of neutral proteases in neutrophilic polymorphonuclear leukocytes, *J. Exp. Med.*, 141, 709, 1975.

254. Ohlsson, K., Olsson, I., and Spitznagel, J. K., Localization of chymotrypsin-like cationic protein, collagenase and elastase in azurophil granules of human neutrophilic polymorphonuclear leukocytes, *Hoppe-Seyler's Z. Physiol. Chem.*, 358, 361, 1977.

255. Ohlsson, K. and Olsson, I., The neutral proteases of human granulocytes. Isolation and partial characterization of granulocyte elastases, *Eur. J. Biochem.*, 42, 519, 1974.

256. Ohlsson, K., Olsson, I., Delshammar, M., and Schiessler, H., Elastases from human and canine granulocytes. I. Some proteolytic and esterolytic properties, *Hoppe-Seyler's Z. Physiol. Chem.*, 357, 1245, 1976.

257. Vassalli, J-D., Granelli-Piperno, A., Griscelli, C., and Reich, E., Specific protease deficiency in polymorphonuclear leukocytes of Chediak-Higashi syndrome and beige mouse, *J. Exp. Med.*, 147, 1285, 1978.

258. Rausch, P. G., Pryzwansky, B. S., and Spitznagel, J. K., Immunocytochemical identification of azurophilic and specific granule markers in the giant granules of Chediak-Higashi neutrophils, *N. Engl. J. Med.*, 298, 693, 1978.

259. Feinstein, G. and Janoff, A., A rapid method of purification of human granulocyte cationic neutral proteases: purification and further characterization of human granulocyte elastase, *Biochim. Biophys. Acta*, 403, 493, 1975.

260. Baugh, R. J. and Travis, J., Human leukocyte granule elastase: rapid isolation and characterization, *Biochemistry*, 15, 836, 1976.

261. Twumasi, D. Y. and Liener, I. E., Proteases from purulent sputum. Purification and properties of the elastase and chymotrypsin-like enzymes, *J. Biol. Chem.*, 252, 1917, 1977.

262. Martodam, R. R., Baugh, R. J., Twumasi, D. Y., and Liener, I. E., A rapid procedure for the large scale purification of elastase and cathepsin G from sputum, *Prep. Biochem.*, 9, 15, 1979.

263. Senior, R. M., Bielefeld, D. R., and Starcher, B. C., A comparison of the elastolytic effects of human leukocyte elastase and porcine pancreatic elastase, *Biochem. Biophys. Res. Commun.*, 72, 1327, 1976.

264. Huebner, P., unpublished.

265. Campbell, E. J., White, R. R., Senior, R. M., Rodriguez, R. J., and Kuhn, C., Receptor mediated binding and internalization of leukocyte elastase by alveolar macrophages in vitro, *J. Clin. Invest.*, 64, 824, 1979.

266. McDonald, J. A., Baum, B. J., Rosenberg, D. M., Kelman, J. A., Brin, S. C., and Crystal, R. G., Destruction of a major extracellular adhesive glycoprotein (fibronectin) of human fibroblasts by neutral proteases from polymorphonuclear leukocyte granules, *Lab. Invest.*, 40, 350, 1979.

267. Blondin, J. and Janoff, A., The role of lysosomal elastase in the digestion of *Escherichia coli* proteins by human polymorphonuclear leukocytes. Experiments with living leukocytes, *J. Clin. Invest.*, 58, 971, 1976.

268. Odeberg, H. and Olsson, I., Microbicidal mechanisms of human granulocytes: synergistic effects of granulocyte elastase and myeloperoxidase or chymotrypsin-like cationic protein, *Infect. Immun.*, 14, 1276, 1976.

269. Vischer, T. L., Bretz, U., and Baggiolini, M., In vitro stimulation of lymphocytes by neutral proteases from human polymorphonuclear leukocyte granules, *J. Exp. Med.*, 144, 863, 1976.

270. Johnson, U., Ohlsson, K., and Olsson, I., Effects of granulocyte neutral proteases on complement components, *Scand. J. Immunol.*, 5, 421, 1976.

271. Taylor, J. C., Crawford, I. P., and Hugli, T. E., Limited degradation of the third component (C3) of human complement by human leukocyte elastase (LE): partial characterization of C3 fragments, *Biochemistry*, 16, 3390, 1977.

272. Brozna, J. P., Senior, R. M., Kreutzer, D. L., and Ward, P. A., Chemotactic factor inactivators of human granulocytes, *J. Clin. Invest.*, 60, 1280, 1977.

273. Galdston, M., Janoff, A., and Davis, A. L., Familial variation of leukocyte lysosomal protease and serum alpha$_1$-antitrypsin as determinants in chronic obstructive pulmonary disease, *Am. Rev. Respir. Dis.*, 107, 718, 1973.

274. Lam, S., Abboud, R. T., Chan-Yeung, M., and Rushton, J-M., Neutrophil elastase and pulmonary function in subjects with intermediate alpha-1-antitrypsin deficiency (MZ phenotype), *Am. Rev. Respir. Dis.,* 119, 941, 1979.

275. Klayton, R., Fallat, R., and Cohen, A. B., Determinants of chronic obstructive pulmonary disease in patients with intermediate levels of alpha$_1$-antitrypsin, *Am. Rev. Respir. Dis.,* 112, 71, 1975.

276. Kidokoro, Y., Kravis, T. C., Moser, K. M., Taylor, J. C., and Crawford, I. P., Relationship of leukocyte elastase concentration to severity of emphysema in homozygous α_1-antitrypsin-deficient persons, *Am. Rev. Respir. Dis.,* 115, 793, 1977.

277. Galdston, M., Melnick, E. L., Goldring, R. M., Levytska, V., Curasi, C. A., and Davis, A. L., Interactions of neutrophil elastase, serum trypsin inhibitory activity, and smoking history as risk factors for chronic obstructive pulmonary disease in patients with MM, MZ, and ZZ phenotypes for alpha$_1$-antitrypsin, *Am. Rev. Respir. Dis.,* 116, 837, 1977.

278. Rodriguez, J. R., Seals, J. E., Radin, A., Lin, J. S., Mandl, I., and Turino, G. M., Neutrophil lysosomal elastase activity in normal subjects and in patients with chronic obstructive pulmonary disease, *Am. Rev. Respir. Dis.,* 119, 409, 1979.

279. Werb, Z., Biochemical actions of glucocorticoids on macrophages in culture: specific inhibition of elastase collagenase and plasminogen activator secretion, *J. Exp. Med.,* 147, 1695, 1978.

280. Rifkin, D. B. and Crowe, R. M., A sensitive assay for elastase employing radioactive elastin coupled to sepharose, *Anal. Biochem.,* 79, 268, 1977.

281. Green, M. R., Lin, J. S., Berman, L. B., Osman, J. M., Mandl, I., and Turino, G. M., Elastolytic activity of alveolar macrophages in normal dogs and human subjects, *J. Lab. Clin. Med.,* 94, 549, 1979.

282. Rodriguez, R. J., White, R. R., Senior, R. M., and Levine, E. A., Elastase release from human alveolar macrophages. Comparison between smokers and non-smokers, *Science,* 198, 313, 1977.

283. Banda, M. J. and Werb, Z., Mouse macrophage elastase purification and characterization as a metalloproteinase, *Biochem. J.,* 193, 589, 1981.

284. McLaughlin, R. F. and Tueller, E. E., Anatomic and histologic changes of early emphysema, *Chest,* 59, 592, 1971.

285. Martin, R. R. and Warr, G. A., Cigarette smoking and human pulmonary macrophages, *Hosp. Pract.,* 12, 97, 1977.

286. Niewoehner, D. E., Kleinerman, J., and Rice, D. B., Pathologic changes in the peripheral airways of young cigarette smokers, *N. Engl. J. Med.,* 291, 755, 1974.

287. White, R., White, J., and Janoff, A., Effects of cigarette smoke on elastase secretion by murine macrophages, *J. Lab. and Clin. Med.,* 94, 489, 1979.

288. Fine, R. and Collins, J. F., Elastase secretion by alveolar macrophages from smoking baboons, *Clin. Res.,* 27, 397a, 1979.

289. Coudon, W. L. and Harris, J. O., Human alveolar macrophage proteolytic enzyme activities in chronic obstructive pulmonary disease: lack of correlation with functional abnormalities, *Chest,* 73, 364, 1978.

290. Legrand, Y., Caen, J. P., Robert, L., and Wantier, J. L., Platelet elastase and leukocyte elastase are two different entities, *Thromb. Hemostasis,* 37, 580, 1977.

291. Legrand, Y., Pignaud, G., and Caen, J., Purification of platelet proteases: activation of proelastase by a trypsin-like enzyme, *FEBS Lett.,* 76, 294, 1977.

292. Weissmann, G., Leukocytes as secretory organs of inflammation, *Hosp. Pract.,* 13, 53, 1978.

293. Unanue, E. R., Secretory function of mononuclear phagocytes, *Am. J. Pathol.,* 83, 396, 1976.

293a. Wright, D. G. and Gallin, J. I., A functional differentiation of human neutrophil granules: generation of C5a by a specific (secondary) granule product and inactivation of C5a by azurophil (primary) granule products, *J. Immunol.,* 119, 1068, 1977.

294. Gordon, S. and Werb, Z., Secretion of macrophage neutral proteinase is enhanced by colchicine, *Proc. Natl. Acad. Sci. U.S.A.,* 73, 872, 1976.

295. Smolen, J. E. and Weissmann, G., The granulocyte: metabolic properties and mechanisms of lysosomal enzyme release in *Neutral Proteases of Human Polymorphonuclear Leukocytes,* Havemann, K. and Janoff, A., Eds., Urban and Schwarzenberg, Baltimore, 1978, 56.

296. Blue, M-L. and Janoff, A., Possible mechanisms of emphysema in cigarette smokers: release of elastase from human polymorphonuclear leukocytes by cigarette smoke condensate "in vitro," *Am. Rev. Respir. Dis.,* 117, 317, 1978.

297. Hunninghake, G. W., Gallin, J. I., and Fauci, A. S., Immunologic reactivity of the lung: the "in vivo" and "in vitro" generation of a neutrophil chemotactic factor by alveolar macrophages, *Am. Rev. Respir. Dis.,* 117, 15, 1978.

298. Hunninghake, G. W., Gadek, J. E., and Crystal, R. G., Human alveolar macrophage chemotactic factor for neutrophils: stimuli and partial characterization, submitted for publication.

299. Merrill, W. W., Naegel, G. P., Matthay, R. A., and Reynolds, H. Y., Production of chemotactic factor(s) by in vivo cultured human alveolar macrophages, *Chest,* 75, 224, 1979.

300. **Cohn, Z. A.**, Macrophage physiology, *Fed. Proc. Fed. Am. Soc. Exp. Med.*, 34, 1725, 1975.

301. **Gordon, S.**, Macrophage neutral proteinases and defense of the lung, *Fed. Proc. Fed. Am. Soc. Exp. Med.*, 36, 2707, 1977.

302. **Werb, Z., Foley, R., and Yunck, A.**, Glucocorticoid receptors and glucocorticoid-sensitive secretion of neutral proteinases in a macrophage line, *J. Immunol.*, 121, 115, 1978.

303. **Werb, Z.**, unpublished.

304. **Ohlsson, K., Olsson, I., and Tynelius-Bratthall, G.**, Neutrophil leukocyte collagenase, elastase and serum protease inhibitors in human gingival crevices, *Acta Odontol. Scand.*, 31, 51, 1973.

305. **Olsson, I., Olofsson, T., Ohlsson, K., and Gustavsson, A.**, Serum and plasma myeloperoxidase, elastase and lactoferrin content in acute myeloid leukaemia, *Scand. J. Haematol.*, 22, 397, 1979.

306. **Egbring, R., Schmidt, W., Fuchs, G., and Havemann, K.**, Demonstration of granulocytic proteases in plasma of patients with acute leukemia and septicemia with coagulation defects, *Blood*, 49, 219, 1977.

307. **Ohlsson, K.**, Collagenase and elastase released during peritonitis are complexed by plasma protease inhibitors, *Surgery*, 76, 652, 1976.

308. **Bierman, H. R., Kelly, K. H., and Cordes, F. L.**, The sequestration and visceral circulation of leukocytes in man, *Ann. N.Y. Acad. Sci.*, 59, 850, 1955.

309. **Wittels, E. H., Coalson, J. J., Welch, M. H., and Guenter, C. A.**, Pulmonary intravascular leukocyte sequestration: a potential mechanism of lung injury, *Am. Rev. Respir. Dis.*, 109, 502, 1974.

310. **Cohen, A. B., Batra, G., Petersen, R., Podany, J., and Nguyen, D.**, Size of the pool of alveolar neutrophils in normal rabbit lungs, *J. Appl. Physiol.*, 47, 440, 1979.

311. **Heimburger, N., Haupt, H., and Schwick, H. G.**, Proteinase inhibitors of human plasma, in *Proc. Int. Res. Conf. on Proteinase Inhibitors*, Fritz, H., and Tschesche, H., Eds., W. deGruyter, Berlin, 1971, 1.

312. **Woolley, D. E., Roberts, D. R., and Evanson, J. M.**, Small molecular weight β_1 serum protein which specifically inhibits human collagenases, *Nature (London)*, 261, 325, 1976.

313. **Weinbaum, G., Takamoto, M., Slodan, B., and Kimbel, P.**, Lung antiproteinase: a potential defense against emphysema development, *Am. Rev. Respir. Dis.*, 113, 245, 1976.

314. **Hochstrasser, K., Haendle, H., Reichert, R., Werle, E., and Schwarz, S.**, Über Vorkommen und Eigenschaften eines Proteaseninhibitors in menschlichen Nasensekret, *Hoppe-Seyler's Z. physiol. Chem.*, 352, 954, 1971.

315. **Schiessler, H., Hochstrasser, K., and Ohlsson, K.**, Acid-stable inhibitors of granulocyte neutral proteases in human mucous secretions: biochemistry and possible biological function, in *Neutral Proteases of Human Polymorphonuclear Leukocytes. Biochemistry, Physiology and Clinical Significance*, Havemann, K. and Janoff, A., Eds., Urban and Schwarzenberg, Baltimore, 1978, 195.

316. **Hochstrasser, K., Reichert, R., and Heimberger, N.**, Antigenic relationship between the human bronchial mucus inhibitor and plasma inter-α-trypsin inhibitor, *Hoppe-Seyler's Z. Physiol. Chem.*, 354, 587, 1973.

317. **Ohlsson, K. and Tegner, H.**, Inhibition of elastase from granulocytes by the low molecular weight bronchial protease inhibitor, *Scand. J. Clin. Lab. Invest.*, 36, 437, 1976.

318. **Tegner, H. and Ohlsson, K.**, Localization of a low molecular weight protease inhibitor to tracheal and maxillary sinus mucosa, *Hoppe-Seyler's Z. Physiol. Chem.*, 358, 425, 1977.

319. **Ganrot, P. O., Laurell, C. B., and Ohlsson, K.**, Concentration of trypsin inhibitors of different molecular size and of albumin and haptoglobin in blood and lymph of various organs in the dog, *Acta Physiol. Scand.*, 79, 280, 1970.

320. **Reynolds, H. Y. and Newball, H. H.**, Analysis of proteins and respiratory cells obtained from human lungs by bronchial lavage, *J. Lab. Clin. Med.*, 84, 559, 1974.

321. **Olsen, G. N., Harris, J. O., Castle, J. R., Waldman, R. H., and Karmgard, H. J.**, Alpha-1-antitrypsin content in the serum, alveolar macrophages, and alveolar lavage fluid of smoking and non-smoking normal subjects, *J. Clin. Invest.*, 55, 427, 1975.

322. **Warr, G. A., Martin, R. R., Sharp, P. M., and Rosen, R.**, Normal human bronchial immunoglobulins and proteins: effect of cigarette smoking, *Am. Rev. Respir. Dis.*, 116, 25, 1977.

323. **Low, R. B., Davis, G. S., and Giancola, M. S.**, Biochemical analyses of bronchoalveolar lavage fluids of healthy human volunteer smokers and non-smokers, *Am. Rev. Respir. Dis.*, 118, 863, 1978.

324. **Bell, D. Y. and Hook, G. E. R.**, Pulmonary alveolar proteinosis: analysis of airway and alveolar proteins, *Am. Rev. Respir. Dis.*, 119, 979, 1979.

325. **Tuttle, W. C. and Jones, P. K.**, Fluorescent antibody studies of alpha$_1$-antitrypsin in adult human lung, *Am. J. Clin. Pathol.*, 64, 477, 1975.

326. **Maran, A. G. and Kueppers, F.**, Pulmonary arteriovenous differences in serum antiprotease activity during experimental pneumonitis, *Am. Rev. Respir. Dis.*, 112, 527, 1975.

327. **James, H. L. and Cohen, A. B.**, Mechanism of inhibition of porcine elastase by human alpha-1-antitrypsin, *J. Clin. Invest.*, 62, 1344, 1978.

328. Johnson, D. and Travis, J., Structural evidence for methionine at the reactive site of human α-1-proteinase inhibitor, *J. Biol. Chem.*, 253, 7142, 1978.

329. Johnson, D. and Travis, J., The oxidative inactivation of human α-1-proteinase inhibitor, *J. Biol. Chem.*, 254, 4022, 1979.

330. Chowdhury, P. and Louria, D. B., Influence of cadmium and other trace metals on human α₁-antitrypsin: an in vitro study, *Science*, 191, 480, 1976.

331. Glaser, C. B., Karic, L., Huffaker, T., and Fallat, R. J., Influence of cadmium on human alpha-1-antitrypsin: a reexamination, *Science*, 196, 556, 1977.

332. Janoff, A. and Carp, H., Possible mechanisms of emphysema in smokers. Cigarette smoke condensate suppresses protease inhibition *in vitro*, *Am. Rev. Respir. Dis.*, 116, 65, 1977.

333. Carp, H. and Janoff, A., Possible mechanisms of emphysema in smokers. *In vitro* suppression of serum elastase-inhibitory capacity by fresh cigarette smoke and its prevention by antioxidants, *Am. Rev. Respir. Dis.*, 118, 617, 1978.

334. Leh, F., Warr, T. A., and Mudd, J. B., Reaction of ozone with protease inhibitors from bovine pancreas, egg white and human serum, *Environ. Res.*, 16, 179, 1978.

335. Carp, H. and Janoff, A., In vitro suppression of serum elastase-inhibitory capacity by reactive oxygen species generated by phagocytosing polymorphonuclear leukocytes, *J. Clin. Invest.*, 63, 793, 1979.

336. Blackwood, C. E., Moret, J. E., Keller, S., Fierer, J. A., and Mandl, I., Alpha-1-antitrypsin concentration in serum of laboratory animals. Changes following proteolytic enzyme injections, *J. Lab. Clin. Med.*, 84, 813, 1974.

337. Harpel, P. C., Studies on human plasma α₂-macroglobulin-enzyme interactions. Evidence for proteolytic modification of the subunit chain structure, *J. Exp. Med.*, 138, 508, 1973.

338. Swenson, R. P. and Howard, J. B., Structural characterization of human α₂-macroglobulin subunits, *J. Biol. Chem.*, 254, 4452, 1979.

339. Barrett, A. J. and Starkey, P. M., The interaction of α₂-macroglobulin with proteinase. Characteristics and specificity of the reaction and a hypothesis concerning its molecular mechanism, *Biochem. J.*, 133, 709, 1973.

340. Baumstark, J. S., Studies on the elastase-serum protein interaction. III. The elastase inhibitors of swine serum with emphasis on the elastase-α₂-macroglobulin interaction, *Biochim. Biophys. Acta*, 309, 181, 1973.

341. Harpel, P. C. and Mosesson, M. W., Degradation of human fibrinogen by plasma α₂-macroglobulin-enzyme complexes, *J. Clin. Invest.*, 52, 2175, 1973.

342. Twumasi, D. Y., Liener, I. E., Gladston, M., and Levystska, V., Activation of human leukocyte elastase by human α₂-macroglobulin, *Nature (London)*, 267, 61, 1977.

343. Mosher, D. F. and Wing, D. A., Synthesis and secretion of α₂-macroglobulin by cultured human fibroblasts, *J. Exp. Med.*, 143, 462, 1976.

344. Mosher, D. F., Saksela, O., and Vaheri, A., Synthesis and secretion of alpha-2-macroglobulin by cultured adherent lung cells. Comparison with cell strains derived from other tissues, *J. Clin. Invest.*, 60, 1036, 1977.

345. Hovi, T., Mosher, D., and Vaheri, A., Cultured human monocytes synthesize and secrete α₂-macroglobulin, *J. Exp. Med.*, 145, 1580, 1977.

346. Ohlsson, K. and Olsson, I., Neutral proteases of human granulocytes. III. Interaction between human granulocyte elastase and plasma protease inhibitors, *Scand. J. Clin. Lab. Invest.*, 34, 349, 1974.

347. Ohlsson, K. and Delshammar, M., Interactions between granulocyte elastase and collagenase and the plasma proteinase inhibitors in vitro and in vivo, in *Dynamics of Connective Tissue Macromolecules*, Burleigh, P. M. C. and Poole, A. R., Eds., North-Holland, Amsterdam, 1975, 259.

348. Ohlsson, K., Elimination of ¹²⁵I-trypsin-macroglobulin. Complexes from blood by reticuloendothelial cells in dog, *Acta Physiol. Scand.*, 81, 269, 1971.

349. Ohlsson, K., α₁-antitrypsin and α₂-macroglobulin interactions with human neutrophil collagenase and elastase, *Ann. N.Y. Acad. Sci.*, 256, 409, 1975.

350. Katayama, K. and Fujita, T., Studies on biotransformation of elastase. III. Effects of elastase-binding proteins in serum on the disappearance of ¹³¹I-labeled elastase from blood, *Biochim. Biophys. Acta*, 336, 165, 1974.

351. Katayama, K. and Fujita, T., Studies on biotransformation of elastase: IV. Tissue distribution of ¹³¹I-labeled elastase and intracellular distribution in liver after intravenous administration in rats, *Biochim. Biophys. Acta*, 336, 178, 1974.

352. Katayama, K. and Fujita, T., Studies on biotransformation of elastase. V. Degradation of injected ¹³¹I-labeled elastase by subcellular particles of rat liver, *Biochim. Biophys. Acta*, 336, 191, 1974.

353. Dolovich, J., Debanne, M. T., and Bell, R., The role of alpha-1-antitrypsin and alpha macroglobulins in the uptake of proteinase by rabbit alveolar macrophages, *Am. Rev. Respir. Dis.*, 112, 521, 1975.

354. Kaplan, J. and Nielsen, M. L., Analysis of macrophage surface receptors. I. Binding of α-macroglobulin-protease complexes to rabbit alveolar macrophages, *J. Biol. Chem.*, 254, 7323, 1976.

355. Kaplan, J. and Nielsen, M. L., Analysis of macrophage surface receptors. II. Internalization of α-macroglobulin-trypsin complexes by rabbit alveolar macrophages, *J. Biol. Chem.*, 254, 7329, 1979.

356. Cohen, A. B., Interrelationships between the human alveolar macrophage and alpha-1-antitrypsin, *J. Clin. Invest.*, 52, 2793, 1973.

357. Gupta, P. K., Frost, J. K., Geddes, S., Aracil, B., and Davidovski, F., Morphological identification of alpha-1-antitrypsin in pulmonary macrophages, *Hum. Pathol.*, 10, 345, 1979.

358. Michaeli, D. and Fudenberg, H. H., Antibodies to collagen in patients with emphysema, *Clin. Immunol. Immunopathol.*, 3, 187, 1974.

359. Laros, C. D., Kuyper, C. M. A., and Janssen, H. M. J., The Chemical composition of fresh human lung parenchyma, *Respiration*, 29, 458, 1972.

360. Laros, C. D., The pathogenesis of emphysema, *Respiration*, 29, 442, 1972.

361. King, G. S., Mohan, V. S., and Starcher, B., Radioimmunoassay for desmosine and isodesmosine, *Connective Tissue Res.*, 7, 263, 1980.

362. Golde, D. W., Finley, T. N., and Cline, M. J., Production of colony stimulating factor by human macrophages, *Lancet*, 2, 1397, 1972.

363. West, J. B., Regional differences in the lung, *Chest*, 74, 426, 1978.

364. Starkey, P. M., Barrett, A. J., and Burleigh, M. C., The degradation of articular cartilage by neutrophil proteinases, *Biochim. Biophys. Acta*, 483, 386, 1977.

365. Keiser, H., Greenwald, R. A., Feinstein, G., and Janoff, A., Degradation of cartilage proteoglycan by human leukocyte granule neutral proteases — a model of joint injury. II. Degradation of isolated bovine nasal cartilage proteoglycan, *J. Clin. Invest.*, 57, 625, 1976.

366. Janoff, A., Human granulocyte elastase. Further delineation of its role in connective tissue damage, *Am. J. Pathol.*, 68, 579, 1972.

367. Gramse, M., Bigenheimer, C., Schmidt, W., Egbring, R., and Havemann, K., Degradation products of fibrinogen by elastase-like neutral protease from human granulocytes. Characterization and effects on blood coagulation in vitro, *J. Clin. Invest.*, 61, 1027, 1978.

368. Solomon, A., Schmidt, W., and Havemann, K., Bence Jones proteins and light chains of immunoglobulins. XIII. Effect of elastase-like and chymotrypsin-like neutral proteases derived from human granulocytes on Bench Jones proteins, *J. Immunol.*, 117, 1010, 1976.

369. Orr, F. W., Varani, J., Kreutzer, D. L., Senior, R. M., and Ward, P. A., Digestion of the fifth component of complement by leukocyte enzymes, *Am. J. Pathol.*, 94, 75, 1979.

Index

INDEX

A

Abnormalitis of connective tissue, II: 162

Abnormal levels of inhibitors, II: 36

Accumulation
  of basic amines, I: 172—175
  of foreign compounds, I: 169—177
  of nutrophil, II: 41
  of phagocyte, I: 235
  steady-state, I: 170, 171

Acetaldehyde, I: 254, 263

C-Acetate, II: 105

Acetylcholine, I: 257, 258; II: 74, 78—79

Acetylcysteine, I: 258

N-Acetylcysteine, I: 257

Acetylene, I: 254

Acetylouabain, I: 258

Acid phosphatase, I: 135; II: 38

Acrolein, I: 255; II: 43, 44

ACTH, see Adrenocorticotropic hormone

Actin, I: 135

Activated macrophages, II: 21, 22

Activated mediators, II: 70, 89

Activated oxygen, II: 86, 106

Activated phagocytes, I: 231, 235

Activity median aerodynamic diameter (AMAD)
  of particles, I: 33

Activity median diameter (AMD) of particles, I: 31

Activity median diffusive diameter (AMDD) of
  particles, I: 33

Acute bronchitis, II: 46—47

Acute pancreatitis, II: 78

Adenosine diphosphate (ADP), II: 76

Adenosine triphosphate (ATP), II: 71, 105

ADH, see Antidiuretic hormone

ADP, see Adenosine diphosphate

α-Adrenergic blocking agents, I: 259

β-Adrenergic blocking agents, I: 170

Adrenergic effectors, I: 263

β-Adrenergic system, II: 130

Adrenocorticotropic hormone (ACTH), II: 67, 69, 80

Adult respiratory distress syndrome (ARDS), II: 77

Adventitia, see Tunica adventitia

Aerodynamic diameter of particles, I: 32, 33, 49—51, 59

Aerodynamic properties of particles, I: 31—33, 41

Aerodynamic separation, I: 49

Aerodynamic size of particles, I: 41

Aerosol hair spray, I: 253

Aerosols, I: 254, 255
  coagulation rate for, I: 33
  defined, I: 29
  dispersion characteristics of, I: 33—34
  hydrolytic, I: 64
  monodisperse, I: 47, 50, 53, 56
  polydisperse, I: 53, 56

properties of, I: 29—35

Aflatoxin B_1, II: 92

AHH, see Aryl hydrocarbon hydroxylase

Air-blood barrier, I: 79, 93, 97, 123, 151, 220

Airflow, I: 41—47
  patterns of in airway, I: 65
  resistance in, I: 4

Air pollution, I: 59, 248; II: 14, 15, 164

Air tissue-lymph interface, I: 146

Airway branching, I: 4
  angles of, I: 4, 5, 38, 39
  irregularity in, I: 5
  patterns in, I: 39

Airways, I: 213, 223, 260
  airflow patterns in, I: 65
  branching in, see Airway branching
  cell death and renewal in, I: 189—218
  epithelium of, I: 6—10
  geometry of, I: 4, 35—41
  models of, I: 40—41
  morphometry of, I: 4—5, 35—40, 50, 51
  organization of, I: 6—11
  resistance in, II: 162, 171

Albumin distribution volume, I: 222

Alkalosis, II: 74—75, 89—91

Alkylation products, II: 95

Allergic bronchopulmonary aspergillosis, II: 50—51

Aluminum silicate, II: 13

Alveolar air spaces, I: 123, 139, 147, 150, 151, 236; II: 4, 7, 10, 42, 52, 191

Alveolar atrophy, II: 173

Alveolar basement membranes, II: 4

Alveolar bronchiolization, I: 207

Alveolar capillaries, I: 78, 81, 93, 97, 127, 150, 151, 190, 231; II: 49

Alveolar-capillary membrane, see also Air-blood barrier, I: 220, 231

Alveolar cells, I: 207
  morphometry of, I: 204

Alveolar clearance, I: 59—61

Alveolar deposition, I: 51

Alveolar ducts, I: 38, 91, 131; II: 11, 12, 47, 67, 76, 174, 175, 178

Alveolar edema, I: 220, 232; II: 11, 42

Alveolar epithelial cells, I: 174, 176; II: 99
  permeability of, I: 229
  Type I, I: 16; II: 48, 105
  Type II, I: 16; II: 48, 105

Alveolar epithelium, II: 191—196, 228, 230—233; II: 4, 49, 177, 178, 194

Alveolar flooding, see also Pulmonary edema, I: 222, 223

Alveolar forces, I: 228

Alveolar hemorrhage, II: 96

Alveolar hypoxia, II: 77

Alveolar interstitium, II: 125, 128

Alveolar lymphatic vessels, I: 127

Alveolar macrophage collagenase, II: 35

Alveolar macrophages, I: 190, 209, 211, 223;

C

F

G

K

L

Q

R

S